Household Safety Sourcebook

Hypertension Sourcebook

Immune System Disorders Sourcebook

Infant & Toddler Health Sourcebook

Infectious Diseases Sourcebook

Injury & Trauma Sourcebook

Kidney & Urinary Tract Diseases &
Disorders Sourcebook

Learning Disabilities Sourcebook,
2nd Edition

Leukemia Sourcebook

Liver Disorders Sourcebook

Lung Disorders Sourcebook

Medical Tests Sourcebook, 2nd Edition

Men's Health Concerns Sourcebook,
2nd Edition

Mental Health Disorders Sourcebook,
3rd Edition

Mental Retardation Sourcebook

Movement Disorders Sourcebook

Muscular Dystrophy Sourcebook

Obesity Sourcebook

Osteoporosis Sourcebook

Pain Sourcebook, 2nd Edition

Pediatric Cancer Sourcebook

Physical & Mental Issues in Aging
Sourcebook

Podiatry Sourcebook

Pregnancy & Birth Sourcebook,
2nd Edition

Prostate Cancer

Public Health Sourcebook

Reconstructive & Cosmetic Surgery
Sourcebook

Rehabilitation Sourcebook

Respiratory Diseases & Disorders
Sourcebook

Sexually Transmitted Diseases
Sourcebook, 2nd Edition

Skin Disorders Sourcebook

Sleep Disorders Sourcebook,
2nd Edition

Smoking Concerns Sourcebook

Sports Injuries Sourcebook, 2nd Edition

Stress-Related Disorders Sourcebook

Stroke Sourcebook

Substance Abuse Sourcebook

Surgery Sourcebook

Thyroid Sourcebook

Transplantation Sourcebook

Traveler's Health Sourcebook

Vegetarian Sourcebook

Women's Health Concerns Sourcebook,
2nd Edition

Workplace Health & Safety Sourcebook

Worldwide Health Sourcebook

D1016898

Teen Health Series

Alcohol Information for Teens

Asthma Information for Teens

Cancer Information for Teens

Diet Information for Teens

Drug Information for Teens

Eating Disorders Information
for Teens

Fitness Information for Teens

Mental Health Information
for Teens

Sexual Health Information
for Teens

Skin Health Information for
Teens

Sports Injuries Information
for Teens

Suicide Information for Teens

Urinary Tract and Kidney
Diseases and Disorders
SOURCEBOOK

Second Edition

Health Reference Series

Second Edition

Urinary Tract and Kidney
Diseases and Disorders
SOURCEBOOK

*Basic Consumer Health Information about the
Urinary System, Including the Bladder, Urethra,
Ureters, and Kidneys, with Facts about Urinary Tract
Infections, Incontinence, Congenital Disorders, Kidney
Stones, Cancers of the Urinary Tract and Kidneys,
Kidney Failure, Dialysis, and Kidney Transplantation*

*Along with Statistical and Demographic Information,
Reports on Current Research in Kidney and Urologic
Health, a Summary of Commonly Used Diagnostic
Tests, a Glossary of Related Terms, and a Directory of
Resources for Additional Help and Information*

Edited by
Ivy L. Alexander

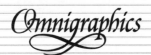

Omnigraphics

615 Griswold Street • Detroit, MI 48226

Bibliographic Note

Because this page cannot legibly accommodate all the copyright notices, the Bibliographic Note portion of the Preface constitutes an extension of the copyright notice.

Edited by Ivy L. Alexander

Health Reference Series

Karen Bellenir, *Managing Editor*
David A. Cooke, M.D., *Medical Consultant*
Elizabeth Barbour, *Research and Permissions Coordinator*
Cherry Stockdale, *Permissions Assistant*
Dawn Matthews, *Verification Assistant*
Laura Pleva Nielsen, *Index Editor*
EdIndex, Services for Publishers, *Indexers*

* * *

Omnigraphics, Inc.

Matthew P. Barbour, *Senior Vice President*
Kay Gill, *Vice President—Directories*
Kevin Hayes, *Operations Manager*
Leif Gruenberg, *Development Manager*
David P. Bianco, *Marketing Director*

* * *

Peter E. Ruffner, *Publisher*

Frederick G. Ruffner, Jr., *Chairman*

Copyright © 2005 Omnigraphics, Inc.

ISBN 0-7808-0750-2

Library of Congress Cataloging-in-Publication Data

Urinary tract and kidney diseases and disorders sourcebook / edited by Ivy L. Alexander. -- 2nd ed.
   p. cm. -- (Health reference series)
   "Basic consumer health information about the urinary system, including the bladder, urethra, ureters, and kidneys, with facts about urinary tract infections, incontinence, congenital disorders, kidney stones, cancers of the urinary tract and kidneys, kidney failure, dialysis, and kidney transplantation, along with statistical and demographic information, reports on current research in kidney and urologic health, a summary of commonly used diagnostic tests, a glossary of related terms, and a directory of resources for additional help and information."
   Summary: "Provides basic consumer health information about causes, and treatment of diseases and related disorders of the urinary system and kidneys. Includes index, glossary of related terms, and other resources"--Provided : by publisher.
   Includes index.
   ISBN 0-7808-0750-2 (hardcover : alk. paper)
   1. Urinary organs--Popular works. 2. Urinary organs--Diseases--Popular works. 3. Kidneys --Diseases--Popular works. 4. Consumer education.   I. Alexander, Ivy L. II. Series: Health reference series (Unnumbered)
   RC900.U745 2005
   616.6--dc22
                                                                                    2005024064

This book is printed on acid-free paper meeting the ANSI Z39.48 Standard. The infinity symbol that appears above indicates that the paper in this book meets that standard.

Printed in the United States

Table of Contents

Visit www.healthreferenceseries.com to view *A Contents Guide to the Health Reference Series*, a listing of more than 10,000 topics and the volumes in which they are covered.

Part II: Urinary Tract Infections and Bladder Disorders

Part III: Urinary Incontinence

Part IV: Disorders of the Ureters, Urethra, and Genitals

Part V: Disorders of the Kidneys

Part VI: Cancers of the Urinary Tract and Kidneys

Part VIII: Additional Help and Information

Preface

About This Book

Millions of Americans experience difficulties involving the kidneys, ureters, bladder, and urethra—the components of the urinary system. Problems can be caused by illness, injury, genetics, or aging and include such disorders as incontinence, urinary tract infections, cancers of the urinary tract, kidney stones, kidney disease, and kidney failure. According to statistics available from the National Institute of Diabetes and Digestive and Kidney Diseases:

- 10 to 20 million people in the U.S. may have kidney disease, but most don't know it. An estimated 7.4 million adults have less than half the kidney function of a healthy young adult, and nearly 400,000 are being treated for end-stage renal disease (kidney failure).

- 61.4 million adults report having experienced at least one occurrence of a urinary tract infection or cystitis; 6.2 million report experiencing a bladder infection that lasted more than three months.

- 13 million men and women in the U.S. suffer from urinary incontinence.

Although these types of disorders can have a significant impact on a person's physical, emotional, and social well-being, recent medical advances offer the promise of more effective treatments, and they provide the means by which those affected can learn to cope more successfully with related challenges. Additionally, by understanding the risk factors associated with kidney disease and other disorders of the urinary system, people can make lifestyle adjustments and take preventative measures to preserve urological health.

Urinary Tract and Kidney Diseases and Disorders Sourcebook, Second Edition provides information about the causes, symptoms, diagnosis, and treatment of problems that impact the body's urinary system, including bladder control problems, kidney and urinary stones, cancers, infections, prostate enlargement, glomerular diseases, nephropathies, and kidney failure. It describes risk factors, offers statistical information, explains the different types of dialysis, and provides facts about kidney transplantation. Reports on current research initiatives, a glossary of related terms, and a directory of additional resources are also included.

How to Use This Book

This book is divided into parts and chapters. Parts focus on broad areas of interest. Chapters are devoted to single topics within a part.

Part I: Understanding the Urinary System describes the organs, tubes, and muscles that work together to make, move, store, and release urine—processes vital for keeping the body healthy. It explains the risk factors for kidney and urologic disorders and includes facts about racial and ethnic groups with disproportionately high incidences of related diseases. Information on how high blood pressure, obesity, age, and medications can affect kidney health is included along with updates about current clinical trials, research initiatives, and other medical advances.

Part II: Urinary Tract Infections and Bladder Disorders explains the causes, symptoms, diagnosis, treatment, and prevention of urinary tract infections. It includes chapters covering issues specific to urinary tract infections in pregnancy and in children. Conventional medical treatments, including drug therapy, are described and self-care options are explained. Other bladder disorders, including bladder stones, fallen bladder, and conditions which result from injuries or trauma are also discussed.

Part III: Urinary Incontinence explains the loss of bladder control and related underlying medical conditions. Causes, diagnosis, and treatment options for incontinence are discussed. Individual chapters focus on issues specific to children, men, and women.

Part IV: Disorders of the Ureters, Urethra, and Genitals pays particular attention to problems of the genitals and urinary tract which may be present before birth (congenital), inherited from a parent, or caused later in life by infection, injury, or trauma. Symptoms, diagnostic tests, and available treatments are discussed. Prostate problems and treatments are also discussed.

Part V: Disorders of the Kidneys focuses on diseases and disorders affecting the kidneys, including genetic, congenital, and acquired disorders. Facts about symptoms, diagnostic procedures, and treatment options are included.

Part VI: Cancers of the Urinary Tract and Kidneys describes the causes, symptoms, diagnosis, and treatment of various cancers that can affect the different components of the urinary system, including bladder cancer, urethral cancer, and prostate cancer. Tests used in the staging process (the careful attempt to determine where and how a cancer has spread) are also explained.

Part VII: Kidney Failure: End-Stage Renal Disease explains treatments used to replace the work of failed kidneys and related ongoing health maintenance issues, including diet, nutrition, exercise, and working with a dietitian. The advantages and disadvantages of the types of dialysis are presented, along with detailed information on kidney transplantation and financial help for the treatment of kidney failure.

Part VIII: Additional Help and Information offers a glossary of important terms and a directory of government agencies and private organizations that provide help and information to patients with urinary tract and kidney diseases and disorders. A suggested list of organizations and websites which provide materials and information for further reading is also provided.

Bibliographic Note

This volume contains documents and excerpts from publications issued by the following U.S. government agencies: Centers for Disease Control and Prevention (CDC) and its Office of Minority Health; Centers for Medicare and Medicaid Services; National Cancer Institute (NCI); National Council of Complimentary and Alternative Medicines

(NCCAM); National Institute of Diabetes and Digestive and Kidney Diseases (NIDDK); National Institutes of Health (NIH); National Institutes of Health Clinical Center; National Kidney Disease Education Program (NKDEP); and the National Women's Health Information Center (NWHIC).

In addition, this volume contains copyrighted documents from the following organizations and individuals: A.D.A.M., Inc.; American Academy of Family Physicians; American Pregnancy Association; American Society of Radiologic Technologists; American Urological Association; Cincinnati Children's Hospital Medical Center; Cleveland Clinic; Healthcommunities.com, Inc.; HealthDay/ScoutNews; IgA Nephropathy Support Group; Johns Hopkins Bloomberg School of Public Health; Life Options Rehabilitation Program; March of Dimes; National Kidney Foundation; Nemours Center for Children's Health Media; Oxalosis and Hyperoxaluria Foundation; Prostate Cancer Research Institute; Tulane University; and University of Michigan Health System.

Full citation information is provided on the first page of each chapter. Every effort has been made to secure all necessary rights to reprint the copyrighted material. If any omissions have been made, please contact Omnigraphics to make corrections for future editions.

Acknowledgements

Thanks go to the many organizations, agencies, and individuals who have contributed materials for this *Sourcebook* and to medical consultant Dr. David Cooke, verification assistant Dawn Matthews, and document engineer Bruce Bellenir. Special thanks go to managing editor Karen Bellenir and permissions specialist Liz Barbour for their help and support.

About the Health Reference Series

The *Health Reference Series* is designed to provide basic medical information for patients, families, caregivers, and the general public. Each volume takes a particular topic and provides comprehensive coverage. This is especially important for people who may be dealing with a newly diagnosed disease or a chronic disorder in themselves or in a family member. People looking for preventive guidance, information about disease warning signs, medical statistics, and risk factors for health problems will also find answers to their questions in the *Health Reference Series*. The *Series*, however, is not intended to serve as a tool for diagnosing illness, in prescribing treatments, or as a substitute for the physician/patient relationship. All people concerned about medical symptoms or the possibility of disease are encouraged to seek professional care from an appropriate health care provider.

Locating Information within the Health Reference Series

The *Health Reference Series* contains a wealth of information about a wide variety of medical topics. Ensuring easy access to all the fact sheets, research reports, in-depth discussions, and other material contained within the individual books of the *Series* remains one of our highest priorities. As the *Series* continues to grow in size and scope, however, locating the precise information needed by a reader may become more challenging.

A Contents Guide to the Health Reference Series was developed to direct readers to the specific volumes that address their concerns. It presents an extensive list of diseases, treatments, and other topics of general interest compiled from the Tables of Contents and major index headings. To access *A Contents Guide to the Health Reference Series*, visit www.healthreferenceseries.com.

Medical Consultant

Medical consultation services are provided to the *Health Reference Series* editors by David A. Cooke, M.D. Dr. Cooke is a graduate of Brandeis University, and he received his M.D. degree from the University of Michigan. He completed residency training at the University of Wisconsin Hospital and Clinics. He is board-certified in Internal Medicine. Dr. Cooke currently works as part of the University of Michigan Health System and practices in Ann Arbor, MI. In his free time, he enjoys writing, science fiction, and spending time with his family.

Our Advisory Board

We would like to thank the following board members for providing guidance to the development of this *Series*:

- Dr. Lynda Baker,
  Associate Professor of Library and Information Science,
  Wayne State University, Detroit, MI

- Nancy Bulgarelli,
  William Beaumont Hospital Library, Royal Oak, MI

- Karen Imarisio,
  Bloomfield Township Public Library, Bloomfield Township, MI

- Karen Morgan,
  Mardigian Library, University of Michigan-Dearborn,
  Dearborn, MI

- Rosemary Orlando,
  St. Clair Shores Public Library, St. Clair Shores, MI

Health Reference Series *Update Policy*

The inaugural book in the *Health Reference Series* was the first edition of *Cancer Sourcebook* published in 1989. Since then, the *Series* has been enthusiastically received by librarians and in the medical community. In order to maintain the standard of providing high-quality health information for the layperson the editorial staff at Omnigraphics felt it was necessary to implement a policy of updating volumes when warranted.

Medical researchers have been making tremendous strides, and it is the purpose of the *Health Reference Series* to stay current with the most recent advances. Each decision to update a volume is made on an individual basis. Some of the considerations include how much new information is available and the feedback we receive from people who use the books. If there is a topic you would like to see added to the update list, or an area of medical concern you feel has not been adequately addressed, please write to:

Editor
Health Reference Series
Omnigraphics, Inc.
615 Griswold Street
Detroit, MI 48226
E-mail: editorial@omnigraphics.com

Part One

Understanding the
Urinary System

Chapter 1

Your Urinary System and How It Works

The organs, tubes, muscles, and nerves that work together to create, store, and carry urine are the urinary system. The urinary system includes two kidneys, two ureters, the bladder, two sphincter muscles, and the urethra.

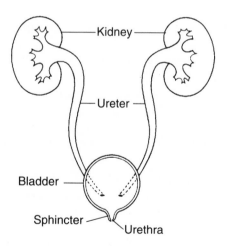

Figure 1.1. *Front view of urinary tract.*

National Kidney and Urologic Diseases Information Clearinghouse (NKUDIC), a service of the National Institute of Diabetes and Digestive and Kidney Diseases (NIDDK), National Institutes of Health (NIH), Pub. No. 04-3195, September 2004.

How does the urinary system work?

Your body takes nutrients from food and uses them to maintain all bodily functions including energy and self-repair. After your body has taken what it needs from the food, waste products are left behind in the blood and in the bowel. The urinary system works with the lungs, skin, and intestines—all of which also excrete wastes—to keep the chemicals and water in your body balanced. Adults eliminate about a quart and a half of urine each day. The amount depends on many factors, especially the amounts of fluid and food a person consumes and how much fluid is lost through sweat and breathing. Certain types of medications can also affect the amount of urine eliminated.

The urinary system removes a type of waste called urea from your blood. Urea is produced when foods containing protein, such as meat, poultry, and certain vegetables, are broken down in the body. Urea is carried in the bloodstream to the kidneys.

The kidneys are bean-shaped organs about the size of your fists. They are near the middle of the back, just below the rib cage. The kidneys remove urea from the blood through tiny filtering units called nephrons. Each nephron consists of a ball formed of small blood capillaries, called a glomerulus, and a small tube called a renal tubule. Urea, together with water and other waste substances, forms the urine as it passes through the nephrons and down the renal tubules of the kidney.

From the kidneys, urine travels down two thin tubes called ureters to the bladder. The ureters are about 8 to 10 inches long. Muscles in the ureter walls constantly tighten and relax to force urine downward away from the kidneys. If urine is allowed to stand still, or back up, a kidney infection can develop. Small amounts of urine are emptied into the bladder from the ureters about every 10 to 15 seconds.

The bladder is a hollow muscular organ shaped like a balloon. It sits in your pelvis and is held in place by ligaments attached to other organs and the pelvic bones. The bladder stores urine until you are ready to go to the bathroom to empty it. It swells into a round shape when it is full and gets smaller when empty. If the urinary system is healthy, the bladder can hold up to 16 ounces (two cups) of urine comfortably for two to five hours.

Circular muscles called sphincters help keep urine from leaking. The sphincter muscles close tightly like a rubber band around the opening of the bladder into the urethra, the tube that allows urine to pass outside the body.

Nerves in the bladder tell you when it is time to urinate (empty your bladder). As the bladder first fills with urine, you may notice a feeling that you need to urinate. The sensation to urinate becomes stronger as the bladder continues to fill and reaches its limit. At that point, nerves from the bladder send a message to the brain that the bladder is full, and your urge to empty your bladder intensifies.

When you urinate, the brain signals the bladder muscles to tighten, squeezing urine out of the bladder. At the same time, the brain signals the sphincter muscles to relax. As these muscles relax, urine exits the bladder through the urethra. When all the signals occur in the correct order, normal urination occurs.

What causes problems in the urinary system?

Problems in the urinary system can be caused by aging, illness, or injury. As you get older, changes in the kidneys' structure cause them to lose some of their ability to remove wastes from the blood. Also, the muscles in your ureters, bladder, and urethra tend to lose some of their strength. You may have more urinary infections because the bladder muscles do not tighten enough to empty your bladder completely. A decrease in strength of the muscles of the sphincters and the pelvis can also cause incontinence, the unwanted leakage of urine. Illness or injury can also prevent the kidneys from filtering the blood completely or block the passage of urine.

How are problems in the urinary system detected?

Urinalysis is a test that studies the content of urine for abnormal substances such as protein or signs of infection. This test involves urinating into a special container and leaving the sample to be studied.

Urodynamic tests evaluate the storage of urine in the bladder and the flow of urine from the bladder through the urethra. Your doctor may want to do a urodynamic test if you are having symptoms that suggest problems with the muscles or nerves of your lower urinary system and pelvis (ureters, bladder, urethra, and sphincter muscles).

Urodynamic tests measure the contraction of the bladder muscle as it fills and empties. The test is done by inserting a small tube called a catheter through your urethra into your bladder to fill it either with water or a gas. Another small tube is inserted into your rectum to measure the pressure put on your bladder when you strain or cough. Other bladder tests use x-ray dye instead of water so that x-ray pictures can be taken when the bladder fills and empties to detect any abnormalities in the shape and function of the bladder. These tests take about an hour.

What are some disorders of the urinary system?

Disorders of the urinary system range in severity from easy-to-treat to life-threatening.

Benign prostatic hyperplasia (BPH) is a condition in men that affects the prostate gland, which is part of the male reproductive system. The prostate is located at the bottom of the bladder and surrounds the urethra. BPH is an enlargement of the prostate gland that can interfere with urinary function in older men. It causes blockage by squeezing the urethra, which can make it difficult to urinate. Men with BPH frequently have other bladder symptoms including an increase in frequency of bladder emptying both during the day and at night. Most men over age 60 have some BPH, but not all have problems with blockage. There are many different treatment options for BPH.

Interstitial cystitis (IC) is a chronic bladder disorder also known as painful bladder syndrome and frequency-urgency-dysuria syndrome. In this disorder, the bladder wall can become inflamed and irritated. The inflammation can lead to scarring and stiffening of the bladder, decreased bladder capacity, pinpoint bleeding, and, in rare cases, ulcers in the bladder lining. The cause of IC is unknown at this time.

Kidney stones is the term commonly used to refer to stones, or calculi, in the urinary system. Stones form in the kidneys and may be found anywhere in the urinary system. They vary in size. Some stones cause great pain while others cause very little. The aim of treatment is to remove the stones, prevent infection, and prevent recurrence. Both nonsurgical and surgical treatments are used. Kidney stones affect men more often than women.

Prostatitis is inflammation of the prostate gland that results in urinary frequency and urgency, burning or painful urination (dysuria), and pain in the lower back and genital area, among other symptoms. In some cases, prostatitis is caused by bacterial infection and can be treated with antibiotics. But the more common forms of prostatitis are not associated with any known infecting organism. Antibiotics are often ineffective in treating the nonbacterial forms of prostatitis.

Proteinuria is the presence of abnormal amounts of protein in the urine. Healthy kidneys take wastes out of the blood, but leave in protein. Protein in the urine does not cause a problem by itself. But it may be a sign that your kidneys are not working properly.

Renal (kidney) failure results when the kidneys are not able to regulate water and chemicals in the body or remove waste products from your blood. Acute renal failure (ARF) is the sudden onset of kidney failure. This can be caused by an accident that injures the kidneys, loss of a lot of blood, or some drugs or poisons. ARF may lead to permanent loss of kidney function. But if the kidneys are not seriously damaged, they may recover. Chronic kidney disease (CKD) is the gradual reduction of kidney function that may lead to permanent kidney failure, or end-stage renal disease (ESRD). You may go several years without knowing you have CKD.

Urinary tract infections (UTIs) are caused by bacteria in the urinary tract. Women get UTIs more often than men. UTIs are treated with antibiotics. Drinking lots of fluids also helps by flushing out the bacteria.

The name of the UTI depends on its location in the urinary tract. An infection in the bladder is called cystitis. If the infection is in one or both of the kidneys, the infection is called pyelonephritis. This type of UTI can cause serious damage to the kidneys if it is not adequately treated.

Urinary incontinence, loss of bladder control, is the involuntary passage of urine. There are many causes and types of incontinence, and many treatment options. Treatments range from simple exercises to surgery. Women are affected by urinary incontinence more often than men.

Urinary retention, or bladder-emptying problems, is a common urological problem with many possible causes. Normally, urination can be initiated voluntarily and the bladder empties completely. Urinary retention is the abnormal holding of urine in the bladder. Acute urinary retention is the sudden inability to urinate, causing pain and discomfort. Causes can include an obstruction in the urinary system, stress, or neurologic problems. Chronic urinary retention refers to the persistent presence of urine left in the bladder after incomplete emptying. Common causes of chronic urinary retention are bladder muscle failure, nerve damage, or obstructions in the urinary tract. Treatment for urinary retention depends on the cause.

Who can help me with a urinary problem?

Your primary doctor can help you with some urinary problems. Your pediatrician may be able to treat some of your child's urinary problems. But some problems may require the attention of a urologist, a doctor who specializes in treating problems of the urinary system and the male reproductive system. A gynecologist is a doctor who specializes in the female reproductive system and may be able to help with some urinary problems. A urogynecologist is a gynecologist who specializes in the female urinary system. A nephrologist specializes in treating diseases of the kidney.

Chapter 2

Your Kidneys and How They Work

Your two kidneys are vital organs that perform many functions to keep your blood clean and chemically balanced. Understanding how your kidneys work can help you to keep them healthy.

What do my kidneys do?

Your kidneys are bean-shaped organs, each about the size of your fist. They are located near the middle of your back, just below the rib cage. The kidneys are sophisticated reprocessing machines. Every day, your kidneys process about 200 quarts of blood to sift out about two quarts of waste products and extra water. The waste and extra water become urine, which flows to your bladder through tubes called ureters. Your bladder stores urine until you go to the bathroom.

The wastes in your blood come from the normal breakdown of active tissues and from the food you eat. Your body uses the food for energy and self-repair. After your body has taken what it needs from the food, waste is sent to the blood. If your kidneys did not remove these wastes, the wastes would build up in the blood and damage your body.

The actual filtering occurs in tiny units inside your kidneys called nephrons. Every kidney has about a million nephrons. In the nephron,

National Kidney and Urologic Diseases Information Clearinghouse (NKUDIC), a service of the National Institute of Diabetes and Digestive and Kidney Diseases (NIDDK), National Institutes of Health (NIH), Pub. No. 03-4241, July 2003.

9

a glomerulus—which is a tiny blood vessel, or capillary—intertwines with a tiny urine-collecting tube called a tubule. A complicated chemical exchange takes place, as waste materials and water leave your blood and enter your urinary system.

At first, the tubules receive a combination of waste materials and chemicals that your body can still use. Your kidneys measure out chemicals like sodium, phosphorus, and potassium and release them back to the blood to return to the body. In this way, your kidneys regulate the body's level of these substances. The right balance is necessary for life, but excess levels can be harmful.

In addition to removing wastes, your kidneys release three important hormones:

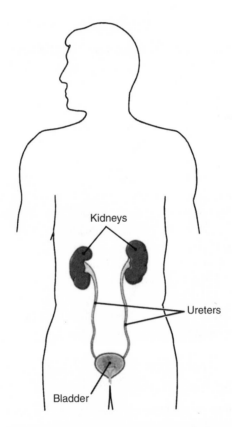

Figure 2.1. *The kidneys remove wastes and extra water from the blood to form urine. Urine flows from the kidneys to the bladder through the ureters.*

- erythropoietin (eh-RITH-ro-POY-eh-tin), or EPO, which stimulates the bone marrow to make red blood cells

- renin (REE-nin), which regulates blood pressure

- the active form of vitamin D, which helps maintain calcium for bones and for normal chemical balance in the body

What is renal function?

Your healthcare team may talk about the work your kidneys do as renal function. If you have two healthy kidneys, you have 100 percent of your renal function. This is more renal function than you really need. Some people are born with only one kidney, and these people

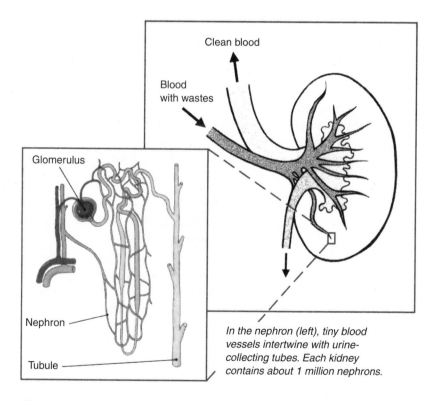

Clean blood

Blood with wastes

Glomerulus

Nephron

Tubule

In the nephron (left), tiny blood vessels intertwine with urine-collecting tubes. Each kidney contains about 1 million nephrons.

Figure 2.2. *In the nephron, tiny blood vessels intertwine with urine-collecting tubes. Each kidney contains about one million nephrons.*

are able to lead normal, healthy lives. Many people donate a kidney for transplantation to a family member or friend. Small declines in renal function may not cause a problem.

But many people with reduced renal function have a kidney disease that will get worse. You will have serious health problems if you have less than 25 percent of your renal function. If your renal function drops below 10 to 15 percent, you cannot live long without some form of renal replacement therapy—either dialysis or transplantation.

Why do kidneys fail?

Most kidney diseases attack the nephrons, causing them to lose their filtering capacity. Damage to the nephrons may happen quickly, often as the result of injury or poisoning. But most kidney diseases destroy the nephrons slowly and silently. Only after years, or even decades, will the damage become apparent. Most kidney diseases attack both kidneys simultaneously.

The two most common causes of kidney disease are diabetes and high blood pressure. If your family has a history of any kind of kidney problems, you may be at risk for kidney disease.

Diabetic nephropathy: Diabetes is a disease that keeps the body from using glucose (sugar) as it should. If glucose stays in your blood instead of breaking down, it can act like a poison. Damage to the nephrons from unused glucose in the blood is called diabetic nephropathy. If you keep your blood glucose levels down, you can delay or prevent diabetic nephropathy.

High blood pressure: High blood pressure can damage the small blood vessels in your kidneys. The damaged vessels cannot filter wastes from your blood as they are supposed to.

Your doctor may prescribe blood pressure medication. Blood pressure medicines called angiotensin-converting enzyme (ACE) inhibitors and angiotensin receptor blockers (ARBs) have been found to protect the kidneys even more than other medicines that lower blood pressure to similar levels. The National Heart, Lung, and Blood Institute (NHLBI), one of the National Institutes of Health, recommends that people with diabetes or reduced kidney function should keep their blood pressure below 130/80 mm Hg.

Glomerulonephritis: Several different types of kidney disease are grouped together under this category. Protein, blood, or both in the urine are often the first signs of these diseases. They can slowly destroy kidney function. Blood pressure control is important, and different treatments for the different types of glomerulonephritis may be used.

Inherited and congenital kidney diseases: Some kidney diseases result from hereditary factors. Polycystic kidney disease (PKD), for example, is a genetic disorder in which many cysts grow in the kidneys. PKD cysts can slowly replace much of the mass of the kidneys, reducing kidney function and leading to kidney failure.

Some kidney problems may show up when a child is still developing in the womb. Examples include autosomal recessive PKD, a rare form of PKD, and other developmental problems that interfere with the normal formation of the nephrons. The signs of kidney disease in children vary. A child may grow unusually slowly, may vomit often, or may have back or side pain. Some kidney diseases may be "silent" for months or even years.

If your child has a kidney disease, your child's doctor should find it during a regular checkup. Be sure your child sees a doctor regularly. The first sign of a kidney problem may be high blood pressure, a low number of red blood cells (anemia), or blood or protein in the child's urine. If the doctor finds any of these problems, further tests may be necessary, including additional blood and urine tests or radiology studies. In some cases, the doctor may need to perform a biopsy—removing a tiny piece of the kidney to examine under a microscope.

Some hereditary kidney diseases may not be detected until adulthood. The most common form of PKD was once called "adult PKD" because the symptoms of high blood pressure and renal failure usually do not occur until patients are in their twenties or thirties. But with advances in diagnostic imaging technology, doctors have found cysts in children and adolescents before any symptoms appear.

Other causes of kidney disease: Poisons and trauma, for example a direct and forceful blow to your kidneys, can lead to kidney disease.

Some over-the-counter medicines can be poisonous to your kidneys if taken regularly over a long period of time. Products that combine aspirin, acetaminophen, and other medicines such as ibuprofen have been found to be the most dangerous to the kidneys. If you take pain-killers regularly, check with your doctor to make sure you are not putting your kidneys at risk.

How do kidneys fail?

Many factors that influence the speed of kidney failure are not completely understood. Researchers are still studying how protein in the diet and cholesterol levels in the blood affect kidney function.

Acute renal failure: Some kidney problems happen quickly, like an accident that injures the kidneys. Losing a lot of blood can cause sudden kidney failure. Some drugs or poisons can make your kidneys stop working. These sudden drops in kidney function are called acute renal failure (ARF).

ARF may lead to permanent loss of kidney function. But if your kidneys are not seriously damaged, acute renal failure may be reversed.

Chronic kidney disease: Most kidney problems, however, happen slowly. You may have "silent" kidney disease for years. Gradual loss of kidney function is called chronic kidney disease (CKD) or chronic renal insufficiency. People with CKD may go on to permanent kidney failure. They also have a high risk of dying from a stroke or heart attack.

End-stage renal disease: The condition of total or nearly total and permanent kidney failure is called end-stage renal disease (ESRD). People with ESRD must undergo dialysis or transplantation to stay alive.

What are the signs of kidney disease?

People in the early stages of kidney disease usually do not feel sick at all.

If your kidney disease gets worse, you may need to urinate more often or less often. You may feel tired or itchy. You may lose your appetite or experience nausea and vomiting. Your hands or feet may swell or feel numb. You may get drowsy or have trouble concentrating. Your skin may darken. You may have muscle cramps.

What can I do about kidney disease?

Unfortunately, chronic kidney disease often cannot be cured. But if you are in the early stages of a kidney disease, you may be able to make your kidneys last longer by taking certain steps. You will also want to be sure that risks for heart attack and stroke are minimized, since CKD patients are susceptible to these problems.

- If you have diabetes, watch your blood glucose closely to keep it under control. Consult your doctor for the latest in treatment.

- Avoid pain pills that may make your kidney disease worse. Check with your doctor before taking any medicine.

Blood pressure: People with reduced kidney function (a high creatinine level in the blood or a low creatinine clearance) should have their blood pressure controlled, and an ACE inhibitor or an ARB should be one of their medications. Many people will require two or more types of medication to keep the blood pressure below 130/80 mm Hg. A diuretic is an important addition to the ACE inhibitor or ARB.

Diet: People with reduced kidney function need to be aware that some parts of a normal diet may speed their kidney failure.

Protein is important to your body. It helps your body repair muscles and fight disease. Protein comes mostly from meat. As discussed in an earlier portion of this text, healthy kidneys take wastes out of the blood but leave protein. Impaired kidneys may fail to separate the protein from the wastes. Some doctors tell their kidney patients to limit the amount of protein they eat so that the kidneys have less work to do. But you cannot avoid protein entirely. You may need to work with a dietitian to find the right food plan.

Another problem that may be associated with kidney failure is too much cholesterol (koh-LES-tuh-rawl) in your blood. High levels of cholesterol may result from a high-fat diet. Cholesterol can build up on the inside walls of your blood vessels. The buildup makes pumping blood through the vessels harder for your heart and can cause heart attacks and strokes.

Smoking not only increases the risk of kidney disease, it contributes to deaths from strokes and heart attacks in people with CKD. You should try your best to stop smoking.

Sodium is a chemical found in salt and other foods. Sodium in your diet may raise your blood pressure, so you should limit foods that contain high levels of sodium. High-sodium foods include canned or processed foods like frozen dinners and hot dogs.

Potassium is a mineral found naturally in many fruits and vegetables, like potatoes, bananas, dried fruits, dried beans and peas, and nuts. Healthy kidneys measure potassium in your blood and remove excess amounts. Diseased kidneys may fail to remove excess potassium, and with very poor kidney function, high potassium levels can affect the heart rhythm.

Treating anemia: Anemia is a condition in which the blood does not contain enough red blood cells. These cells are important because they carry oxygen throughout the body. If you are anemic, you will feel tired and look pale. Healthy kidneys make the hormone EPO, which stimulates the bones to make red blood cells. Diseased kidneys may not make enough EPO. You may need to take injections of a manmade form of EPO.

Preparing for end-stage renal disease: As your kidney disease progresses, you will need to make several decisions. You will need to learn about your options for treating ESRD so that you can make an informed choice between hemodialysis, peritoneal dialysis, and transplantation.

What happens if my kidneys fail completely?

Complete and irreversible kidney failure is sometimes called end-stage renal disease, or ESRD. If your kidneys stop working completely, your body fills with extra water and waste products. This condition is called uremia. Your hands or feet may swell. You will feel tired and weak because your body needs clean blood to function properly.

Untreated uremia may lead to seizures or coma and will ultimately result in death. If your kidneys stop working completely, you will need to undergo dialysis or kidney transplantation.

Dialysis: The two major forms of dialysis are hemodialysis and peritoneal dialysis. In hemodialysis, your blood is sent through a machine that filters away waste products. The clean blood is returned to your body. Hemodialysis is usually performed at a dialysis center three times per week for three to four hours.

In peritoneal dialysis, a fluid is put into your abdomen. This fluid, called dialysate, captures the waste products from your blood. After a few hours, the dialysate containing your body's wastes is drained away. Then, a fresh bag of dialysate is dripped into the abdomen. Patients can perform peritoneal dialysis themselves. Patients using continuous ambulatory peritoneal dialysis (CAPD), the most common form of peritoneal dialysis, change dialysate four times a day. Another form of peritoneal dialysis, however, can be performed at night with a machine that drains and refills the abdomen automatically.

Transplantation: A donated kidney may come from an anonymous donor who has recently died or from a living person, usually a relative. The kidney that you receive must be a good match for your body. The more the new kidney is like you, the less likely your immune system is to reject it. Your immune system protects you from disease by attacking anything that is not recognized as a normal part of your body. So your immune system will attack a kidney that appears too "foreign." You will take special drugs to help trick your immune system so it does not reject the transplanted kidney.

Hope through Research

As our understanding of the causes of kidney failure increases, so will our ability to predict and prevent these diseases. Recent studies have shown that intensive control of diabetes and high blood pressure can prevent or delay the onset of kidney disease.

In the area of genetics, researchers supported by the National Institute of Diabetes and Digestive and Kidney Diseases (NIDDK) have located two genes that cause the most common form of PKD and learned that a person must have two defective copies of the *PKD1* gene to develop PKD. Researchers have also found a gene in the roundworm that is identical to the *PKD1* gene. This new knowledge will be used in the search for effective therapies to prevent or treat PKD.

In the area of transplantation, new drugs to help the body accept foreign tissue increase the likelihood that a transplanted kidney will survive and function properly. Scientists at NIDDK are also developing new techniques to induce tolerance for foreign tissue in patients before they receive transplanted organs. This technique will eliminate or reduce the need for immunosuppressive drugs and thereby reduce expense and complications. In the distant future, scientists may develop an artificial kidney for implantation.

Chapter 3

Protect Your Kidneys from Common Risks

Chapter Contents

Section 3.1

You Have the Power to Prevent Kidney Disease

National Kidney Disease Education Program (NKDEP), National Institute of Diabetes and Digestive and Kidney Diseases (NIDDK), National Institutes of Health (NIH). Reviewed April 26, 2005.

What to Ask Your Doctor or Healthcare Professional

1. Based on my medical and family history, am I at risk for kidney disease?

2. Would lowering my blood pressure help reduce my risk of developing kidney disease?

3. Do my blood and urine tests show signs of kidney disease?

4. How can I prevent or control kidney disease?

Learn the Risks

Kidney disease is a growing problem in the United States. It is a problem that affects adults of all ages and races. People with diabetes, high blood pressure, or a family member with kidney failure are more likely to develop kidney disease. African Americans with any of these risk factors have an even greater chance of developing this disease.

- African Americans are four times more likely to get kidney failure than whites.

- Diabetes and high blood pressure are the two leading causes of kidney failure in African Americans.

- Many African Americans know they have diabetes or high blood pressure, but do not know that they may also have kidney disease.

Healthy kidneys filter your blood. They remove waste and extra water. They help control the amount of certain chemicals in your blood like sodium, phosphorus, and potassium. The right balance of these chemicals helps your body work well. Healthy kidneys help keep this balance.

When kidneys are diseased they slowly stop doing these jobs. If not treated, kidney disease can lead to kidney failure. When that happens, dialysis or a kidney transplant are the only options for keeping a person alive.

Are You at Risk for Kidney Disease?

- Do you have diabetes?
- Do you have high blood pressure?
- Did your mother, father, sister, or brother ever have kidney disease or failure?
- Has a doctor ever told you that you had protein in your urine?

If you answered "yes" to any of these questions, you are at risk for kidney disease. Now is the time to talk to your doctor or healthcare professional about getting tested. It could save your life.

Stop a Disease that Comes Without Warning

Early kidney disease is a silent problem, like high blood pressure. Kidney disease can become kidney failure with little or no warning, and is usually discovered right before the kidneys fail. If you have diabetes, high blood pressure, or a family member with kidney failure, a doctor or healthcare professional should test your blood and urine for early signs of kidney disease. You can take steps to keep your kidneys working if the tests show kidney disease.

Steps to Protect Your Kidneys

1. Control your blood pressure and diabetes.
2. Ask your doctor or healthcare professional to test your blood and urine for kidney disease.
3. If these tests show kidney disease, special medicines called ACE-inhibitors or ARBs [angiotensin receptor blockers] can help. Talk to your doctor about these medications.

Tips for Talking with Your Doctor or Healthcare Professional

- Know as much as you can about your family's medical history.

- Take a copy of this document with you so you don't forget what to ask.

- Write down the answers you get and ask more questions if you need to.

- Bring someone else with you for support and to help you remember what you learn.

Section 3.2

Diabetes and Kidney Disease

"Kidney Disease of Diabetes," National Kidney and Urologic Diseases Information Clearinghouse (NKUDIC), a service of the National Institute of Diabetes and Digestive and Kidney Diseases (NIDDK), National Institutes of Health (NIH), Pub. No. 04-3925, November 2003.

Each year in the United States, nearly 100,000 people are diagnosed with kidney failure, a serious condition in which the kidneys fail to rid the body of wastes. Kidney failure is the final stage of a slow deterioration of the kidneys, a process known as nephropathy.

Diabetes is the most common cause of kidney failure, accounting for more than 40 percent of new cases. Even when drugs and diet are able to control diabetes, the disease can lead to nephropathy and kidney failure. Most people with diabetes do not develop nephropathy that is severe enough to cause kidney failure. About 17 million people in the United States have diabetes, and over 100,000 people are living with kidney failure as a result of diabetes.

People with kidney failure undergo either dialysis, which substitutes for some of the filtering functions of the kidneys, or transplantation to receive a healthy donor kidney. Most U.S. citizens who develop kidney failure are eligible for federally funded care. In 2000, care for patients with kidney failure cost the nation nearly $20 billion.

African Americans, American Indians, and Hispanic Americans develop diabetes, nephropathy, and kidney failure at rates higher than average. Scientists have not been able to explain these higher rates. Nor can they explain fully the interplay of factors leading to diabetic nephropathy—factors including heredity, diet, and other medical conditions, such as high blood pressure. They have found that high blood pressure and high levels of blood glucose increase the risk that a person with diabetes will progress to kidney failure.

Two Types of Diabetes

There are two types of diabetes. In patients with either type, the body does not properly process and use food. The human body normally converts food to glucose, the simple sugar that is the main source of energy for the body's cells. To enter cells, glucose needs the help of insulin, a hormone produced by the pancreas. When a person does not make enough insulin, or the body does not respond to the insulin that is present, the body cannot process glucose, and it builds up in the bloodstream. High levels of glucose in the blood lead to a diagnosis of diabetes. Both types of diabetes can lead to kidney disease.

Type 1 Diabetes

Only about 1 in 20 people with diabetes has type 1 diabetes, which tends to occur in young adults and children. Type 1 used to be known as insulin-dependent diabetes mellitus (IDDM) or juvenile diabetes. In type 1 diabetes, the body stops producing insulin. People with type 1 diabetes must take daily insulin injections or use an insulin pump. They also control blood glucose levels with meal planning and physical activity. Type 1 diabetes is more likely to lead to kidney failure. Twenty to 40 percent of people with type 1 diabetes develop kidney failure by the age of 50. Some develop kidney failure before the age of 30.

Type 2 Diabetes

About 95 percent of people with diabetes have type 2 diabetes, once known as non-insulin-dependent diabetes mellitus (NIDDM) or adult-onset diabetes. Many people with type 2 diabetes do not respond normally to their own or to injected insulin—a condition called insulin resistance. Type 2 diabetes occurs more often in people over the age of 40, and many people with type 2 are overweight. Many also are not aware that they have the disease. Some people with type 2 control their blood glucose with meal planning and physical activity. Others must take pills that stimulate production of insulin, reduce insulin resistance, decrease the liver's output of glucose, or slow absorption of carbohydrate from the gastrointestinal tract. Still others require injections of insulin. Between 1993 and 1997, more than 100,000 people in the United States were treated for kidney failure caused by type 2 diabetes.

The Course of Kidney Disease

Diabetic kidney disease takes many years to develop. In some people, the filtering function of the kidneys is actually higher than normal in the first few years of their diabetes. This process has been called hyperfiltration.

Over several years, people who are developing kidney disease will have small amounts of the blood protein albumin begin to leak into their urine. At its first stage, this condition has been called microalbuminuria. The kidney's filtration function usually remains normal during this period.

As the disease progresses, more albumin leaks into the urine. Various names are attached to this interval of the disease such as overt diabetic nephropathy or macroalbuminuria. As the amount of albumin in the urine increases, filtering function usually begins to drop. The body retains various wastes as filtration falls. Creatinine is one such waste, and a blood test for creatinine can measure the decline in kidney filtration. As kidney damage develops, blood pressure often rises as well.

Overall, kidney damage rarely occurs in the first 10 years of diabetes, and usually 15 to 25 years will pass before kidney failure occurs. For people who live with diabetes for more than 25 years without any signs of kidney failure, the risk of ever developing it decreases.

Effects of High Blood Pressure

High blood pressure, or hypertension, is a major factor in the development of kidney problems in people with diabetes. Both a family history of hypertension and the presence of hypertension appear to increase chances of developing kidney disease. Hypertension also accelerates the progress of kidney disease where it already exists. See Section 3.3 for additional information about hypertension.

Preventing and Slowing Kidney Disease

Blood Pressure Medicines

Any medicine that helps patients achieve a blood pressure target of 130/80 or lower provides benefits. Patients with even mild hypertension or persistent microalbuminuria should consult a physician about the use of antihypertensive medicines.

Moderate-Protein Diets

In people with diabetes, excessive consumption of protein may be harmful. Experts recommend that people with kidney disease of diabetes consume the recommended dietary allowance (RDA) for protein, but avoid high-protein diets. For people with greatly reduced kidney function, a diet containing reduced amounts of protein may help delay the onset of kidney failure. Anyone following a reduced-protein diet should work with a dietitian to ensure adequate nutrition.

Intensive Management of Blood Glucose

Antihypertensive drugs and low-protein diets can slow kidney disease when significant nephropathy is present. A third treatment, known as intensive management of blood glucose or glycemic control, has shown great promise for people with type 1 and type 2 diabetes, especially for those in early stages of nephropathy.

Intensive management is a treatment regimen that aims to keep blood glucose levels close to normal. The regimen includes testing blood glucose frequently, administering insulin frequently throughout the day on the basis of food intake and exercise, following a diet and exercise plan, and consulting a healthcare team frequently. Some people use an insulin pump to supply insulin throughout the day.

A number of studies have pointed to the beneficial effects of intensive management. Two such studies, funded by the National Institute of Diabetes and Digestive and Kidney Diseases (NIDDK) of the National Institutes of Health, are the Diabetes Control and Complications Trial (DCCT) and a trial led by researchers at the University of Minnesota Medical School. A third study, conducted in the United Kingdom, is the U.K. Prospective Diabetes Study (UKPDS).

The DCCT, conducted from 1983 to 1993, involved 1,441 participants who had type 1 diabetes. Researchers found a 50 percent decrease in both development and progression of early diabetic kidney disease in participants who followed an intensive regimen for controlling blood glucose levels. The intensively managed patients had average blood glucose levels of 150 milligrams per deciliter—about 80 milligrams per deciliter lower than the levels observed in the conventionally managed patients.

In the Minnesota Medical School trial, researchers examined kidney tissues of people with long-standing diabetes who received healthy kidney transplants. After five years, patients who followed an intensive regimen developed significantly fewer lesions in their glomeruli than did patients not following an intensive regimen. This result, along with findings of the DCCT and studies performed in Scandinavia, suggests that any program resulting in sustained lowering of blood glucose levels will be beneficial to patients in the early stages of diabetic nephropathy.

The UKPDS—a 20-year trial conducted in England, Ireland, and Scotland—tested the effects of intensive glucose and blood pressure control in people with type 2 diabetes and found similar benefits for this group.

Dialysis and Transplantation

When people with diabetes experience kidney failure, they must undergo either dialysis or a kidney transplant. As recently as the 1970s, medical experts commonly excluded people with diabetes from dialysis and transplantation, in part because the experts felt damage caused by diabetes would offset benefits of the treatments. Today, because of better control of diabetes and improved rates of survival following treatment, doctors do not hesitate to offer dialysis and kidney transplantation to people with diabetes.

Currently, the survival of kidneys transplanted into patients with diabetes is about the same as survival of transplants in people without diabetes. Dialysis for people with diabetes also works well in the short run. Even so, people with diabetes who receive transplants or dialysis experience higher morbidity and mortality because of coexisting complications of the diabetes—such as damage to the heart, eyes, and nerves.

Good Care Makes a Difference

If you have diabetes:

- Have your doctor measure your A1C level at least twice a year. The test provides a weighted average of your blood glucose level for the previous three months. Aim to keep it at less than seven percent.

- Work with your doctor regarding insulin injections, medicines, meal planning, physical activity, and blood glucose monitoring.

- Have your blood pressure checked several times a year. If blood pressure is high, follow your doctor's plan for keeping it near normal levels. Aim to keep it at less than 130/80.

- Ask your doctor whether you might benefit from taking an ACE inhibitor or ARB.

- Have your urine checked yearly for microalbumin and protein. If there is protein in your urine, have your blood checked for elevated amounts of waste products such as creatinine. The doctor should provide you with an estimate of your kidney's filtration based on the blood creatinine level.

- Ask your doctor whether you should reduce the amount of protein in your diet. Ask for a referral to see a registered dietitian to help you with meal planning.

Hope through Research

The incidences of both diabetes and kidney failure caused by diabetes have been rising. Some experts predict that diabetes soon might account for half the cases of kidney failure. In light of the increasing morbidity and mortality related to diabetes and kidney failure, patients, researchers, and healthcare professionals will continue to benefit by addressing the relationship between the two diseases. NIDDK is a leader in supporting research in this area.

Several areas of research supported by NIDDK hold great potential. Discovery of ways to predict who will develop kidney disease may lead to greater prevention, as people with diabetes who learn they are at risk institute strategies such as intensive management and blood pressure control. Discovery of better anti-rejection drugs will improve results of kidney transplantation in patients with diabetes who develop kidney failure. For some people with type 1 diabetes, advances in transplantation—especially transplantation of insulin-producing cells of the pancreas—could lead to a cure for both diabetes and the kidney disease of diabetes.

Section 3.3

High Blood Pressure and Kidney Disease

National Kidney and Urologic Diseases Information Clearinghouse (NKUDIC), a service of the National Institute of Diabetes and Digestive and Kidney Diseases (NIDDK), National Institutes of Health (NIH), Pub. No. 03-4572, July 2003.

Your kidneys play a key role in keeping your blood pressure in a healthy range, and blood pressure, in turn, can affect the health of your kidneys. High blood pressure, also called hypertension, can damage the kidneys.

What is high blood pressure?

Blood pressure measures the force of blood against the walls of your blood vessels. Blood pressure that remains high over time is called hypertension. Extra fluid in your body increases the amount of fluid in your blood vessels and makes your blood pressure higher. Narrow or clogged blood vessels also raise blood pressure. If you have high blood pressure, see your doctor regularly.

How does high blood pressure hurt my kidneys?

High blood pressure makes your heart work harder and, over time, can damage blood vessels throughout your body. If the blood vessels in your kidneys are damaged, they may stop removing wastes and extra fluid from your body. The extra fluid in your blood vessels may then raise blood pressure even more. It's a dangerous cycle.

High blood pressure is one of the leading causes of kidney failure, also commonly called end-stage renal disease (ESRD). People with kidney failure must either receive a kidney transplant or go on dialysis. Every year, high blood pressure causes more than 15,000 new cases of kidney failure in the United States.

How will I know whether I have high blood pressure?

Most people with high blood pressure have no symptoms. The only way to know whether your blood pressure is high is to have a health professional measure it with a blood pressure cuff. The result is expressed as two numbers. The top number, which is called the systolic pressure, represents the pressure when your heart is beating. The bottom number, which is called the diastolic pressure, shows the pressure when your heart is resting between beats. Your blood pressure is considered normal if it stays below 120/80 (expressed as "120 over 80"). People with a systolic blood pressure of 120 to 139 or a diastolic blood pressure of 80 to 89 are considered pre-hypertensive and should adopt health-promoting lifestyle changes to prevent diseases of the heart and blood vessels.

How will I know whether I have kidney damage?

Kidney damage, like hypertension, can be unnoticeable and detected only through medical tests. Blood tests will show whether your kidneys are removing wastes efficiently. Your doctor may refer to tests for serum creatinine and BUN, which stands for blood urea nitrogen. Having too much creatinine and urea nitrogen in your blood is a sign that you have kidney damage.

Another sign is proteinuria, or protein in your urine. Proteinuria has also been shown to be associated with heart disease and damaged blood vessels. [For more information, see Chapter 37 "Proteinuria" which has been reprinted from the National Institute of Diabetes and Digestive and Kidney Diseases (NIDDK).]

How can I prevent high blood pressure from damaging my kidneys?

If you have kidney damage, you should keep your blood pressure below 130/80. The National Heart, Lung, and Blood Institute (NHLBI), one of the National Institutes of Health (NIH), recommends that people with kidney disease use whatever therapy is necessary, including lifestyle changes and medicines, to keep their blood pressure below 130/80.

NHLBI has found that five lifestyle changes can help control blood pressure:

- Maintain your weight at a level close to normal. Choose fruits, vegetables, grains, and low-fat dairy foods.

- Limit your daily sodium (salt) intake to 2,000 milligrams or lower if you already have high blood pressure. Read nutrition labels on packaged foods to learn how much sodium is in one serving. Keep a sodium diary.

- Get plenty of exercise, which means at least 30 minutes of moderate activity, such as walking, most days of the week.

- Avoid consuming too much alcohol. Men should limit consumption to two drinks (two 12-ounce servings of beer or two 5-ounce servings of wine or two 1.5-ounce servings of "hard" liquor) a day. Women should have no more than a single serving on a given day because metabolic differences make women more susceptible.

- Limit caffeine intake.

Are there medicines that can help?

Many people need medicine to control high blood pressure. Two groups of medications called ACE (angiotensin-converting enzyme) inhibitors and ARBs (angiotensin receptor blockers) lower blood pressure and have an added protective effect on the kidney in people with diabetes. Additional studies have shown that ACE inhibitors and ARBs also reduce proteinuria and slow the progression of kidney damage in people who do not have diabetes. You may need to take a combination of two or more blood pressure medicines to stay below 130/80.

What groups are at risk for kidney failure related to high blood pressure?

All racial groups have some risk of developing kidney failure from high blood pressure. African Americans, American Indians, and Alaska Natives, however, are more likely than whites to have high blood pressure and to develop kidney problems from it—even when their blood pressure is only mildly elevated. In fact, African Americans are six times more likely than whites to develop hypertension-related kidney failure.

People with diabetes also have a substantially increased risk for developing kidney failure. People who are at risk both because of their race and because of diabetes should have early management of high blood pressure.

The National Institute of Diabetes and Digestive and Kidney Diseases (NIDDK), also part of the National Institutes of Health (NIH), sponsored the African American Study of Kidney Disease and Hypertension (AASK) to find effective ways to prevent high blood pressure and kidney failure in this population. The results, released in 2003, showed that an ACE inhibitor was better at slowing the progression of kidney disease in African Americans than either of two other drugs.

Hope through Research

In recent years, researchers have learned a great deal about kidney disease. NIDDK sponsors several programs aimed at understanding kidney failure and finding treatments to stop its progression. NIDDK's Division of Kidney, Urologic, and Hematologic Diseases supports basic research into normal kidney function and the diseases that impair normal function at the cellular and molecular levels, including diabetes, high blood pressure, glomerulonephritis, and polycystic kidney disease.

Section 3.4

Obesity Can Increase Your Risk for Kidney Disease

What is obesity?

People who are obese have an excess amount of body fat. In contrast, people who are overweight have an excess amount of body weight that includes muscle, bone, fat, and water. Some people, such as body-builders or other athletes with a lot of muscle can be overweight without being obese. Men with more than 25 percent body fat and women with more than 30 percent body fat are considered obese. More than 60 percent of Americans aged 20 and older are overweight, and 25 percent are also obese.

How is obesity measured?

Different methods have been used to measure if someone is overweight and obese. Today, body mass index (BMI) has become the standard. BMI uses a formula based on your height and weight. Most

31

doctors agree that people with a BMI of 30 or more can improve their health through weight loss.

Can obesity cause health problems?

Yes. According to the National Institutes of Health, 280,000 adult deaths each year in the U.S. are related to obesity. People who are overweight or obese have an increased health risk for chronic diseases like type 2 diabetes, high blood pressure, kidney disease, stroke, and heart disease.

Does obesity increase your risk for diabetes?

Yes. Obesity has been directly linked to the growing number of cases of type 2 diabetes in the U.S. type 2 is the most common type of diabetes, accounting for more than 90 percent of all cases. As diabetes is the number one cause of chronic kidney disease, obesity is also an important factor in chronic kidney disease.

Type 2 diabetes has been increasing in all groups, but especially among African Americans, Hispanic Americans, Asian Americans, and American Indians. This is due in large part to the growing number of obese people in these communities.

Type 2 diabetes used to occur mostly in individuals over 45. Now, the disease is becoming more common in younger people. This is a very serious problem because it could cause complications such as heart disease and chronic kidney disease to happen at an earlier age. The increasing number of type 2 diabetes cases in younger people is also linked to increasing obesity in people under 45.

Does obesity increase your risk for high blood pressure?

Yes. Being overweight or obese increases your risk of developing high blood pressure. Nearly 50 million Americans have high blood pressure, and many are not aware of it. Losing excess weight helps to lower your risk of developing high blood pressure. In addition, losing excess weight can help to reduce your blood pressure if it is already high. High blood pressure is the second leading cause of chronic kidney disease.

Does obesity increase your risk for chronic kidney disease?

Yes. Because diabetes and high blood pressure are the leading causes of chronic kidney disease, your chance of developing kidney disease is greater if you are overweight or obese.

Does it matter where my excess weight is located?

Yes. Doctors are concerned not only with how much fat a person has, but also where the fat is located on the body. Women typically collect fat around their hips, giving them a pear shape. Men usually build up fat around their bellies giving them more of an apple shape. If you carry fat mainly around your waist, you are more likely to develop obesity-related health problems. Women whose waists measure more than 35 inches or men whose waists measure more than 40 inches have a higher health risk because of their fat distribution.

Does obesity run in families?

Obesity tends to run in families, suggesting that genetics may play a role. However, lifestyle behaviors—such as diet and level of physical activity—also strongly influence obesity.

Can losing excess weight improve my health?

Yes. A weight loss of five to ten percent can help to improve health by lowering blood pressure and cholesterol levels. Weight control is considered the single most important factor in the prevention of high blood pressure. In addition, recent research has shown that a weight loss of five to seven percent can prevent type 2 diabetes in people at high risk for the disease.

Are there any tips to help me lose weight?

You can lower your risk for chronic diseases such as diabetes, high blood pressure, and chronic kidney disease by losing excess weight. Some tips to help change your eating and exercise habits include:

- Learning how to make healthier food choices. Speak to a dietitian if you need help.

- Learning to recognize and control things that make you want to eat even when you are not hungry, such as inviting smells.

- Being more physically active. Most people need to exercise about 45 minutes on most days of the week. Activities like brisk walking can help you get in shape. You should always set a checklist with your doctor before starting an exercise program.

- Keeping daily logs of what you eat, and your physical activity.

Is there anything else I should know?

Chronic kidney disease is often "silent" in its early stages, meaning that you may not see or feel any symptoms. It is important for people who have an increased risk of developing kidney disease to have a test for protein in their urine and a blood test to estimate their level of kidney function (glomerular filtration rate or GFR). Kidney disease can often be successfully treated when detected early. Speak to your doctor about getting tested if you:

- have diabetes.
- have high blood pressure.
- have a family history of chronic kidney disease.
- are older.
- are an African American, Hispanic American, Asian or Pacific Islander or American Indian.

More than 20 million Americans—one in nine adults—has chronic kidney disease, and most don't even know it. More than 20 million others are at increased risk. The National Kidney Foundation, a major voluntary health organization, seeks to prevent kidney and urinary tract diseases, improve the health and well-being of individuals and families affected by these diseases, and increase the availability of all organs for transplantation. Through its 51 affiliates nationwide, the foundation conducts programs in research, professional education, patient and community services, public education, and organ donation. The work of the National Kidney Foundation is funded by public donations.

The National Kidney Foundation provides a free community-based health program called the Kidney Early Evaluation Program (KEEP). This includes tests for the early detection of chronic kidney disease.

Section 3.5

Aging Increases Risk of Urinary and Kidney Disorders

"Aging Changes in the Kidneys," © 2005 A.D.A.M., Inc. Reprinted with permission. Updated October 26, 2004.

Background

The kidneys filter the blood. Wastes are removed and excess fluid is disposed of as urine. The kidneys also play an important role in the chemical balance of the body. As with other organs, kidney function may be slightly reduced with aging.

The urinary system also includes the ureters and the bladder. Bladder control can be affected by muscle changes and changes in the reproductive system.

Aging Changes

As the kidney ages, the number of filtering units (nephrons) is reduced. Nephrons filter waste material from the blood.

In addition to this filtering tissue, the overall amount of kidney tissue is reduced. The blood vessels supplying the kidney can become hardened. The kidneys filter blood more slowly.

The bladder wall changes with age. The elastic tissue is replaced with tough fibrous tissue, and the bladder becomes less "stretchy" (distensible). Muscles weaken, and the bladder may not empty completely when going to the bathroom.

In men, the urethra may become blocked by an enlarged prostate gland. In women, weakened muscles can allow the bladder or vagina to "fall" out of position (prolapse), which can block the urethra.

Effect of Changes

The kidneys have a built-in extra capacity. Under usual conditions, kidney function remains normal in an aging person, although sometimes they function more slowly than the kidneys of a younger person.

However, decreased efficiency occurs when the kidneys are under an increased workload. Illness, medications, and other conditions can increase kidney workload.

The changes in the kidneys may affect an elderly person's ability to concentrate urine and hold onto water. The response to changes in fluids and electrolytes taken in is slowed. Dehydration occurs more readily because older people frequently have less of a sense of thirst.

Dehydration can also be aggravated if an older person reduces fluid intake in an attempt to reduce bladder control problems (urinary incontinence).

Common Problems

Aging increases the risk for urinary disorders including acute kidney failure and chronic kidney failure. Bladder infections and other urinary tract infections are more common in the elderly. In part, this is related to incomplete emptying. It is also related to changes in the chemical balance of the urinary membranes.

Urinary retention (inability to completely drain the bladder, which can back up into the kidneys and damage them) is more common in the elderly. Many older people experience problems with bladder control (urinary incontinence).

Urinary system cancers are more common in the elderly, especially prostate cancer (men) and bladder cancer.

In both men and women, urinary changes are closely related to changes in the reproductive system. For example, men may experience problems because of an enlarged prostate (benign prostatic hypertrophy). Women may experience vaginal infections (vaginitis) and subsequent bladder infections.

Section 3.6

Analgesics and Kidney Health

Many analgesic medicines (pain relievers) are available over the counter. These medicines are generally safe when taken as directed. However, their heavy or long-term use may harm the kidneys. Up to an estimated three to five percent of the new cases of chronic kidney failure each year may be caused by chronic overuse of these medicines. It is important to realize that, while helpful, these medicines are not completely without risk, and they should be used carefully. Kidney disease related to analgesics is preventable.

What are analgesics?

Analgesics are medicines that help to control pain and reduce fever. Examples of analgesics that are available over the counter are: aspirin, acetaminophen, ibuprofen, ketoprofen, and naproxen sodium. Some analgesics contain a combination of ingredients in one pill, such as aspirin, acetaminophen, and caffeine.

Can analgesics hurt kidneys?

Generally, when used according to directions, over-the-counter analgesics are safe. However, heavy or long-term use of these medicines, especially those that contain a mixture of painkilling ingredients—such as aspirin, acetaminophen, and caffeine—in one pill, have been linked to chronic kidney disease in European studies. The warning labels on over-the-counter analgesics tell you not to use these medicines more than ten days for pain and more than three days for fever. If you have pain and/or fever for a longer time, you should see your doctor. The doctor can check for possible medical problems and advise you about what medications you should take.

Is aspirin safe for regular use?

When taken as directed, regular use of aspirin does not seem to increase the risk of kidney disease in people who have normal kidney function. However, taking doses that are too large (usually more than six or eight tablets a day) may temporarily reduce kidney function. In people with kidney disease, aspirin may increase the tendency to bleed. People who already have reduced kidney function or other health problems, such as liver disease or severe heart failure, should not use aspirin without speaking to their doctor.

My doctor recommended that I take an aspirin every day to prevent heart attacks. Will this hurt my kidneys?

No. There is no risk to the regular use of aspirin in the small doses recommended for prevention of heart attacks.

What analgesics are safe for people who have kidney disease?

Acetaminophen remains the drug of choice for occasional use in patients with kidney disease because of bleeding complications that may occur when these patients use aspirin. However, kidney patients who need to use acetaminophen habitually should be supervised by their doctors.

What are NSAIDs? Are they safe to take?

Nonsteroidal anti-inflammatory drugs (NSAIDs) are a specific group of pain relievers. Some NSAIDs are available over the counter. This includes different brands of ibuprofen, naproxen sodium, and ketoprofen.

NSAIDs are safe for occasional use when taken as directed. However, these medications should only be used under a doctor's care by patients with kidney disease, heart disease, high blood pressure or liver disease or by people who are over 65 or who take diuretic medications. In these people, NSAIDs may cause an increased risk of sudden kidney failure and even progressive kidney damage.

I have arthritis. What pain relievers can I take that won't hurt my kidneys?

You should speak to your doctor about the best choice for you. In addition, if you have any of the medical conditions listed in the previous question, you should only use nonsteroidal anti-inflammatory drugs (NSAIDs) under your doctor's supervision.

How do I know if analgesics have affected my kidneys?

Your doctor can check your kidneys by doing simple blood tests like BUN (blood urea nitrogen) and serum creatinine level. These tests measure the amount of waste products in your blood that are normally removed by your kidneys. If your kidneys are not working as well as they should, these levels will be increased in your blood. A urine test for the presence of protein may also be done. Persistent protein in the urine may be an early indication of kidney damage. The results of the serum creatinine test can be used to estimate your glomerular filtration rate (GFR), which tells your doctor how much kidney function you have.

Are there other side effects from taking aspirin and NSAIDs?

Yes. The development of stomach ulcers and gastrointestinal bleeding has been the most common serious side effect from taking NSAIDs and aspirin.

What can I do to keep my kidneys healthy?

Kidney disease caused by analgesics is preventable. Here are some things you can do to help keep your kidneys healthy.

- Do not use over-the-counter pain relievers more than ten days for pain or more than three days for fever. If you have pain or fever for a longer time, you should see your doctor.

- Avoid prolonged use of analgesics that contain a mixture of painkilling ingredients, like aspirin, acetaminophen, and caffeine mixtures in one pill.

- If you are taking analgesics, increase the amount of fluid you drink to six to eight glasses a day.

- If you have kidney disease, consult your doctor before choosing an analgesic.

- Use NSAIDs under your doctor's supervision if you have heart disease, high blood pressure, kidney disease or liver disease or if you take diuretic medications or are over 65 years of age.

- Make sure your doctor knows about all medicines you are taking, even over-the-counter medicines.

- Make sure you read the warning label before using any over-the-counter analgesics.

Chapter 4

Statistical and Demographic Information about Kidney and Urologic Health

Chapter Contents

Section 4.1

Kidney and Urologic Diseases Statistics for the United States

National Kidney and Urologic Diseases Information Clearinghouse (NKUDIC), a service of the National Institute of Diabetes and Digestive and Kidney Diseases (NIDDK), National Institutes of Health (NIH), Pub. No. 04-3895, February 2004. The complete text of this document, including sources, is available online at http://kidney.niddk.nih.gov/kudiseases/pubs/kustats/index.htm.

Kidney Problems

Kidney Disease

Prevalence (1988–1994): An estimated 4.5 percent of adults 20 years of age and older have physiological evidence of chronic kidney disease (7.4 million adults) determined as a moderately or severely reduced glomerular filtration rate.

End-Stage Renal Disease (ESRD)

Prevalence (2001): 392,023 U.S. residents were under treatment during the calendar year resulting from these primary diseases.

- Diabetes: 138,483
- Hypertension: 91,636
- Glomerulonephritis: 60,888
- Cystic kidney: 17,112
- All other: 83,904

Incidence (2001): 93,327 U.S. residents were new beneficiaries of treatment resulting from these primary diseases.

- Diabetes: 41,312
- Hypertension: 24,942
- Glomerulonephritis: 7,687

- Cystic kidney: 2,143
- All other: 17,243

Mortality (2001): Among U.S. residents, there were 177.6 deaths per 1,000 patient years and 76,584 deaths in all patients undergoing ESRD treatment.

Costs for the ESRD Program (2001): $22.8 billion in public and private spending.

Dialysis Treatment (2001): 287,494 U.S. residents with ESRD received dialysis.

- In-center hemodialysis: 259,538
- Home hemodialysis: 1,122
- Peritoneal dialysis: 26,834
    - CAPD (continuous ambulatory peritoneal dialysis): 11,794
    - CCPD (continuous cycler-assisted peritoneal dialysis): 12,014
    - Other PD (peritoneal dialysis): 445
- Uncertain dialysis: 2,581

Kidney Transplants: Number of kidney transplants performed:

- 2001: 15,331
- 2000: 14,680
- 1999: 13,770
- 1998: 13,532
- 1988: 9,655

Organ Donors (2001): Source of organ donations for kidney transplants performed:

- From cadaver: 9,078
- From living related donor: 3,480
- From living unrelated donor: 1,130

Waiting Lists: Number of people awaiting transplants as of December 18, 2003:

- Kidney (only): 56,598
- Kidney and pancreas: 2,444

Dialysis Survival: Probability of patients surviving, from day 91 of ESRD, unadjusted:

- 1 year (2000–2001): 77.8
- 2 years (1999–2001): 62.9
- 5 years (1996–2001): 31.9
- 10 years (1991–2001): 9.0

Patient Survival following Cadaver Transplant: Probability of recipients surviving, from day one of transplantation, unadjusted:

- 1 year (2000–2001): 93.7
- 2 years (1999–2001): 91.6
- 5 years (1996–2001): 80.6
- 10 years (1991–2001): 58.9

Patient Survival following Living-Donor Transplant: Probability of recipients surviving, from day one of transplantation, unadjusted:

- 1 year (2000–2001): 97.6
- 2 years (1998–2001): 96.4
- 5 years (1996–2001): 90.4
- 10 years (1991–2001): 77.8

Urologic Problems

Interstitial Cystitis: Prevalence: 1988–1994

- An estimated 3.6 percent of adults aged 20 or older (6.2 million) self-report having had a bladder infection that lasted more than three months (2.1 percent of men and 5.0 percent of women reported a history of this problem).
- An estimated 847,000 adults aged 20 or older self-report having been diagnosed with interstitial cystitis: 94 percent of affected adults were women.

Urinary Stones

Prevalence of Kidney Stones: The percent of adults aged 20–74 who self-reported ever having had kidney stones:

- 1988–1994: 5.2 percent of adults (6.3 percent of men and 4.1 percent of women)
- 1976–1980: 3.2 percent of adults (4.9 percent of men and 2.8 percent of women)

Hospital Discharges: The estimated number of hospital discharges among adults aged 20 years or older with "calculus of kidney and ureters" as a primary diagnosis:

- 2001: 177,509 discharges
- 2000: 168,564 discharges

Doctor Visits: The estimated number of doctor visits by adults aged 20 years or older with "calculus of kidney and ureters" as a listed diagnosis:

- 2000: 2.2 million visits
- 1999: 1.8 million visits

Cost (1993): $1.83 billion expended (direct and indirect) for evaluation and treatment.

Urinary Tract Infections (UTIs)

Prevalence (1988–1994): An estimated 34 percent of adults aged 20 or older (61.4 million) self-reported having had at least one occurrence of a urinary tract infection or cystitis.

- 13.9 percent (11.7 million) of men have had a UTI or cystitis
- 53.5 percent (49.7 million) of women have had a UTI or cystitis

Incidence (1988–1994): 794 per 10,000 adults aged 20 years or older have at least one occurrence of a urinary tract infection or cystitis.

Hospital Discharges: The estimated number of hospital discharges among adults aged 20 years or older with urinary tract infection or cystitis listed as a diagnosis:

- 2001: 1.78 million discharges (0.49 million men; 1.29 million women)

- 2000: 1.69 million discharges (0.47 million men; 1.22 million women)

Doctor Visits: The estimated number of doctor visits by patients aged 20 years or older, with urinary tract infection or cystitis listed as a diagnosis:

- 2000: 9.1 million visits (1.3 million men; 7.9 million women)

- 1999: 7.9 million visits (0.9 million men; 7.0 million women)

Urinary Incontinence

Prevalence (2001): In community dwelling adults, urinary incontinence affects an estimated 35 percent of women 65 years or older and 10 percent of women younger than 65 years and an estimated 22 percent of men 65 years or older and 1.5 percent of men younger than 65 years. Approximately 30 to 50 percent of institutionalized adults 65 years or older have urinary incontinence.

Costs (1995): $16.3 billion annually in direct expenditures for routine care, evaluations, and treatments in persons aged 15 years and older.

Other Related Problems

Enlarged Prostate: Benign Prostatic Hyperplasia (BPH)

Prevalence (1999–2000): 9.0 percent of men aged 30 years and older (6.3 million men) self-reported having been told by a physician that their prostate gland was enlarged and the enlargement was benign. BPH prevalence estimates for different ages are as follows:

- 30–54: 2.2 percent

- 55–74: 19.6 percent

- 75–up: 36.3 percent

Hospital Discharges: The estimated number of hospital discharges among men aged 20 years or older with a discharge diagnosis of "hyperplasia of the prostate":

- 2001: 402,000 discharges
- 2000: 398,000 discharges

Doctor Visits: The estimated number of doctor visits by men aged 20 years or older with "hyperplasia of the prostate" as a listed diagnosis:

- 2000: 6.4 million visits
- 1999: 6.0 million visits

Erectile Dysfunction: Impotence

Prevalence (2000–2002): 20 percent to 46 percent of men aged 40-69 years in community surveys self-reported moderate or complete erectile dysfunction.

Incidence (2000): 26 new cases per 1,000 population of men 40–69 years of age.

Prostate Cancer

Incidence (1996–2000): 975 cases per 100,000 population for men 65 years or older; 57 cases per 100,000 population for men under 65 years old.

Mortality (1996–2000): 245 deaths per 100,000 population for men 65 years or older; 2 deaths per 100,000 population for men under 65 years old.

Lifetime Prevalence (2000): The number of living men who have had a diagnosis of prostate cancer is 1.6 million.

Section 4.2

Few Americans Are Aware They Have Chronic Kidney Disease

National Institute of Diabetes and Digestive and Kidney Diseases
(NIDDK), National Institutes of Health (NIH), NIH News Press Release,
December 17, 2004.

Ten to 20 million people in the United States have kidney disease but most don't know it, according to researchers at the National Institute of Diabetes and Digestive and Kidney Diseases (NIDDK) at the National Institutes of Health, the Johns Hopkins Bloomberg School of Public Health, and the National Center for Health Statistics (NCHS) at the Centers for Disease Control and Prevention. The findings are in the *Journal of the American Society of Nephrology.*

Over the past decade the number of people with kidney failure doubled and the number starting dialysis or having a first kidney transplant increased by 50 percent, so that more than 400,000 Americans are now being treated for kidney failure at a cost of $25 billion annually. In contrast to these dramatic increases, the study also found that the number of people with earlier stages of kidney disease remained stable. About 7.4 million people have less than half the kidney function of a healthy young adult. Another 11.3 million have at least half of what's considered normal function, but they also have persistent protein in their urine, a sign of kidney disease. The researchers can't explain the paradox between stable prevalence of kidney disease and rising incidence of kidney failure, but they suggest that fewer patients may be dying and more may be progressing faster to dialysis.

"Given the high prevalence of chronic kidney disease, we need to increase awareness, diagnosis, and treatment if we are going to reduce the rate of progression and complications. Most critical are control of diabetes and hypertension," said Josef Coresh, M.D., Ph.D., lead author of the study and professor of epidemiology, medicine, and biostatistics at the Bloomberg School of Public Health in Baltimore.

Coresh and his colleagues estimated awareness of chronic kidney disease among 4,101 people in the United States from 1999 to 2000 and compared disease prevalence in those years with that from 1988 to 1994, when 15,488 people were surveyed. Data were from two National Health and Nutrition Examination Surveys by NCHS of nationally representative, non-institutionalized adults.

In the most recent survey, participants were asked: "Have you ever been told by a doctor or other health professional that you had weak or failing kidneys (excluding kidney stones, bladder infections, or incontinence)?" Less than ten percent of adults with moderately decreased kidney function (one-half to one-quarter the filtering capacity of a young healthy adult) reported being told they had weakened or failing kidneys. Awareness was low in all but the most severe stages of kidney disease. Women with moderately decreased kidney function were significantly less aware of their illness compared to similarly affected men. The researchers determined actual kidney function from blood and urine tests and estimated glomerular filtration rate (GFR), a measure of how well the kidneys are filtering waste from the blood.

Lack of awareness may be due in part to doctors' sole reliance on the blood level of a substance known as creatinine. Because muscle mass and other person-to-person variables can alter creatinine levels, a "normal" reading can provide a false sense of security. Instead, creatinine should be considered along with a patient's age, gender, and race to estimate GFR.

"Kidney disease can be well advanced before it's found with creatinine alone. GFR is a more accurate gauge of how well the kidneys work, and our free calculator makes finding the rate a snap," said Thomas H. Hostetter, M.D., senior author of the study and director of NIDDK's National Kidney Disease Education Program (NKDEP). "The earlier we identify kidney disease the sooner we can treat it," said Hostetter.

NKDEP is asking labs to streamline the process for identifying kidney disease. "The GFR calculator is a great tool, but it's still one more step for busy doctors' offices. We are really pleased that several major labs have agreed to automatically report estimated GFR whenever creatinine is measured, removing a potential barrier to finding kidney disease early," said Hostetter. "We are still working quite hard to standardize tests for kidney disease by all labs."

People with chronic kidney disease are at high risk for premature death, heart attacks, and strokes as well as hypertension, anemia, bone disease, and malnutrition. NKDEP strives to increase awareness about kidney disease and offers the GFR calculator and other free tools at http://www.nkdep.nih.gov.

Section 4.3

African Americans Unaware of High Kidney Disease Risk

National Institute of Diabetes and Digestive and Kidney Diseases (NIDDK), National Institutes of Health (NIH), NIH News Press Release, March 8, 2004.

Although kidney failure and its leading causes disproportionately affect African Americans, they are largely unaware of their high risk and of preventive measures, according to the first NIH study to assess the group's knowledge and awareness about kidney disease.

While 90 percent of African Americans surveyed by the National Kidney Disease Education Program (NKDEP) had heard about kidney disease, only 15 percent felt their personal risk for developing the disease was higher than average and fewer knew specifically how to prevent it. This gap in awareness raises serious concern, especially because 44 percent of them had at least one major risk factor for kidney disease—diabetes, high blood pressure or a blood relative with the disease. In addition, only 17 percent named kidney disease as a consequence of diabetes and only 8 percent named it as a consequence of hypertension. These two diseases are the leading causes of kidney failure in the United States and account for 70 percent of kidney failure among African Americans.

"We clearly need to work closely within our community to provide the facts about kidney disease," said Janice Lea, M.D., spokesperson for Atlanta's NKDEP coalition. "One step we are taking is asking dialysis patients to encourage relatives and friends who are at high risk to take the disease seriously and be tested while they can still do something about it."

The poll also found that 52 percent of people knew at least one major cause of kidney disease, but 48 percent were unable to name any cause and others named incorrect causes such as drinking sodas. When asked about symptoms of early kidney disease, 13 percent correctly said that there are none, while 64 percent expected early symptoms to include difficulty urinating, general pain, and frequent urination.

"Kidney disease is a silent killer. People find themselves in the emergency room, on dialysis, before they even know they have a problem," said Dr. Lea. "That's why it is so important to control diabetes and high blood pressure and have your blood and urine regularly tested for kidney disease once you know you are at risk."

While anyone can develop kidney disease, African Americans are hit especially hard. An estimated 36 in 100,000 African Americans versus 11 in 100,000 whites were treated for kidney failure in 2001. African Americans have four times the risk of kidney failure and those with diabetes have up to six times the risk compared to white counterparts. But the biggest disparity is among African American men ages 25 to 44, who are 20 times more likely to develop kidney failure compared to corresponding whites.

Epidemic numbers of people—roughly 20 million—have kidney disease and another 400,000 or more are already on dialysis or have a kidney transplant because their kidneys failed. The cost to taxpayers, insurers, and patients was an estimated $22.8 billion in 2001 alone.

NKDEP polled more than 2,000 African Americans aged 30 and older living in Atlanta; Baltimore; Cleveland; and Jackson, Mississippi, in April 2003, shortly before local coalitions launched a year-long pilot program, "You Have the Power to Prevent Kidney Disease." The study was repeated in May to measure changes in knowledge and awareness.

"Seeing an increased awareness in our pilot cities would be a good indication that the program is working," said Thomas H. Hostetter, M.D., a kidney specialist and national director of NKDEP. "What we learn will help us fine-tune the program, but we definitely plan to expand it nationally and to other people at high risk. We think all segments of the population, not only African Americans, are largely unaware of the risks."

Section 4.4

Ten Facts about African Americans and Kidney Disease

"Ten Facts about African-Americans and Kidney Disease" is reprinted with permission from the National Kidney Foundation, http://www.kidney.org, © 2003. All rights reserved. Updated January 2005.

Due to high rates of diabetes, high blood pressure, and glomerulo-nephritis, African Americans have an increased risk of developing kidney failure, which requires dialysis treatments or a kidney transplant to sustain life. African Americans need to have an increased awareness of these risk factors and visit their doctor or clinic regularly to check their blood sugar, blood pressure, urine protein, and kidney function. Following are ten facts about African Americans and chronic kidney disease:

1. African Americans suffer from kidney failure disproportionately. In 2002, the incidence of kidney failure per million population was 982 in African Americans, compared with 256 in white Americans.[1] African Americans constitute about 33 percent of all patients treated for kidney failure in the U.S., but only about 13 percent of the overall U.S. population.[1]

2. African Americans also develop kidney failure at an earlier age than white Americans. In 2002, the mean age for African Americans at the start of treatment for kidney failure was 60 years, compared with 65 in white Americans.[1]

3. Diabetes is the leading cause of kidney failure in African Americans, accounting for 43 percent of their new cases of kidney failure each year.[1] The prevalence of diabetes in African Americans is much higher than in white Americans. Among those aged 40 to 74 years, the rate is 11.2 percent for white Americans, compared with 18.2 percent for African Americans.[2]

4. Approximately 13 percent of all African Americans (2.8 million) have diabetes. On average, African Americans are twice

as likely to have diabetes as white Americans of similar age. Among African Americans 20 years or older, the overall rate of diabetes is 11.8 percent for women and 8.5 percent for men. The prevalence of diabetes is highest (32 percent) among African American women aged 60 to 74 years.[2]

5. National surveys conducted over the past 35 years show that the number of cases of diabetes among African Americans has doubled. Yet, about a third of the diabetes cases among African Americans are undiagnosed.[2]

6. The most common type of diabetes in African Americans is type 2 diabetes. The risk factors for this type of diabetes include: family history, impaired glucose tolerance, diabetes during pregnancy, hyperinsulinemia and insulin resistance, obesity, and physical inactivity.[2]

7. African Americans with diabetes are more likely to develop complications of diabetes and to have greater disability from these complications than white Americans. African Americans experience kidney failure about four times more often than white Americans with diabetes. They are also more likely to develop other serious complications such as heart disease and strokes and to experience greater disability than white Americans with diabetes. Death rates associated with diabetes are 20 percent higher for African American men and 40 percent higher for African American women, compared with their white counterparts.[2]

8. High blood pressure is the second leading cause of kidney failure among African Americans, accounting for 34 percent of the new cases each year.[1] However, high blood pressure remains the leading cause of death overall in African Americans because of its link with heart attacks and strokes.[2]

9. It is not known for sure why African Americans are more prone to develop high blood pressure. However, some research points to a particular gene that may make African Americans much more sensitive to salt.[3]

10. While the incident rates for white patients with diabetic ESRD have declined 46 percent for patients aged 20 to 29 and 9 percent for those aged 30 to 39, since 1992 black patients have grown 27 percent and 62 percent, respectively.[1]

When high blood pressure and diabetes are detected and controlled early, serious complications can often be avoided. Some evidence also suggests that these diseases may be preventable in some cases. By eating a healthy diet, staying trim, and exercising regularly, individuals may be able to decrease their risk of developing diabetes and high blood pressure. Since African Americans who are also sensitive to large amounts of salt in their diet, keeping salt intake down may help to control existing high blood pressure and may even play a role in prevention in this population. The National Kidney Foundation and its 49 affiliates comprise the major voluntary health organization in the United States dedicated to the eradication of kidney and urologic diseases.

Sources of Facts and Statistics

1. U.S. Renal Data System 2004 Annual Data Report (http://www.usrds.org).

2. "Diabetes in African Americans," from the National Kidney and Urologic Diseases Information Clearinghouse (http://www.niddk.nih.gov).

3. American Heart Association Meeting Report (http://www.americanheart.org).

4. "Early Identification of Renal Disease Among African Americans: A Continuing Problem," M. Thornhill-Joynes and M. Moore, *Nephrology News & Issues*, November 1995, p.16-18.

Section 4.5

Reducing Racial and Ethnic Disparities in Chronic Kidney Disease and Kidney Failure

"Highlights in Minority Health 3/04: Reducing Racial and Ethnic Disparities in Chronic Kidney Disease and Kidney Failure," Centers for Disease Control and Prevention (CDC), Office of Minority Health (OMH), January 2005.

Chronic kidney disease (CKD) reduces the body's ability to filter blood, remove waste and extra water, and keep beneficial electrolytes in balance. Left untreated, CKD can lead to kidney failure requiring kidney replacement treatment (dialysis or transplantation) to maintain life. In 2001, approximately 10.9 million U.S. residents had CKD, 406,081 were receiving kidney replacement therapy for kidney failure, 96,295 new cases of kidney failure were diagnosed, and 99,000 deaths from kidney failure were recorded. Annual death rates from cardiovascular diseases are increased 10–100 times among persons with kidney failure.

CKD, kidney failure, and related disability, premature death, and economic costs are growing public health problems that disproportionately affect racial and ethnic minority populations in the United States. African Americans, American Indians, Hispanics, and Asians are respectively 4.5, 3.6, 2, and 1.6 times more likely to develop kidney failure than are whites. The ongoing epidemics of CKD and kidney failure are due mainly to increased prevalence of type 2 diabetes, poor control of diabetes and hypertension, and delayed detection and treatment of the early stages of CKD. In addition, racial and ethnic disparities in CKD, kidney failure, and kidney replacement therapy (dialysis and transplantation) are caused by a combination of biological, clinical, economic, social, and cultural forces which lead to disproportionate burdens of suffering among racial and ethnic minorities.

Effective clinical methods of early diagnosis and treatment for CKD are available, not used often enough, and not equally accessible to all patients who need them. Experts recommend tight control of blood sugar in people with diabetes, lowering of blood pressure below targets set for persons with hypertension who do not have kidney disease, screening for early signs of CKD, and low protein diets to prevent progression of CKD to kidney failure.

Organized public health programs are also in place to support actions taken by clinicians and individuals. Since 2000, the National Institute of Diabetes and Digestive and Kidney Diseases (NIDDK), Council of American Kidney Societies (CAKS), and other public and private groups have conducted the National Kidney Disease Education Program (NKDEP) to increase awareness, motivate action among healthcare providers, policy makers, and populations at high risk for CKD. To reduce extreme racial disparities in CKD, kidney failure, and renal replacement therapy, the NKDEP has targeted African Americans with hypertension, diabetes, and a family history of kidney failure. The NKDEP is conducting pilot projects to develop educational materials and methods in selected cities (Atlanta, GA; Baltimore, MD; Jackson, MS; and Cleveland, OH).

Chapter 5

Kidney and Urologic Tests

Chapter Contents

Section 5.1

Urinalysis

© 2005 A.D.A.M., Inc. Reprinted with permission.
Updated August 18, 2003.

Alternative names: Urine appearance and color; routine urine test

Definition: A urinalysis is an examination of the urine by physical or chemical means. Urinalysis comprises a battery of chemical and microscopic tests that help to screen for urinary tract infections, renal disease, and diseases of other organs that result in abnormal metabolites (break-down products) appearing in the urine.

How the Test Is Performed

Collect a "clean-catch" (midstream) urine sample. To do so, men or boys should wipe clean the head of the penis. Women or girls need to wash the area between the lips of the vagina with soapy water and rinse well. As you start to urinate, allow a small amount to fall into the toilet bowl (this clears the urethra of contaminants). Then, in a clean container, catch about one to two ounces of urine, and remove the container from the urine stream. Give the container to the health-care provider or assistant.

For an infant, thoroughly wash the area around the urethra. Open a urine collection bag (a plastic bag with an adhesive paper on one end), and place it on your infant. For boys, the entire penis can be placed in the bag and the adhesive attached to the skin. For girls, the bag is placed over the labia. Place a diaper over the infant (bag and all).

Check your baby frequently and remove the bag after the infant has urinated into it. For active infants, this procedure may take a couple of attempts—lively infants can displace the bag, causing an inability to obtain the specimen. The urine is drained into a container for transport back to the healthcare provider.

The tests should be performed within 15 minutes after the urine is collected. Various tests can be conducted from the sample. Most of the screening urinalysis tests are measured by a reagent "dipstick" which contains little pads of chemicals that change color when they come in contact with the substances of interest. There are several types of reagent strips, and it depends on the type of strip as to what tests can be performed. The urine can also be analyzed in the laboratory.

Gross and Chemical Exam

- Urine appearance and color (for example, clear, cloudy, turbid, layered; pale yellow, dark yellow, red, green, blue)
- Bilirubin, urine (a degradation product of hemoglobin)
- Glucose (a sugar)
- Hemoglobin (an indication of hemolysis)
- Urine ketones (a byproduct of fat metabolism and present in starvation and diabetes)
- Nitrite (an indication of urinary tract infection)
- Urine pH (the acidity or alkalinity of the urine)
- Urine protein
- Urine specific gravity (that is, how concentrated or dilute the urine is)
- Urobilinogen (a degradation product of bilirubin)

Microscopic Exam

- Bacteria and other microorganisms (not normally present) or see urine culture (clean catch)
- Casts
- Crystals
- Fat
- Mucous
- Red blood cells (an indication of damage to the tubules)
- Renal tubular cells
- Transitional epithelial cells
- White blood cells (an indication of urinary tract infection)

How to Prepare for the Test

Collect a urine sample. The first morning urine is the most concentrated, and it is more likely to show abnormalities. Some drugs and medications can affect the test. These will be monitored or discontinued (see the "Special Considerations" heading in this section).

If the collection is being taken from an infant, a couple of extra collection bags may be necessary.

How the Test Will Feel

The test involves only normal urination, and there is no discomfort.

Why the Test Is Performed

This may be done as a general screening to check for early signs of disease. It may also be used to monitor diabetes or kidney disease. It may be used to check for a urinary tract infection or blood in the urine.

Normal Values

- Normal urine may vary in color from almost colorless to dark yellow. Some foods (like beets and blackberries) may color the urine red.

- The urine specific gravity ranges between 1.006 and 1.030 (higher numbers mean a higher concentration). The specific gravity varies depending on the time of day, amount of food and liquids consumed, and the amount of recent exercise.

- The urine pH is also influenced by a number of factors. Generally the normal pH range is from 4.6 to 8.0, with an average of 6.0.

- There is usually no detectable urine glucose, urine ketones, or urine protein.

- There are usually no red blood cells in urine.

- Hemoglobin is not normally found in the urine.

- Bilirubin is normally not detected in the urine. There may be a trace of urobilinogen in the urine.

- Nitrites and white blood cells (leukocytes) are not normally present in the urine.

What Abnormal Results Mean

Urine appearance and color: If the urine is of an unusual color that cannot be accounted for by food intake or medication (and the urinalysis is positive), consult the healthcare provider.

Urine specific gravity: If the specific gravity is higher or lower than the normal range, or if it does not vary (the concentration of the urine depends on the time of day, the amount of food and fluids you have had, and the amount of exercise you have had recently), it may indicate a kidney problem, and you should consult the healthcare provider.

Urine pH: In some situations, an alkaline urine is good. Kidney stones are less likely to form and some antibiotics are more effective in the alkaline urine. There may be times when the acidic urine may help prevent some kinds of kidney stones and may prevent growth of certain types of bacteria. If the pH is very acidic or alkaline, you may want to discuss it with the healthcare provider.

Urine sugar: When blood levels of glucose are very high, some of the glucose may show up in the urine. The glucose and the ketones tests are usually done together. Large amounts of ketones may be present in uncontrolled diabetes. Consult the healthcare provider.

Urine protein: Finding protein in the urine is probably the best test for screening for kidney disease, although there may be a number of causes for an increased protein level in the urine. Consult the healthcare provider.

When blood is found in the urine, it may indicate a urinary tract disease or bleeding from the kidneys. However, the cause may also be vigorous physical exercise. If there is no association between exercise and the positive blood findings, consult the healthcare provider.

Other: Bilirubin in the urine is a sign of a liver or bile duct disease, and you should consult the healthcare provider. Urobilinogen is found in small traces in the urine. If there are large amounts, you should discuss it with the healthcare provider.

Nitrites and white blood cells are an indication that a urinary tract infection is present, and you should contact the healthcare provider.

Any vitamin C that the body does not need is excreted in the urine. If there are measurable amounts of vitamin C in the urine, it may interfere with the other urine tests. One may receive false positives and false negatives on the results.

Special Considerations

If a home test is used, the person reading the results must not have impaired color vision, as the results are interpreted using a color chart.

Some drugs change the color of urine, but this does not indicate disease. Some of these are chloroquine, iron supplements, levodopa, nitrofurantoin, phenazopyridine, phenothiazines, phenytoin, riboflavin, and triamterene.

Section 5.2

Urodynamic Tests

"Urodynamic Testing," National Kidney and Urologic Diseases Information Clearinghouse (NKUDIC), a service of the National Institute of Diabetes and Digestive and Kidney Diseases (NIDDK), National Institutes of Health (NIH), Pub. No. 04-5106, August 2004.

If you have a problem with urine leakage or blocked urine flow, your doctor or nurse can help. One of the first steps may be urodynamic testing to find precisely what the problem is.

Urodynamics is the study of how the body stores and releases urine. Urodynamic tests help your doctor or nurse see how well your bladder and sphincter muscles work and can help explain symptoms such as the following:

- incontinence
- frequent urination
- sudden, strong urges to urinate
- problems starting a urine stream
- painful urination

- problems emptying your bladder completely
- recurrent urinary tract infections

These tests may involve imaging equipment that films urination or may be as simple as urinating behind a curtain while a doctor or nurse listens.

Seeing Your Doctor or Nurse

The first step in solving a urinary problem is to talk to your doctor or nurse. He or she should ask you about your general medical history, including any major illnesses or surgeries. You should talk about the medicines you take, both prescription and nonprescription, because they might be part of the problem. You should talk about how much fluid you drink a day and whether you use alcohol or caffeine. Give as many details as you can about the problem and when it started. The doctor or nurse may ask you to keep a voiding diary, which

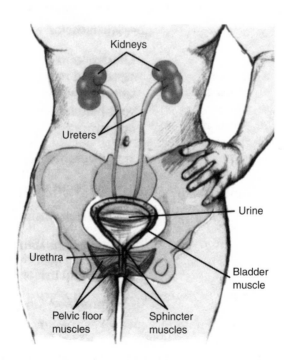

Figure 5.1. Urinary tract.

is a record of fluid intake and trips to the bathroom, plus any episodes of leakage.

If leakage is the problem, a pad test is a simple way to measure how much urine seeps out. You will be given a number of absorbent pads and plastic bags of a standard weight. You will be told to wear the pad for one or two hours and then seal it in a bag. Your healthcare team will then weigh the bags to see how much urine has been caught in the pad. A simpler but less precise method is to change pads as often as you need to and keep tract of how many pads you use in a day.

A physical exam will also be performed to rule out other causes of urinary problems, such as weakening pelvic muscles or prostate enlargement.

Preparing for the Test

If the doctor or nurse recommends bladder testing, usually no special preparations are needed, but make sure you understand any instructions you do receive. Depending on the test, you may be asked to come with a full bladder or an empty one. Also, ask whether you should change your diet or skip your regular medicines and for how long.

Taking the Test

Any procedure designed to provide information about a bladder problem can be called a urodynamic test. The type of test you take depends on your problem.

Most urodynamic testing focuses on the bladder's ability to empty steadily and completely. It can also show whether the bladder is having abnormal contractions that cause leakage. Your doctor will want to know whether you have difficulty starting a urine stream, how hard you have to strain to maintain it, whether the stream is interrupted, and whether any urine is left in your bladder when you are done (postvoid residual). Urodynamic tests can range from simple observation to precise measurement using sophisticated instruments.

Uroflowmetry: Measurement of Urine Speed and Volume

A uroflowmeter automatically measures the amount of urine and the flow rate (how fast the urine comes out). You may be asked to urinate privately into a toilet that contains a collection device and scale. This equipment creates a graph that shows changes in flow rate from second to second so the doctor or nurse can see the peak flow rate and how many seconds it took to get there. Results of this test will be abnormal if the bladder muscle is weak or urine flow is obstructed.

Your doctor or nurse can also get some idea of your bladder function by using a stopwatch to time you as you urinate into a graduated container. The volume of urine is divided by the time to see what your average flow rate is. For example, 330 milliliters (mL) of urine in 30 seconds means that your average flow rate is 11 mL per second.

Measurement of Postvoid Residual

After you have finished, you may still have some urine, usually only an ounce or two, remaining in your bladder. To measure this postvoid residual, the doctor or nurse may remove it with a catheter, a thin tube that can be gently guided into the urethra. Ultrasound equipment that uses harmless sound waves to create a picture of the bladder can also be used. A postvoid residual of more than 200 mL, about half a pint, is a clear sign of a problem. Even 100 mL, about half a cup, requires further evaluation. However, the amount of postvoid residual can be different each time you urinate.

Cystometry: Measurement of Bladder Pressure

A cystometrogram (CMG) measures how much your bladder can hold, how much pressure builds up inside your bladder as it stores urine, and how full it is when you feel the urge to urinate. The doctor or nurse will use a catheter to empty your bladder completely. Then a special, smaller catheter with a pressure-measuring tube called a cystometer will be used to fill your bladder slowly with warm water. Another catheter may be placed in the rectum to record pressure there as well. You will be asked how your bladder feels and when you feel the need to urinate. The volume of water and the bladder pressure will be recorded. You may be asked to cough or strain during this procedure. Involuntary bladder contractions can be identified.

Measurement of Leak Point Pressure

While your bladder is being filled for the CMG, it may suddenly contract and squeeze some water out without warning. The cystometer will record the pressure at the point when the leakage occurred. This reading may provide information about the kind of bladder problem you have. You may also be asked to try to exhale while holding your nose and mouth to apply abdominal pressure to the bladder or cough or shift positions. These actions help the doctor or nurse evaluate your sphincter muscles.

Pressure Flow Study

After the CMG, you will be asked to empty your bladder so that the catheter can measure the pressures required to urinate. This pressure flow study helps to identify bladder outlet obstructions that men may experience with prostate enlargement. Bladder outlet obstruction is less common in women, but can occur with a fallen bladder or rarely after a surgical procedure for urinary incontinence. Some catheters can be used for both CMG and pressure flow studies.

Electromyography: Measurement of Nerve Impulses

If your doctor or nurse thinks that your urinary problem is related to nerve damage, you may be given an electromyography. This test measures the muscle activity in the urethral sphincter using sensors placed on the skin near the urethra and rectum. Sometimes the sensors are on the urethral or rectal catheter. Muscle activity is recorded on a machine. The patterns of the impulses will show whether the messages sent to the bladder and urethra are coordinated correctly.

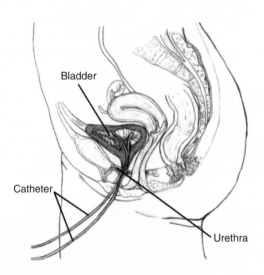

Figure 5.2. *Cystometry in a female patient.*

Video Urodynamics

Urodynamic tests may be performed with or without equipment to take pictures of the bladder during filling and emptying. The imaging equipment may use x-rays or sound waves. If x-ray equipment is used, the liquid used to fill the bladder may be a contrast medium that will show up on the x-ray. The pictures and videos show the size and shape of the urinary tract and help your doctor or nurse understand your problem.

After the Test

You may have mild discomfort for a few hours after these tests. Drinking two eight-ounce glasses of water each hour for two hours should help. Ask your doctor whether you can take a warm bath, if not, you may be able to hold a warm, damp washcloth over the urethral opening to relieve discomfort.

Your doctor may give you an antibiotic to take for one or two days to prevent an infection. If you have signs of infection—including pain, chills, or fever—call your doctor at once.

Getting the Results

Results for simple tests can be discussed with your doctor or nurse immediately after the test. Results of other tests may take a few days. You will have the chance to ask questions about the results and possible treatments for your problem.

Section 5.3

Cystoscopy and Ureteroscopy

National Kidney and Urologic Diseases Information Clearinghouse (NKUDIC), a service of the National Institute of Diabetes and Digestive and Kidney Diseases (NIDDK), National Institutes of Health (NIH), Pub. No. 04-4800, December 2003.

When you have a urinary problem, your doctor may use a cystoscope to see inside your bladder and urethra. The urethra is the tube that carries urine from the bladder to the outside of the body. The cystoscope has lenses like a telescope or microscope. These lenses let the doctor focus on the inner surfaces of the urinary tract. Some cystoscopes use optical fibers (flexible glass fibers) that carry an image from the tip of the instrument to a viewing piece at the other end. The cystoscope is as thin as a pencil and has a light at the tip. Many cystoscopes have extra tubes to guide other instruments for procedures to treat urinary problems.

Your doctor may recommend cystoscopy for any of the following conditions:

- frequent urinary tract infections

- blood in your urine (hematuria)

- loss of bladder control (incontinence) or overactive bladder

- unusual cells found in urine sample

- need for a bladder catheter

- painful urination, chronic pelvic pain, or interstitial cystitis

- urinary blockage such as prostate enlargement, stricture, or narrowing of the urinary tract

- stone in the urinary tract

- unusual growth, polyp, tumor, or cancer

If you have a stone lodged higher in your urinary tract, the doctor may extend the cystoscope through the bladder and up into the ureter.

The ureter is the tube that carries urine from the kidney to the bladder. When used to view the ureters, the cystoscope is called a ureteroscope. The doctor can then see the stone and remove it with a small basket at the end of a wire inserted through an extra tube in the ureteroscope. The doctor may also use the extra tube in the cystoscope to extend a flexible fiber that carries a laser beam to break the stone into smaller pieces that can then pass out of the body in your urine.

Preparation

Ask your doctor about any special instructions. In most cases, you will be able to eat normally and return to normal activities after the test.

Since any medical procedure has a small risk of injury, you will need to sign a consent form before the test. Do not hesitate to ask your doctor about any concerns you might have.

You may be asked to give a urine sample before the test to check for infection. Avoid urinating for an hour before this part of the test.

You will wear a hospital gown for the examination, and the lower part of your body will be covered with a sterile drape. In most cases, you will lie on your back with your knees raised and apart. A nurse or technician will clean the area around your urethral opening and apply a local anesthetic.

If you are going to have a ureteroscopy, you may receive a spinal or general anesthetic. If you know this is the case, you will want to arrange a ride home after the test.

Test Procedures

The doctor will gently insert the tip of the cystoscope into your urethra and slowly glide it up into the bladder. Relaxing your pelvic muscles will help make this part of the test easier. A sterile liquid (water or saline) will flow through the cystoscope to slowly fill your bladder and stretch it so that the doctor has a better view of the bladder wall.

As your bladder reaches capacity, you will feel some discomfort and the urge to urinate. You will be able to empty your bladder as soon as the examination is over.

The time from insertion of the cystoscope to removal may be only a few minutes, or it may be longer if the doctor finds a stone and decides to remove it. Taking a biopsy (a small tissue sample for examination under a microscope) will also make the procedure last longer.

In most cases, the entire examination, including preparation, will take about 15 to 20 minutes.

After the Test

You may have a mild burning feeling when you urinate, and you may see small amounts of blood in your urine. These problems should not last more than 24 hours. Tell your doctor if bleeding or pain is severe or if problems last more than a couple of days.

To relieve discomfort, drink two eight-ounce glasses of water each hour for two hours. Ask your doctor if you can take a warm bath to relieve the burning feeling. If not, you may be able to hold a warm, damp washcloth over the urethral opening.

Your doctor may give you an antibiotic to take for one or two days to prevent an infection. If you have signs if infection—including pain, chills, or fever—call your doctor.

Section 5.4

Imaging of the Urinary Tract

National Kidney and Urologic Diseases Information Clearinghouse (NKUDIC), a service of the National Institute of Diabetes and Digestive and Kidney Diseases (NIDDK), National Institutes of Health (NIH), Pub. No. 04-5107, March 2004.

What does 'imaging' mean?

In medicine, "imaging" is the general term for any technique used to provide pictures of bones and organs inside the body. Imaging techniques consist of x-rays, ultrasound, magnetic resonance imaging (MRI), and computed axial tomography (CAT or CT) scans. Imaging helps doctors see the causes of medical problems.

What problems could require imaging of the urinary tract?

Imaging may help your doctor find the cause of the following:

- urinary incontinence (unintended leakage of urine)
- frequent, urgent urination
- blockage of urine
- abdominal mass
- pain in the groin or lower back
- blood in the urine
- high blood pressure
- kidney failure

One symptom could have several possible causes. Your doctor can use imaging techniques to determine, for example, whether a urinary stone or an enlarged prostate is blocking urine flow. Imaging can also help clarify kidney diseases, tumors, urinary reflux (backward flow of urine), urinary tract infections, incomplete emptying, and small bladder capacity.

What other factors will my doctor consider before ordering tests?

The first step in solving a urinary problem is to talk to your doctor. You will be asked about your general medical history, including any major illnesses or surgeries, so you should be prepared to give as many details as you can about the problem and when it started. You should mention all the medicines you take, both prescription and nonprescription, because they might be part of the problem. You should also talk about how much fluid you drink a day and whether the beverages you drink contain alcohol or caffeine.

Why does the doctor choose one imaging technique instead of another?

Your doctor will look at several factors to decide what imaging technique to use. Each has advantages and disadvantages. Convenience and cost effectiveness are also factors.

Conventional radiology: Doctors have used x-ray machines to diagnose diseases for about a century. X-rays of the urinary tract can help highlight a kidney stone or tumor that could block the flow of urine and cause pain. An x-ray can also show the size and shape of the prostate. Two x-ray procedures involve the use of contrast medium, which is a liquid that acts like a dye and shows the shape of the urinary tract as it passes through the tract. Conventional x-rays do involve some exposure to ionizing radiation.

In an intravenous pyelogram (IVP), the contrast medium is injected into a vein, usually in the arm. The radiologist takes a series of snapshots as the medium circulates through the blood and reaches the kidneys. The structure of the kidneys shows up clearly on the x-rays as the contrast medium is filtered from the blood and passes through the kidneys to the ureters.

In a voiding cystourethrogram (VCUG), a catheter inserted in the urethra is used to fill the bladder with the contrast medium. The x-ray machine then captures a video of the contrast medium during urination. This procedure allows the doctor to see things such as whether urine is backing up into the ureters when it should be traveling the other way, down through the urethra, or whether urine outflow through the urethra is blocked. VCUG is often used with children who have recurrent infections to determine whether a defect in the urinary tract is causing the infections. It can also show blockages from an enlarged prostate in men or abnormal bladder position in women.

Ultrasound: In ultrasound, or sonography, a technician holds a device, called a transducer, that sends harmless sound waves into the body and catches them as they bounce back off the internal organs to create a picture on a monitor. Different angles make it possible to examine different organs.

In abdominal ultrasound, the technician applies a gel to the patient's belly and holds the transducer against the skin. The gel allows the transducer to glide easily, and it improves the transmission of the signals. Abdominal ultrasounds are well known for taking pictures of fetuses in the womb and of a woman's ovaries and uterus, but this approach can also be used to evaluate the size and shape of the kidneys.

Transrectal ultrasound is most often used to examine the prostate. The transducer is inserted into the patient's rectum so that it is right next to the prostate. The ultrasound image shows the size and shape of the prostate and any irregularity that might be a tumor. To determine whether an abnormal-looking area is in fact a tumor, the doctor can use the transducer and the ultrasound images to guide a biopsy needle to the suspected tumor. The needle collects a few pieces of prostate tissue for examination under a microscope.

MRI: MRI machines use radio waves and magnets to produce detailed pictures of internal organs and tissues. No exposure to radiation occurs. With most MRI machines, the patient lies on a table that

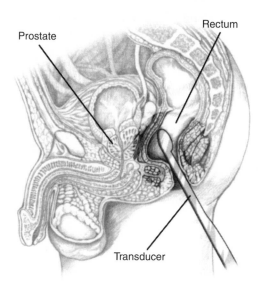

Figure 5.3. *Transrectal ultrasound.*

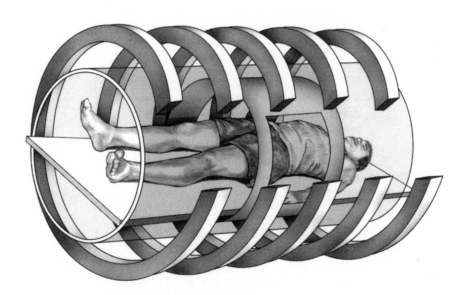

Figure 5.4. *Magnetic resonance angiogram (MRA).*

slides into a tunnel that may be open-ended or closed at one end. Some newer machines are designed to allow the patient to lie in a more open space. During an MRI, the patient is awake but must remain perfectly still while the images are being taken, usually only a few minutes. A sequence of images may be needed to create a detailed picture of the organ. During the sequencing, the patient will hear mechanical knocking and humming noises.

A magnetic resonance angiogram (MRA) provides the most detailed view of renal arteries. It can show renal artery stenosis, which is a narrowing of vessels that causes poor blood flow to the kidney and can cause high blood pressure and lead to reduced kidney function and eventually to kidney failure.

CAT (or CT) scan: CAT scans use a combination of x-rays and computer technology to create three-dimensional images. Like MRIs, CAT scans require the patient to lie on a table that slides into a tunnel. CAT scans can help identify stones in the urinary tract, infections, cysts, tumors, and traumatic injury to the kidneys and ureters.

How do I prepare for an imaging examination?

How you prepare will depend on the purpose of the examination and the type of equipment to be used. You should listen to your doctor's

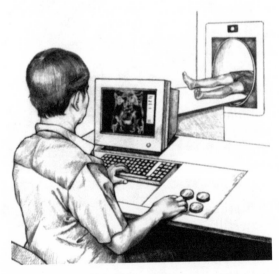

Figure 5.5. CAT (or CT) scan.

instructions carefully and ask questions if you do not understand something that is said.

- Your doctor needs to know if you have any allergies to foods or medications and if you have had any recent illnesses or medical conditions.

- Your doctor may tell you not to eat or drink anything for 12 hours before the test. For some ultrasound examinations, however, you may be instructed to drink several glasses of water two hours before the examination so that your bladder will be full.

- You may be given a laxative to clear the colon before the examination. If you are having a transrectal ultrasound, you will be given an enema about four hours before the examination.

- If you are having an MRI or MRA, talk with the technical staff about any implanted devices—such as heart pacemakers, intrauterine devices (IUDs), hip replacements, and implanted ports for catheterization—which may have metal parts that will affect the images. Metal plates, pins, screws, and surgical staples, as well as any bullets or shrapnel you might have in your body, may cause a problem if they have been in place for less than four to six weeks.

- If you feel uneasy in enclosed spaces, you may need to have a sedative before an MRI or a CAT scan.

What are the test procedures like?

Most procedures for imaging the urinary tract are performed as the patient lies on a table.

- For an IVP, dye is injected into a vein, and x-ray pictures are taken at 0, 5, 10, and 15 minutes to see the progression of the contrast medium through the kidneys and ureters. The dye makes the kidneys and urine visible on the x-ray and shows any narrowing or blockage in the urinary tract. This procedure can help identify problems in the kidneys, ureters, or bladder that may have resulted from urine retention or backup.

- MRI and CAT scans may also require injection of dye. You will be asked to lie still for minutes at a time as the equipment takes pictures from different angles. A computer puts the different views together to create a three-dimensional model of your urinary tract. Some patients find it uncomfortable to lie in the small imaging tunnel, and others find the equipment noises annoying or unsettling. Knowing what to expect helps make these aspects of the test less disturbing.

- VCUG is most often used to evaluate urinary problems in children. The child's bladder is first emptied. The doctor or nurse cleans the area around the urethra, inserts the tip of the catheter, and gently slides it up into the bladder. Contrast medium is slowly dripped into the bladder, by means of gravity, until the bladder is full. X-ray films are then made as the child urinates.

- For a transrectal ultrasound, the doctor or technician inserts a probe slightly larger than a pen into the rectum. The probe directs high-frequency sound waves at the prostate and the echo patterns form an image of the gland on a monitor. Although the image shows the size of the prostate and any irregularities, it cannot definitely identify tumors. To determine whether an abnormal-looking area is in fact a tumor, the doctor can use the probe and the ultrasound images to guide a biopsy needle to the area. The needle collects a few pieces of prostate tissue for examination under a microscope.

- For an abdominal ultrasound exam, a technician will apply gel to your abdomen and sweep a handheld transducer across the area to generate a picture of your urinary tract. Like the IVP, an abdominal ultrasound can show damage or abnormalities in the upper urinary tract.

What should I do after the test?

For most of these tests, you will be able to resume normal activity immediately afterward. If your test involved placing a catheter in the urethra, you may have some mild discomfort. Drinking two eight-ounce glasses of water each hour for two hours should help. Also, you may be able to take a warm bath. Alternatively, holding a warm, damp washcloth over the urethral opening may relieve the discomfort.

You may experience some discomfort after a transrectal ultrasound as well. A prostate biopsy may produce pain in the rectum and the perineum (the area between the rectum and the scrotum).

For catheterization or biopsy, your doctor will sometimes (but not always) give you an antibiotic to take for one or two days to prevent an infection. If you notice signs of infection—including chills, fever, or persistent pain when you urinate—you should call your doctor at once.

When will I get the results?

Results for simple tests can be discussed with your doctor or nurse immediately after the test. Other results may take a few days. You will have the chance to ask questions about the results and possible treatments for your problem.

Section 5.5

Voiding Cystourethrogram

A voiding cystourethrogram is a test which uses x-rays to take pictures of the urinary system. It shows how well the bladder and its connecting tubes (the urethra and the ureters) are working.

Before the Test

Before you come to the hospital, explain to your child what will happen. For young children, use simple words and explain only right before the test.

During the Test

Your child will lie on an x-ray table. A small tube, or catheter, will be placed into the bladder through the opening where urine comes out. A special liquid called x-ray contrast material will be used to fill the bladder through the catheter. When your child's bladder is full, your child will urinate into a urinal or special container while on a table.

While the child is urinating, the x-ray technologist or doctor (radiologist) will take x-ray pictures. Your child will need to lie still while the catheter is being placed and while the x-ray pictures are taken. It is often difficult for young children to hold still for this. If your child is unable to lie still, the hospital staff will assist your child in holding still.

You are encouraged to stay with your child during the test. Children are usually more cooperative and less apprehensive when a loved one is with them. If you are pregnant, you will have to wait outside the room.

It is a good idea for siblings to stay with another caregiver so that you can be with your child. The test usually lasts about 30 minutes.

It is possible that during the procedure your child may experience some discomfort. Please tell the doctor, nurse or technologist if pain occurs.

After the Test

The technologist will let you know when all the x-ray pictures are taken. Your child may return to normal daily activities.

Some discomfort is expected during the procedure. Please tell the doctor, nurse or technologist if pain occurs.

After having the urinary catheter placed for the test, your child's urine may appear pink the first time he or she urinates. This is caused by a small amount of blood in the urine. If this happens more than once or your child has difficulty urinating, call your child's doctor.

Results of the test will be sent to your child's doctor, who will contact you about the results. Results are usually available to your doctor within 24 hours.

Section 5.6

Intravenous Pyelogram (IVP)

Introduction

An intravenous pyelogram (IVP), also called an intravenous urogram, is an x-ray examination of your urinary tract, including the kidneys, ureters, and bladder. This examination is performed when patients experience kidney pain; have several urinary tract infections; when blood is found in the urine; or if a kidney stone, tumor or injury is suspected.

Patient Preparation

For the IVP examination to be successful, your colon must be empty. Your doctor or the radiology department will give you specific instructions, which you should follow closely. You may be asked to drink only clear liquids the day before the exam and use a laxative the night before to help clear your digestive tract. You probably will be asked not eat or drink anything after midnight, although you may take small sips of water. If you have diabetes or take medication daily, tell the person scheduling your exam and ask for special instructions.

Before your examination, a radiographer will explain the procedure to you and answer any questions you might have. A radiographer, also known as a radiologic technologist, is a skilled medical professional who has received specialized education in the areas of radiation protection, patient care, and radiographic positioning and procedures.

You will be asked to remove your clothing and put on a hospital gown. The radiographer will ask you questions about your medical history. It is important to let the radiographer know if you have any allergies to food and medicine or a history of hay fever or asthma. If you are a woman of childbearing age, you should tell the radiographer the date of your last menstrual period and if you are, or believe you may be, pregnant.

During the Examination

Preparation for the examination takes about ten minutes, and the examination itself takes about an hour. You will be asked to lie face up on an x-ray table, and the radiographer will take an image of your abdomen to make sure that your intestines are empty. Next, a contrast agent, which makes your urinary system visible on radiographic images, will be injected into a vein in your arm. As it passes through your bloodstream into your urinary system, you may feel the need to urinate, and you may experience a warm feeling in the pelvic area. You also may feel flushed, notice a slightly metallic taste in your mouth or feel a wave of nausea. These are normal reactions and usually will disappear within a short time. If you begin to itch or feel short of breath, let the radiographer know immediately.

After the contrast is administered, the radiographer will take a series of x-rays. You may be asked to turn from side to side, lie on your stomach, and hold several positions. A light compression band may be placed on your abdomen to hold the contrast material in your kidneys. You will be asked to hold your breath during each exposure and remain still. If you cannot carry out any of the instructions, let the radiographer know.

Next, you may be asked to use the toilet facilities and urinate. Then a final x-ray may be taken to demonstrate the amount of contrast agent that remains in your urinary bladder. This is known as a "post-voiding" study.

Post-Examination Information

A radiologist, a physician who specializes in the diagnostic interpretation of medical images, will review your films and dictate a report of the findings. Your personal physician will receive this information and then will advise you of the results and discuss what further procedures, if any, are needed.

The contrast agent leaves your body as you urinate. It will not discolor your urine or cause discomfort when you urinate. To help eliminate the contrast agent, you should drink more water than usual following the examination. Unless advised otherwise, you can resume normal activities and your usual diet. If you experience any discomfort following the examination, contact your physician.

Please remember that the material presented here is for informational purposes only. If you have specific questions about a medical imaging procedure, contact your physician or the radiology department of the institution where your test will be performed.

Section 5.7

Medical Tests for Prostate Problems

National Kidney and Urologic Diseases Information Clearinghouse (NKUDIC), a service of the National Institute of Diabetes and Digestive and Kidney Diseases (NIDDK), National Institutes of Health (NIH), Pub. No. 04-5105, August 2004.

The prostate is a walnut-sized gland in men that produces fluid that is a component of semen. The gland has two or more lobes—or sections—enclosed by an outer layer of tissue. Located in front of the rectum and just below the bladder, where urine is stored, the prostate surrounds the urethra, which is the canal through which urine passes out of the body.

The most common prostate problem in men under 50 is inflammation or infection, which is called prostatitis. Prostate enlargement is another common problem. Because the prostate normally continues to grow as a man matures, prostate enlargement, also called benign prostatic hyperplasia or BPH, is the most common prostate problem for men over 50. Older men are at risk for prostate cancer as well, but it is much less common than BPH.

Sometimes, different prostate problems have similar symptoms. For example, one man with prostatitis and another with BPH may both have a frequent, urgent need to urinate. Other men with BPH may both have a frequent, urgent need to urinate. Other men with BPH may have different symptoms. For example, one man may have trouble beginning a stream of urine, while another may have to get up to go to the bathroom frequently at night. A man in the early stages of prostate cancer may have no symptoms at all. The confusing array of symptoms makes a thorough medical examination and testing very important. Diagnosing the problem may require a series of tests.

Talking to Your Doctor or Nurse

Letting your doctor or nurse know you have a problem is the first step. Try to give as many details about the problem as you can, including when it began and how often it occurs. Tell the doctor or nurse

81

whether you have had recurrent urinary tract infections or symptoms such as pain after ejaculation or during urination, sudden strong urges, or hesitancy and weak urine stream. You should talk about the medicines you take, both prescription medicines and those you can buy over the counter, because they might be part of the problem. You should also talk about how much fluid you typically drink each day, whether you use caffeine or alcohol, and whether your urine has an unusual color or odor. In turn, the doctor or nurse will ask you about your general medical history, including any major illnesses or surgeries. Other typical questions are as follows:

- Over the past month or so, how often have you had to urinate again in less than two hours?

- Over the past month, from the time you went to bed at night until the time you got up in the morning, how many times a night did you typically get up to urinate?

- Over the past month or so, how often have you had a sensation of not emptying your bladder completely after you finished urinating?

- Over the past month or so, how often have you had a weak urinary stream?

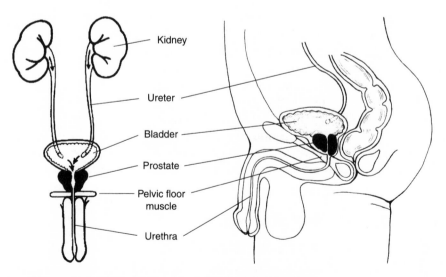

Figure 5.6. Male urinary tract, front and side views.

- Over the past month or so, how often have you had to push or strain to begin urinating?

Your answers to these questions may help your doctor or nurse identify the problem or determine what tests are needed. You may also receive a symptom score evaluation that can be used as a baseline to see how effective later treatments are at relieving those symptoms.

Preparing for the Exam

The common tests your doctor or nurse will perform first require no special preparation. Digital rectal exams (DRE) and blood tests for prostate-specific antigen (PSA) are often included in routine physical examinations for men over 50. For African American men and men with a family history of prostate cancer, it is recommended that tests be given starting at age 40. Some organizations even recommend that these tests be given to all men starting at age 40.

If you have urination problems or if the DRE or PSA test indicates that you might have a problem, you will probably be given additional tests that may require some preparation. Ask your doctor or nurse whether you should change your diet or fluid intake or stop taking any medications. If the tests involve inserting instruments into the urethra or rectum, you may be given antibiotics before and after the test to prevent infection.

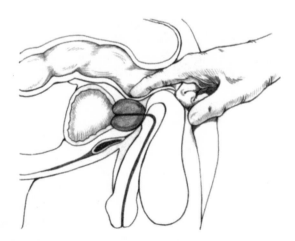

Figure 5.7. Digital rectal exam (DRE).

Procedures

Digital Rectal Exam (DRE)

This exam is usually done first. Many doctors perform a DRE as part of a routine physical exam for any man over 50, some even at 40, whether the man has urinary problems or not. You may be asked to bend over a table or to lie on your side holding your knees close to your chest. The doctor slides a gloved, lubricated finger into the rectum and feels the part of the prostate that lies next to it. You may find the DRE slightly uncomfortable, but it is very brief. This exam tells the doctor whether the gland has any bumps, irregularities, soft spots, or hard spots that require additional tests. If a prostate infection is suspected, the doctor might massage the prostate during the DRE to obtain fluid for examination under a microscope.

Prostate-Specific Antigen (PSA) Blood Test

To rule out cancer, your doctor may recommend a PSA blood test. The amount of PSA, a protein produced by prostate cells, is often higher in the blood of men who have prostate cancer. However, an elevated level of PSA does not necessarily mean you have cancer. The Food and Drug Administration has approved a PSA test for use in conjunction with a DRE to help detect prostate cancer in men age 50 or older and for monitoring men with prostate cancer after treatment. However, much remains unknown about how to interpret the PSA test, its ability to discriminate between cancer and benign prostate conditions, and the best course of action if the PSA is high.

Because so many questions are unanswered, the relative magnitude of the test's potential risks and benefits is unknown. When added to DRE screening, PSA enhances detection, but PSA tests are known to have relatively high false-positive rates, and they also may identify a greater number of medically insignificant tumors.

The PSA test first became available in the 1980s, and its use led to an increase in the detection of prostate cancer between 1986 and 1991. In the mid-1990s, deaths from prostate cancer began to decrease, and some observers credit PSA testing for this trend. Others, however, point out that statistical trends do not necessarily prove a cause-and-effect relationship, and the benefits of screening for prostate cancer are still being studied. The National Cancer Institute is conducting the Prostate, Lung, Colorectal, and Ovarian Cancer Screening Trial, or PLCO Trial, to determine whether certain screening tests reduce the number of deaths from these cancers. DRE and PSA exams are being studied to see whether yearly screening will decrease the risk of dying from prostate cancer.

Until a definitive answer is found, doctors and patients should weigh the benefits of PSA testing against the risks of follow-up diagnostic tests and cancer treatments. The procedures used to diagnose prostate cancer may cause significant side effects, including bleeding and infection. Treatment for prostate cancer often causes erectile dysfunction, or impotence, and may cause urinary incontinence.

Urinalysis

Your doctor or nurse may ask for a urine sample to test with a dipstick or to examine under a microscope. A chemically treated dipstick will change color if the urine contains nitrite, a byproduct of bacterial infection. Traces of blood in the urine may indicate that a kidney stone or infection is present, or the sample might reveal bacteria or infection-fighting white blood cells. You might be asked to urinate into two or three containers to help locate the infection site. If signs of infection appear in the first container but not in the others, the infection is likely to be in the urethra. Your doctor or nurse might ask you to urinate into the first container, then stop the stream for a prostate massage before completing the test. If urine taken after prostate massage or the prostate fluid itself contains significantly more bacteria, it is a strong sign that you have bacterial prostatitis.

Transrectal Ultrasound and Prostate Biopsy

If prostate cancer is suspected, your doctor may recommend transrectal ultrasound. In this procedure, the doctor or technician inserts a probe slightly larger than a pen into the rectum. The probe directs high-frequency sound waves at the prostate, and the echo patterns form an image of the gland on a television monitor. The image shows how big the prostate is and whether there are any irregularities, but cannot unequivocally identify tumors.

To determine whether an abnormal-looking area is indeed a tumor, the doctor can use the probe and the ultrasound images to guide a biopsy needle to the suspected tumor. The needle collects a few pieces of prostate tissue for examination under a microscope.

Magnetic Resonance Imaging (MRI) and Computed Axial Tomography (CAT) Scans

MRI and CAT scans both use computers to create three-dimensional or cross-sectional images of internal organs. These tests can help identify abnormal structures, but they cannot distinguish between cancerous tumors and non-cancerous prostate enlargement. Once a biopsy has confirmed cancer, a doctor might use these imaging techniques to determine how far the cancer has spread. Experts caution, however, that MRI and CAT scans are very expensive and rarely add useful information. They recommend using these techniques only when the PSA score is very high or the DRE suggests an extensive cancer, or both.

Urodynamic Tests

If your problem appears to be related to blockage, your doctor or nurse may recommend tests that measure bladder pressure and urine flow rate. You may be asked to urinate into a special device that measures how quickly the urine is flowing and records how many seconds it takes for the peak flow rate to be reached. Another test measures postvoid residual, the amount of urine left in your bladder when you have finished urinating. A weak stream and difficulty emptying the bladder completely may be signs of urine blockage caused by an enlarged prostate that is squeezing the urethra.

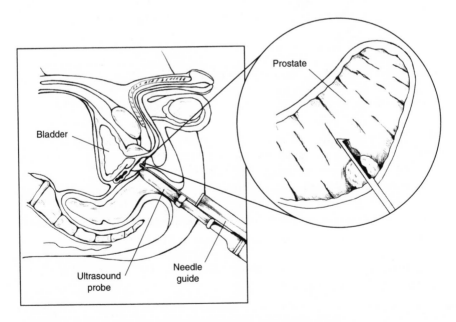

Figure 5.8. Transrectal ultrasound and prostate biopsy.

Intravenous Pyelogram (IVP)

IVP is an x-ray of the urinary tract. In this test, dye is injected into a vein, and x-ray pictures are taken at 0, 5, 10, and 15 minutes to see the progression of contrast through the kidney and ureter. The dye makes the urine visible on the x-ray and shows any narrowing or blockage in the urinary tract. This procedure can help identify problems in the kidneys, ureters, or bladder that may have resulted from urine retention or backup.

Abdominal Ultrasound

For an abdominal ultrasound exam, a technician will apply gel to your lower abdomen and sweep a handheld transducer across the area to receive a picture of your entire urinary tract. Like the IVP, an abdominal ultrasound can show damage in the upper urinary tract that results from urine blockage at the prostate.

Cystoscopy

After a solution numbs the inside of the penis, the doctor inserts a small tube through the urethral opening at the tip of the penis. The tube, called a cystoscope, contains a lens and light system, which allow the doctor to see the inside of the urethra and the bladder. The doctor can then determine the location and degree of the obstruction.

After the Test

You may have mild discomfort for a few hours after urodynamics and cystoscopy. Drinking two eight-ounce glasses of water each hour for two hours should help. Ask your doctor whether you can take a warm bath. If not, you may be able to hold a warm, damp washcloth over the urethral opening to relieve the discomfort. A prostate biopsy may also produce pain in the area of the rectum and the perineum (between the rectum and the scrotum).

Your doctor may give you an antibiotic to take for one or two days to prevent an infection, but not always. If you have signs of infection—including pain, chills, or fever—call your doctor at once.

Getting the Results

Results for simple tests can be discussed with your doctor or nurse immediately after the test. Other tests may take a few days. You will have the chance to ask questions about the results and possible treatments for your problem.

Section 5.8

Medical Tests of Kidney Function

Excerpted from "Your Kidneys and How They Work," National Kidney and Urologic Diseases Information Clearinghouse (NKUDIC), a service of the National Institute of Diabetes and Digestive and Kidney Diseases (NIDDK), National Institutes of Health (NIH), Pub. No. 03-4241, July 2003.

How My Doctor Detects Kidney Disease

Since you can have kidney disease without any symptoms, your doctor may first detect the condition through routine blood and urine tests. The National Kidney Foundation recommends three simple tests to screen for kidney disease: a blood pressure measurement, a spot check for protein or albumin in the urine (proteinuria), and a calculation of glomerular filtration rate (GFR) based on a serum creatinine measurement.

Blood Pressure Measurement

High blood pressure can lead to kidney disease. It can also be a sign that your kidneys are already impaired. The only way to know whether your blood pressure is high is to have a health professional measure it with a blood pressure cuff. The result is expressed as two numbers. The top number, which is called the systolic pressure, represents the pressure when your heart is beating. The bottom number, which is called the diastolic pressure, shows the pressure when your heart is resting between beats. Your blood pressure is considered normal if it stays below 120/80 (expressed as "120 over 80"). The National Heart, Lung, and Blood Institute (NHLBI) recommends that people with kidney disease use whatever therapy is necessary, including lifestyle changes and medicines, to keep their blood pressure below 130/80.

Microalbuminuria and Proteinuria

Healthy kidneys take wastes out of the blood but leave protein. Impaired kidneys may fail to separate blood protein called albumin from the wastes. At first, only small amounts of albumin may leak into the urine, a condition known as microalbuminuria, a sign of deteriorating kidney function. As kidney function worsens, the amount of albumin and other proteins in the urine increases, and the condition is called proteinuria. Your doctor may test for protein using a dipstick in a small sample of your urine taken in the doctor's office. The color of the dipstick indicates the presence or absence of proteinuria.

A more sensitive test for protein or albumin in the urine involves laboratory measurement and calculation of the protein-to-creatinine or albumin-to-creatinine ratio. This test should be used to detect kidney disease in people at high risk, especially those with diabetes. If your first laboratory test shows high levels of protein, another test should be done one to two weeks later. If the second test also shows high levels of protein, you have persistent proteinuria and should have additional tests to evaluate your kidney function.

Glomerular Filtration Rate (GFR) Based on Creatinine Measurement

GFR is a calculation of how efficiently the kidneys are filtering wastes from the blood. A traditional GFR calculation requires an injection into the bloodstream of a substance that is later measured in a 24-hour urine collection. Recently, scientists found they could calculate GFR without an injection or urine collection. The new calculation requires only a measurement of the creatinine in a blood sample.

Creatinine is a waste product in the blood created by the normal breakdown of muscle cells during activity. Healthy kidneys take creatinine out of the blood and put it into the urine to leave the body. When kidneys are not working well, creatinine builds up in the blood.

In the lab, your blood will be tested to see how many milligrams of creatinine are in one deciliter of blood (mg/dL). Creatinine levels in the blood can vary, and each laboratory has its own normal range, usually 0.6 to 1.2 mg/dL. If your creatinine level is only slightly above this range, you probably will not feel sick, but the elevation is a sign that your kidneys are not working at full strength. One formula for estimating kidney function equates a creatinine level of 1.7 mg/dL for most men and 1.4 mg/dL for most women to 50 percent of normal kidney function. But because creatinine values are so variable and can be affected by diet, a GFR calculation is more accurate for determining whether a person has reduced kidney function.

The new GFR calculation uses the patient's creatinine measurement along with weight, age, and values assigned for sex and race. Some medical laboratories may make the GFR calculation when a creatinine value is measured and include it on their lab report. [You can find your own GFR using an online calculator by going to the link provided by the National Institute of Diabetes and Digestive and Kidney Diseases (NIDDK) at http://kidney.niddk.nih.gov/kudiseases/pubs/yourkidneys/index.htm.]

Blood Urea Nitrogen (BUN)

Blood carries protein to cells through the body. After the cells use the protein, the remaining waste product is returned to the blood as urea, a compound that contains nitrogen. Healthy kidneys take urea out of the blood and put it in the urine. If your kidneys are not working well, the urea will stay in the blood.

A deciliter of normal blood contains 7 to 20 milligrams of urea. If your BUN is more than 20 mg/dL, your kidneys may not be working at full strength. Other possible causes of an elevated BUN include dehydration and heart failure.

Additional Tests for Kidney Disease

If blood and urine tests indicate reduced kidney function, your doctor may recommend additional tests to help identify the cause of the problem.

Renal imaging: Methods of renal imaging (taking pictures of the kidneys) include ultrasound, computed tomography (CT scan), and magnetic resonance imaging (MRI). These tools are most helpful in finding unusual growths or blockages to the flow of urine.

Renal biopsy: Your doctor may want to see a tiny piece of your kidney tissue under a microscope. To obtain this tissue sample, the doctor will perform a renal biopsy—a hospital procedure in which the doctor inserts a needle through your skin into the back of the kidney. The needle retrieves a strand of tissue about ½ to ¾ of an inch long. For the procedure, you will lie prone (on your stomach) on a table and receive local anesthetic to numb the skin. The sample tissue will help the doctor identify problems at the cellular level.

Section 5.9

Kidney Biopsy

National Kidney and Urologic Diseases Information Clearinghouse (NKUDIC), a service of the National Institute of Diabetes and Digestive and Kidney Diseases (NIDDK), National Institutes of Health (NIH), Pub. No. 05-4763, January 2005.

A biopsy is a diagnostic test that involves collecting small pieces of tissue, usually through a needle, for examination under a microscope. A kidney biopsy can help find a diagnosis and determine the best course of treatment. Your doctor may recommend a kidney biopsy if you have any of the following conditions:

- hematuria which is blood in your urine
- proteinuria which is excessive protein in your urine
- impaired kidney function which causes excessive waste products in your blood

A pathologist will look at the kidney tissue samples to check for unusual deposits, scarring, or infecting organisms that would explain your condition. The doctor may discover that you have a condition that can be treated and cured. If you have progressive kidney failure, the biopsy may indicate how quickly the disease is advancing. A biopsy can also help explain why a transplanted kidney is not working properly.

Talk with your doctor about what information might be obtained from the biopsy and the risks involved so that you can help make a decision about whether a biopsy is worthwhile in your case.

Preparation

You will have to sign a consent form indicating that you understand the risks involved in this procedure, although they are very slight. Discuss these risks thoroughly with your doctor before you sign the form.

Make sure your doctor is aware of all the medicines you take and any drug allergies you might have. You may be told to avoid food and fluids for eight hours before the test. Shortly before the biopsy, you will give blood and urine samples to make sure you don't have a condition that would make doing a biopsy less desirable.

Test Procedures

Kidney biopsies are usually done in a hospital. You may be fully awake with light sedation, or you may be asleep under general anesthesia. If you are awake, you will be given a local anesthetic before the needle is inserted.

You will lie on your stomach to position the kidneys near the surface of your back. If you have a transplanted kidney, you will lie on your back. The doctor will mark the entry site, clean the area, and inject a local painkiller. For a percutaneous (through the skin) biopsy, your doctor will use a locating needle and x-ray or ultrasound equipment to find the right spot and then a collecting needle to gather the tissue. You will be asked to hold your breath as the doctor inserts the biopsy needle and collects the tissue, usually for about 30 seconds or a little longer for each insertion. Do not exhale until you are told. You may feel a small "popping" sensation as the needle enters the kidney. The doctor may need three or four passes to collect the needed samples.

The entire procedure usually takes about an hour, including time to locate the kidney, clean the biopsy site, inject the local painkiller, and obtain the tissue samples.

Some patients shouldn't have a percutaneous biopsy because they are prone to bleeding problems. These patients may still undergo a kidney biopsy through an open operation in which the surgeon makes an incision and can see the kidney to obtain a biopsy. Another method is the transjugular biopsy. To obtain the tissue sample, the needle is inserted through a catheter that enters the patient's jugular vein at the neck. The needle threads down through the blood vessel to the right kidney in order to obtain the tissue from the inside without puncturing the outside skin of the kidney.

After the Test

You should lie on your back for 12 to 24 hours. During this time, your back will probably feel sore. If you have a transplanted kidney, you will lie on your stomach. You will likely stay in the hospital overnight after the procedure so that staff can check your condition. You may notice some blood in your urine for 24 hours after the test. To detect any problems, your team will monitor your blood pressure and pulse, take blood samples to measure the amount of red cells, and examine the urine that you pass. On rare occasions when bleeding does not stop on its own, it may be necessary to replace lost blood with a transfusion.

A rare complication is infection from the biopsy procedure. Tell your doctor or nurse if you have any of these problems:

- bloody urine more than 24 hours after the test
- inability to urinate
- fever
- worsening pain in the biopsy site
- faintness or dizziness

Getting the Results

After the biopsy, the doctor will inspect the tissue samples in the laboratory under one or more microscopes, perhaps using dyes to identify different substances that may be deposited in the tissue. It usually takes a few days to get the complete biopsy results. If your case is urgent, you may have a preliminary report within a few hours.

Chapter 6

Current Research in Kidney and Urologic Health

Chapter Contents

Section 6.1

Kidney and Urologic Clinical Trials

"Research Updates in Kidney and Urologic Health: Fall 2003," National Kidney and Urologic Diseases Information Clearinghouse (NKUDIC), a service of the National Institute of Diabetes and Digestive and Kidney Diseases (NIDDK), National Institutes of Health (NIH), Fall 2003.

Focus on Chronic Renal Insufficiency, BPH Therapies, and Dialysis Access

The National Institute of Diabetes and Digestive and Kidney Diseases (NIDDK) conducts and supports research on many of the most serious diseases affecting public health. NIDDK's Division of Kidney, Urologic, and Hematologic Diseases (KUH) provides research funding and support for basic science and clinical research studies of the kidney and urinary tract and disorders of the blood and blood-forming organs. The Clinical Trials Program works in concert with other KUH programs to develop and manage cooperative clinical trials to prevent or retard major chronic kidney, urologic, and hematologic diseases. The program coordinates and monitors patient recruitment and adherence to interventions.

Three new clinical trials have begun recruiting patients at participating centers around the country. CRIC [Chronic Renal Insufficiency Cohort], MIST [Minimally Invasive Surgical Therapies], and DAC [Dialysis Access Consortium] are the acronyms that stand for the new programs in chronic renal insufficiency (also called chronic kidney disease), treatments for benign prostatic hyperplasia (BPH), and vascular access for hemodialysis, respectively.

Chronic Renal Insufficiency Cohort (CRIC) Study

End-stage renal disease (ESRD) is an important medical and public health problem in the United States, and it disproportionately affects racial and ethnic minority groups, particularly African Americans, American Indians, and Hispanics. African Americans, and American

96

Indians are four times as likely as whites, and Hispanics are twice as likely as whites, to develop kidney failure, which requires dialysis or kidney transplantation for survival.

In 2000, almost 100,000 people with chronic kidney disease entered ESRD, with the result that approximately 300,000 people were sustained on hemodialysis while 80,000 had functioning transplants. These numbers have doubled since 1990, and they are expected to nearly double again by 2010. The increase in the number of Americans with ESRD is directly proportional to the increase in the number of Americans with type 2 diabetes, a major cause of chronic renal insufficiency. Another major cause is hypertension. The leading cause of death in patients with ESRD is cardiovascular disease.

The factors that contribute to the decline in kidney function and the development of cardiovascular disease in people with chronic renal insufficiency are unknown, and further research is needed before interventions can be evaluated and implemented. To date, few studies have focused on people whose chronic kidney disease has not yet developed into ESRD. Only a small number of studies have been conducted, and all have had significant methodological shortcomings.

One type of study that has played an important role in defining risk factors for a wide range of diseases is the prospective cohort study. To determine the risk factors for rapid decline in kidney function and development of cardiovascular disease, the NIDDK established the CRIC Study, a seven-year prospective, multiethnic, multiracial study of approximately 3,000 patients with chronic renal insufficiency. Participants will reflect the racial, ethnic, and gender composition of the U.S. ESRD population. The data and specimens obtained from people in this study will serve as a national resource for investigating chronic renal as well as cardiovascular disease. Establishing this cohort of patients and following them prospectively will also provide an opportunity to examine genetic, environmental, behavioral, nutritional, quality-of-life, and health resource utilization factors in this population.

Seven clinical centers are participating in the study: University of Pennsylvania, Philadelphia; University of Maryland-Johns Hopkins, Baltimore; University of Illinois at Chicago Clinical Centers; University of Michigan, Ann Arbor; University of California, Kaiser Permanente of Northern California/University of California, San Francisco; Tulane University, New Orleans; and Case Western Reserve University, Cleveland.

Protocol development for the CRIC study began in September 2001. The recruitment stage, begun in 2003, concluded in 2005. The main part of the study will consist of regular clinic visits for follow-up and monitoring of patients so that renal function can be measured and cardiovascular studies and laboratory tests can be performed. In addition, participants will answer questionnaires to assess various demographic, nutritional, and quality-of-life factors. Follow-up and data collection on cohort study participants who develop ESRD will be performed after they start renal replacement therapy (renal transplantation, hemodialysis, or peritoneal dialysis), with modification of data collection, measurements, and follow-up visits as necessary and as described in the protocol. Final data analysis and closeout are scheduled for 2008.

Minimally Invasive Surgical Therapies (MIST) Treatment Consortium for BPH

KUH has had a substantial and longstanding interest in evaluating the effectiveness of strategies for treating BPH. For many years, transurethral resection of the prostate (TURP) has been the surgical standard for this condition; however, over the past decade, a number of technical innovations have allowed the development of new surgical treatments that aim to achieve the same long-term outcomes as TURP but with less morbidity, lower cost, shorter hospital stay, and more rapid recovery. These new, minimally invasive surgical approaches funded by the NIDDK include laser therapy, hyperthermia and thermotherapy, transurethral electrovaporization, microwave therapy, and transurethral needle ablation. New techniques are appearing regularly. The quality of published reports on the outcomes of these minimally invasive therapies is highly variable, and rigorous randomized clinical trials have only rarely been conducted.

To assess the long-term safety and effectiveness of these new therapies, the NIDDK has formed a group of seven collaborative Prostate Evaluation Treatment Centers and a Biostatistical Coordinating Center to develop and conduct randomized, controlled clinical trials that will give a clearer picture of the benefits and risks of these methods. The first trial to be conducted by the MIST consortium will evaluate the safety and effectiveness of transurethral needle ablation (TUNA), transurethral microwave therapy (TUMT), and medical therapy with an alpha-blocker and finasteride combined. The results of this first trial will provide both physicians and patients with the knowledge needed to make the most appropriate choices for long-term management of BPH.

Dialysis Access Consortium (DAC)

Maintenance of vascular access for hemodialysis is one of the major challenges in caring for the hemodialysis patient. Access-related problems are among the most frequent reasons for hospitalization in the ESRD population, and the cost of vascular access placement and repair in the United States exceeds $700 million per year. In fiscal year 2000, NIDDK established the Dialysis Access Consortium, which consists of seven clinical centers and a data coordinating center, to undertake interventional clinical trials to improve outcomes in patients with fistulas and grafts. Two randomized placebo-controlled clinical trials have been designed and have begun recruiting patients. The first trial will evaluate the effects of the antiplatelet agent clopidogrel on prevention of early fistula failure. A second clinical trial will study Aggrenox, with the goal of preventing access stenosis in hemodialysis patients with grafts.

For more information about these trials, call KUH at 301-594-7717 and ask to speak with the project officer.

Section 6.2

Is There a Link between Heart Disease and Kidney Disease?

"Studies Strengthen Kidney and Heart Disease Link," National Institutes of Health (NIH), NIH News Press Release, September 29, 2004.

A pair of new epidemiology studies confirms that chronic kidney disease independently increases the risk of developing cardiovascular disease (CVD), even among people with early kidney disease and after considering other risk factors such as diabetes, hypertension and high cholesterol. The studies appear in the September 23, [2004], *New England Journal of Medicine.*

One of the studies, "Chronic Kidney Disease (CKD) and the Risk of Death, Cardiovascular Events, and Hospitalization," was supported by the National Institute of Diabetes and Digestive and Kidney Diseases (NIDDK) at NIH, part of the Department of Health and Human Services.

These studies "reinforce the importance of early detection of CKD, not only to slow progression to (kidney failure) but also in this case to identify risk factors for cardiovascular disease," says Thomas H. Hostetter, M.D., in an editorial accompanying the papers. Hostetter is a kidney specialist and director of the National Kidney Disease Education Program at NIDDK.

The NIDDK-funded study followed more than 1.1 million adults from the Kaiser Permanente Renal Registry in San Francisco for nearly three years; average age was 52 years. Led by Alan S. Go, M.D., the investigators found that when kidney function (GFR) dropped, the risk of death, cardiovascular events such as heart disease and stroke, and hospitalization increased. Compared to patients whose GFR was at least 60 (ml per min. per 1.73 m2): the increased risk of death ranged from 17 percent in those whose GFR was between 45 and 59 to about 600 percent in those whose GFR was less than 15; the increased risk of CVD events ranged from 43 percent in those whose GFR was between 45 and 59 to 343 percent in those whose GFR was less than 15; and, the increased risk of hospitalization ranged from

14 percent in those whose GFR was between 45 and 59 to 315 percent in those whose GFR was less than 15.

The industry-funded VALIANT study related CKD to deaths from CVD in a two-year drug-treatment trial of more than 14,500 heart-attack patients. The researchers found death rates ranging from 14.1 percent in patients whose GFR was at least 75 to 45.5 percent in those whose GFR was less than 45. The investigators attribute the increased risk of death from CVD in part to complications of kidney disease, including anemia, oxidative stress, changes in calcium and phosphate regulation, inflammation, and conditions promoting clotting. The researchers also suggest that other kidney-related factors such as protein in the urine and elevated blood levels of both homocysteine and uric acid may increase the risk of CVD and death. Furthermore, they found that common CVD therapies such as aspirin and beta-blockers were "curiously underused" in CKD patients with lower kidney function, perhaps inspired by a fatalist mind-set that may be a self-fulfilling prophecy.

An estimated 10 to 20 million people have CKD. While many will never develop kidney failure, others will, joining more than 400,000 people annually treated with dialysis or a kidney transplant. CVD accounts for half of all deaths among people with kidney failure.

An ongoing study supported by NIDDK will help further explain the connection between CKD and CVD and should lead to improved management of these diseases. Investigators in the Chronic Renal Insufficiency Cohort study are looking at earlier kidney disease than most trials have previously studied and are conducting the most thorough review to date of the relative impact of known risk factors for kidney and heart diseases.

NKDEP and its partners recommend regular creatinine testing and the MDRD [Modification of Diet in Renal Disease] equation to estimate GFR in adults at high risk for kidney disease—those with diabetes, high blood pressure, or a family history of kidney problems, especially African Americans, Hispanic Americans, and Native Americans.

Both the Kaiser and VALIANT studies used the MDRD equation to estimate GFR. The formula considers age, sex, race, and the blood level of a substance called creatinine. Creatinine alone is commonly used to test for kidney disease, but up to two-thirds of kidney function may be lost before the test raises suspicions. The MDRD equation was developed in an NIDDK-supported clinical trial completed in the early 1990s and is widely considered the best-validated method for assessing kidney function. However, most labs and doctors still aren't using it.

This is unfortunate, since a simple web-based calculator based on the MDRD equation can compute GFR, [see http://www.nkdep.nih.gov/ healthprofessionals/tools/index.htm], and since creatinine is often measured in standard lab tests, according to Hostetter's editorial. NKDEP is encouraging doctors and labs to use creatinine and the MDRD equation so that patients can be diagnosed and treated earlier. The calculator may also be used on hand-held devices.

Sources

"Chronic Kidney Disease and the Risk of Death, Cardiovascular Events, and Hospitalization," *NEJM* 2004;351:1296-305, http:// content.nejm.org/cgi/content/short/351/13/1296.

"Relation Between Renal Dysfunction and Cardiovascular Outcomes after Myocardial Infarction," *NEJM* 2004;351:1285-95, http:// content.nejm.org/cgi/content/abstract/351/13/1285.

"Chronic Kidney Disease Predicts Cardiovascular Disease," *NEJM* 2004;351:1344-6, http://content.nejm.org/cgi/content/full/351/13/ 1344-a.

Section 6.3

Exploring the Relationship between Cholesterol and Kidney Disease

Researchers at the Johns Hopkins School of Public Health have found that high levels of triglycerides and low levels of high-density (good) cholesterol in the blood predict the onset of chronic kidney disease. In contrast, total cholesterol and low-density lipoprotein (LDL) cholesterol which are important determinants of heart disease risk did not predict kidney disease risk. Individuals who went on to experience an onset of chronic kidney disease were also substantially more likely to be older, black, diabetic, and hypertensive at the start of the study. The study appeared in the June 2000 issue of *Kidney International*.

Five to ten million Americans are estimated to have early stages of chronic kidney disease, having lost at least half of their normal kidney function. Chronic kidney disease shares many common risk factors with heart disease, including hypertension and diabetes, but the role of cholesterol has been less certain. The current study was the first to assess the association between a large number of lipids in the blood and a subsequent decline in kidney function in a large sample of the general population. The findings, which could help identify modifiable risk factors that predict development and progression of kidney disease, suggest that cholesterol treatment for preventing heart disease may not be as effective at preventing kidney disease.

Senior author Josef Coresh, MD, PhD, associate professor, Epidemiology, Biostatistics, and Medicine, Johns Hopkins School of Public Health, noted, "Chronic kidney disease is only beginning to be recognized as a major public health problem. Our goal is to systematically understand why some individuals' kidney function declines more rapidly and why these individuals are at an increased risk of kidney failure and death. Heart and kidney disease share many common risk factors. Understanding the similarities and differences will help us understand why treated kidney disease incidence is increasing while heart disease is decreasing."

The report focused on the risk of declining kidney function over the three years following a baseline examination. A total of 15,792 men and women ages 45 to 64 were followed at three-year intervals since 1987 as participants in the Atherosclerosis Risk in Communities Study. At the baseline examination, participants answered questions about kidney disease risk factors and gave blood samples, which were tested for the following lipid levels: total cholesterol, HDL cholesterol, LDL cholesterol, apolipoproteins A and B, and triglycerides.

Creatinine, a breakdown product of muscle, was used to detect chronic kidney disease. Since a rising level in creatinine in the bloodstream indicates a decline in the kidney's capacity to filter blood, the investigators used an increase of 0.4 milligrams of creatinine per deciliter of blood to indicate a significant decline in kidney function.

The data revealed that higher triglyceride levels were consistently associated with a greater risk of increased creatinine levels, and thus a decrease in kidney function. Similarly, lower levels of high density lipoprotein (HDL or good) cholesterol and apolipoprotein-A (the major protein in HDL cholesterol) were associated with greater risk. In contrast, total cholesterol and low-density lipoprotein cholesterol showed no association with the risk of chronic kidney disease.

Individuals who went on to develop a rise in creatinine had a higher mean age and were substantially more likely to be black, have diabetes, and use anti-hypertensive medications at baseline. For each threefold increase in triglyceride levels, the risk of a rise in creatinine was 2.39 times greater among African Americans and 1.31 times greater among whites. The associations remained when the study was limited to individuals with normal kidney function at baseline.

Lead author Paul Muntner, research assistant, Epidemiology, Johns Hopkins School of Public Health, said, "Among the lipids we investigated, triglycerides had the strongest and most statistically significant association with a future decline in renal function. Individuals with high triglycerides were 1½ times more likely to experience a decline in kidney function compared to individuals with low triglycerides." These associations persisted even after taking into consideration such variables as sex, race, age, systolic blood pressure, diabetes status, and type of blood pressure medication used.

Support for this study was provided by the National Heart, Lung, and Blood Institute; by a training grant from the National Institutes of Health; and by grants from the National Institute of Diabetes, Digestive, and Kidney Disease and the National Center for Research Resources.

Section 6.4

Metabolic Syndrome and Chronic Kidney Disease

"Chronic Kidney Disease Likely in People with Syndrome X," February 2004, is reprinted with permission from the Tulane University Health Sciences Center, Office of Public Relations.

Tulane researchers, published in the February [2004] issue of the *Annals of Internal Medicine*, report that people with metabolic syndrome (syndrome X) are nearly 2.5 times more likely to suffer from chronic kidney disease. Additionally, the more signs they have of syndrome X, the higher their risk of kidney disease.

Syndrome X is a cluster of signs including the following:

• Fat around the waistline

• High blood pressure

• Low levels of HDL "good" cholesterol

• High fasting blood sugar levels

• High triglycerides

If a person has three or more of these signs, they are at higher risk of developing diabetes mellitus and heart disease, as well as kidney disease.

"Our study is the first to find a link between metabolic syndrome and chronic kidney diseases," says Jing Chen, a kidney disease specialist at the Tulane Hypertension and Renal Center of Excellence, and lead author of the article. "However, it looks like earlier, better management of the metabolic syndrome might help prevent kidney disease."

Chronic kidney disease, a major risk factor for kidney failure, heart disease, and early death, affects approximately 8.3 million adults over age 20 in the United States. In addition, 47 million U.S. adults suffer from the metabolic syndrome known as syndrome X.

Data from over 6,000 participants in the National Health and Nutrition Examination Survey was used to assess the association between syndrome X and kidney disease and protein in urine. Protein in the urine is a sign of kidney disease. In addition to discovering a higher risk of chronic kidney disease among people with syndrome X, the researchers also found a higher risk of protein in urine among those with one or more of the signs of syndrome X. The researchers also looked at the individual signs and found that abdominal obesity doubles the risk of chronic kidney disease.

The article is available online at http://www.annals.org.

Section 6.5

Bioartificial Kidneys

"First Human Trial of Bioartificial Kidney Shows Promise for Acute Renal Failure," reprinted with permission from the University of Michigan Health System, http://www.med.umich.edu. Copyright © 2005 Regents of the University of Michigan.

The first test in humans of a bioartificial kidney offers hope of the device's potential to save the lives of people with acute renal failure, researchers at the University of Michigan Health System (UMHS) report.

While the phase I/II study was designed primarily to look at the safety of using this device on humans, the results also suggest improvement in kidney function. The patients enrolled in the trial faced an average 86 percent likelihood of dying at the hospital. Six of those ten patients survived more than 30 days after treatment with the bioartificial kidney. The study appears in the October [2004] issue of the journal *Kidney International*.

"These results showed this type of human adult stem progenitor/ stem cell is well-tolerated by patients with acute renal failure, and resulted in some improvement outcomes of the patients' clinical conditions. It's a small study but it was compelling enough for us and the

FDA to agree to go forward with a full phase II study," says lead study author H. David Humes, M.D., professor of Internal Medicine at the University of Michigan (U-M) Medical School. Humes developed the renal tubule assist device, or RAD, the cell cartridge that is key to the bioartificial kidney.

The RAD is being developed for future commercial applications under license to Nephros Therapeutics Inc.

The phase I/II study enrolled ten patients at UMHS and the Cleveland Clinic Foundation. Patients were seriously ill, with acute renal failure and multiple other illnesses, including sepsis, multiple organ failure, acute respiratory distress syndrome, and postoperative complications.

Each patient received up to 24 hours of treatment with the renal tubule assist device. Several patients were taken off the treatment earlier because of reactions such as hypoglycemia or low platelet counts, or because of complications related to their other medical conditions.

The bioartificial kidney includes a cartridge that filters the blood as in traditional kidney dialysis. That cartridge is connected to a renal tubule assist device, which is made of hollow fibers lined with a type of kidney cell called renal proximal tubule cells. These cells are intended to reclaim vital electrolytes, salt, glucose and water, as well as control production of immune system molecules called cytokines, which the body needs to fight infection.

Conventional kidney dialysis machines remove these important components of blood plasma, along with toxic waste products, and cannot provide the cytokine regulation function of living cells. Traditional therapy for patients with acute or chronic renal failure involves dialysis or kidney transplant, both of which have limitations.

Humes and his colleagues began developing this technology a decade ago, identifying the adult progenitor/stem cells and testing the device in animals. Initial testing in animals, published in the journal *Nature Biotechnology* in April 1999, found the cells in the RAD perform the metabolic and hormonal functions lost in acute renal failure.

Eventually, researchers hope the device can become implantable in patients with acute or chronic renal failure as a long-term replacement for kidney function. More testing is needed before that can become a reality, and any standard use of this therapy is still many years off.

"The long-term goal, if this shows effectiveness in patients with end stage renal disease, is to build a fully implantable device. Our lab is working with engineers at U-M and the Cleveland Clinic to make nanofabricated membranes that can miniaturize the device so it can be implanted and fully replace organ function," Humes says.

A randomized, controlled phase II trial of the RAD in acute renal failure began in 2004 at six academic medical centers under investigational new drug, sponsored by Nephros Therapeutics, Inc. The study was expected to expand to additional centers later in 2004. UMHS researchers also planned, for late 2005, a phase I/II trial to investigate the safety of the RAD for people with end-stage chronic renal failure. Investigators are not looking for volunteers for that trial, and the device is not ready to be implanted in patients.

In addition to Humes, U-M study authors were William Weitzel, M.D., assistant professor of Nephrology; Robert Bartlett, M.D., professor of Surgery; and Fresca Swaniker, M.D., assistant professor of Surgery. Other authors were Emil Paganini, M.D., of the Cleveland Clinic, and Jack Luderer , M.D., and Joseph Sobota , M.D., of Nephros Therapeutics.

Funding for the study was from the National Institutes of Health, the Michigan Life Sciences Corridor Fund and Nephros Therapeutics. The renal assist device technology is owned by the University of Michigan and licensed to Nephros Therapeutics Inc., a biotechnology spin-off company of U-M. Humes, Luderer and Sobota are shareholders in Nephros.

Patients seeking more information about the renal assist device can call 800-742-2300, category 6500.

To learn more about Dr. Humes' research, go to http://www.med .umich.edu/intmed/humes.

—by Nicole Fawcett

Part Two

Urinary Tract Infections and Bladder Disorders

Chapter 7

What Are Urinary Tract Infections?

What is a urinary (yoor-ih-nehr-ee) tract infection (UTI)?

The urinary tract makes and stores urine. Bacteria (bak-teer-ee-uh), a type of germ that gets into your urinary tract, cause a UTI. This infection can happen in parts of your urinary tract, like your kidneys, bladder, or urethra (yuh-ree-thra).

What causes urinary tract infections (UTIs)?

Many things can help to cause UTIs:

- Wiping from back to front after a bowel movement (BM). Germs can get into your urethra, which has its opening in front of the vagina.

- Having sexual intercourse. Germs in the vagina can be pushed into the urethra.

- Waiting too long to pass urine. When urine stays in the bladder for a long time, more germs are made, and the worse a UTI can become.

"Frequently Asked Questions about Urinary Tract Infections," The National Women's Health Information Center, a project of the U.S. Department of Health and Human Services, Office on Women's Health, October 2004.

- Using a diaphragm for birth control, or spermicides with a diaphragm or on a condom.

- Anything that makes it hard to completely empty your bladder, like a kidney stone.

- Having diabetes, which makes it harder for your body to fight other health problems.

- Loss of estrogen and changes in the vagina after menopause. Menopause is when you stop getting your period.

What are the signs of a urinary tract infection (UTI)?

There are signs if you have an infection:

- Pain or stinging when you pass urine

- An urge to pass urine a lot

- Pressure in your lower belly

- Urine that smells bad or looks milky, cloudy, or reddish in color

- Feeling tired or shaky or having a fever

How does a doctor find out I have a urinary tract infection (UTI)?

To find out if you have a UTI, your doctor will ask you to pass urine into a plastic cup. When you open the cup, don't touch the inside of the lid or inside of the cup. Before you pass urine, wipe the area between the labium majora, or outer lips of the vagina, with a special tissue, given to you by your doctor. Then, pass a little bit of urine into the toilet and then into the cup.

How is a urinary tract infection (UTI) treated?

UTIs are treated with antibiotics (an-ty-by-ah-tiks), a medicine that kills the infection. Your doctor will tell you how long you need to take the medicine. Make sure you take all of your medicine, even if you feel better!

If you don't take medicine for a UTI, the UTI can hurt other parts of your body. Also, if you're pregnant and have signs of a UTI, see your doctor right away. A UTI could cause problems in your pregnancy, such as having your baby too early or getting high blood pressure.

Are there steps I can take to help prevent a urinary tract infection (UTI)?

These are steps you can take to try to prevent a UTI. But you may follow these steps and still get a UTI. If you have symptoms of a UTI, call your doctor.

- Urinate when you need to. Don't hold it. Pass urine before and after sex. After you pass urine or have a bowel movement (BM), wipe from front to back.

- Drink water every day and after sex.

- Clean the outer lips of your vagina and anus each day. The anus is the place where a bowel movement leaves your body, located between the buttocks.

- Don't use douches or feminine hygiene sprays.

- If you get a lot of UTIs and use spermicides, or creams the kill sperm, talk to your doctor about using other forms of birth control.

- Wear underwear with a cotton crotch.

Chapter 8

Urinary Tract Infections in Children

Urinary tract infections (UTIs) are common in kids. By 5 years old, about 8% of girls and about 1% to 2% of boys have had at least one UTI. They occur when the kidneys, ureters, bladder, or urethra become infected.

Symptoms of a UTI include:

- pain when urinating.
- changes in frequency, appearance, or smell of urine.
- fever.
- chills.
- loss of appetite.
- nausea.
- vomiting.
- lower abdominal pain.
- lower back pain or discomfort.

Recurrent UTIs can also cause bedwetting in children who were previously dry at night. Infants and young children may only show

This information, from "Recurrent Urinary Tract Infections and Related Conditions," was provided by KidsHealth, one of the largest resources online for medically reviewed health information written for parents, kids, and teens. For more articles like this one, visit www.KidsHealth.org, or www.TeensHealth.org. © 2004 The Nemours Center for Children's Health Media, a division of The Nemours Foundation. Reviewed by Laszlo Hopp, M.D., May 2004.

nonspecific signs such as fever, vomiting, or decreased appetite or activity.

Some children experience UTIs again and again (also called recurrent UTIs). If left untreated, recurrent UTIs can cause kidney damage, especially in children younger than 6. Read on to find out how you can recognize the signs of these repeated infections and get help for your child.

Types of UTIs

Common types of UTIs include:

- **cystitis**, the most common type of UTI, which is a bladder infection that can occur when bacteria move up the urethra (the tube-like structure that allows urine to exit the body from the bladder) and into the bladder.

- **urethritis**, which occurs when bacteria infect the urethra.

- **pyelonephritis**, which is a kidney infection that can occur when infected urine flows backward from the bladder to the kidneys, or when an infection in the bloodstream reaches the kidneys.

Related Urinary Tract Conditions Associated with Recurrent UTIs

Recurrent UTIs are sometimes seen in conjunction with other conditions, such as:

- **vesicoureteral reflux** (VUR), which is found in 30% to 50% of children diagnosed with a UTI and is a congenital condition (it's present at birth) in which urine flows backward from the bladder to the ureters (the thin, tube-like structures that carry urine from the kidney to the bladder) and sometimes reaches the kidneys. If the urine in the bladder is infected with bacteria, VUR can lead to pyelonephritis.

- **hydronephrosis**, which is an enlargement of one or both kidneys due to backup or blockage of urine flow and is usually caused by severe VUR or a blocked ureter. Children with hydronephrosis are sometimes at risk of recurrent UTIs and may need to take daily low doses of antibiotics to prevent UTIs.

But not all cases of recurrent UTIs can be traced back to these body structure-related abnormalities. For example, dysfunctional voiding—

when a child doesn't urinate frequently enough or doesn't relax properly while urinating—is a common cause of UTIs. Unrelated conditions that compromise the body's natural defenses, such as diseases of the immune system, can also lead to recurrent UTIs. In addition, using a nonsterile urinary catheter can introduce bacteria into the urinary tract and cause an infection.

Detecting Kidney and Urinary System Abnormalities

Although UTIs can be treated with antibiotics, it's important for your child's doctor to rule out any underlying abnormalities in the urinary system when these infections occur repeatedly.

Some abnormalities can be detected even before birth. Hydronephrosis, when it occurs as a congenital condition, can be detected in a fetus by ultrasound as early as 16 weeks of gestation. When hydronephrosis poses significant danger to the developing kidneys, surgery may be performed while the baby is in the womb; however, in most cases, doctors wait until after birth before treating the condition because almost half of all cases that are diagnosed prenatally disappear by birth.

Once a baby suspected to have hydronephrosis or another urinary system abnormality is born, the baby's blood pressure will be monitored carefully because some kidney abnormalities can cause high blood pressure. An ultrasound may be used again to get a closer look at the bladder and kidneys.

Approximately 1% of children will have a duplicated, or double, collecting system from one or both kidneys. Some of these children will have an obstruction in one of the two collecting systems, which may result in hydronephrosis. A prenatal ultrasound can detect this condition in many cases.

Diagnosis and Treatment

If your doctor suspects that your child may have an abnormality of the urinary tract, he or she may order tests to make an accurate diagnosis including:

Ultrasound

Using high-frequency sound waves to "echo," or bounce, off the body and create a picture of it, an ultrasound can detect some abnormalities in the kidneys, ureters, and bladder. It can also measure the size and shape of the kidneys. When an ultrasound suggests VUR, a voiding cystourethrogram (VCUG) or a renal scan (see below for descriptions of both) may be performed for further evaluation.

Renal Scan (Nuclear Scan)

Radioactive material is injected into a child's vein and followed through the urinary tract. The material can show the shape of the kidneys, how well the kidneys function, if there is damaged kidney tissue, and the course of the urine. The amount of radiation received is similar to or less than a plain x-ray and the radioactive material leaves the body in the urine.

Voiding Cystourethrogram (VCUG or Cystogram)

A catheter (a hollow, soft tube) is used to inject an opaque dye into the bladder. This x-ray test can identify problems with the bladder or urethra and can also diagnose VUR.

Cystoscopy

A cystoscope uses lenses and a light source within a tube inserted through the urethra to directly view the inside of the bladder. It's used when other tests or symptoms indicate a possible bladder abnormality.

Intravenous Pyelogram

Opaque dye is injected into a child's vein and then x-rays are taken to follow the course of the dye through the urinary system. Although this test is still used sometimes, the renal ultrasound and renal scan have replaced the intravenous pyelogram in most cases.

Because VUR can lead to kidney infection (pyelonephritis) and subsequent kidney damage, children with the condition must be monitored closely. Usually, surgery isn't necessary because 75% of children will outgrow the condition. Even for kids who don't outgrow it, surgery may be unnecessary because antibiotics are usually successful in warding off UTIs and preventing or limiting damage to the kidneys.

The most common type of surgery to correct VUR is ureteral reimplantation, in which one or both ureters are reattached to the bladder to decrease backflow of urine from the bladder to the ureters and kidneys. Although the success of ureteral reimplantation is greater than 90%, only those who have recurrent UTIs while on antibiotic prophylaxis (or preventive therapy) will be considered for surgery.

Blockages can interfere with normal urine flow, which serves to wash bacteria out of the urinary tract. Because severe blockages in the ureter or the urethra may ultimately lead to repeated kidney infections and kidney damage, they may require surgical intervention. Kidney stones are another source of blockage that may obstruct the path of urine.

When anatomical defects have been ruled out, antibiotics may be prescribed for months or even years to prevent recurrent infections and kidney damage. Fortunately, the problems often vanish when the child enters puberty because of the child's growth and development.

The Future for Managing Recurrent UTIs

Doctors have started to use a less invasive way to correct VUR. The procedure involves the injection of such materials as Teflon, Delflux, or collagen into the bladder through a cystoscope. This procedure was considered experimental a few years ago, but is rapidly gaining wider acceptance.

A recent National Institutes of Health (NIH) study has linked recurrent UTIs with certain blood types. Further research is in progress, but researchers hope to use this information to identify those who may be at high risk.

Additional studies have found that women and children who get recurrent UTIs may lack certain immunoglobins (a group of proteins that fight infections). Some researchers are optimistic that a vaccine may be developed that could help boost a person's production of antibodies that fight UTIs. The most promising vaccine would protect against *E. coli* (the most common bacterium that causes UTIs), but it's still in the experimental stage.

Helping Your Child

As soon as you suspect a UTI in your child, it's important to contact your child's doctor.

Although most recurrent UTIs won't cause long-term health problems, in a small portion of patients—primarily those who have had several undiagnosed and untreated UTIs—permanent kidney damage can happen.

If your child suffers from recurrent UTIs, seek out a pediatric nephrologist or urologist who can perform a thorough evaluation and, if necessary, order tests for urinary system abnormalities. In the meantime, follow your child's doctor's instructions for treating a UTI.

Here are some additional things to consider to help prevent recurrent UTIs in your child:

Diet Modifications

Encourage your child to drink 8 to 10 glasses of water and other fluids per day. Cranberry juice is often suggested because it may prevent

E. coli from attaching to the walls of the bladder. Always ask your child's doctor, though, if your child should drink cranberry juice because it can interfere with some medicines.

Multivitamins

Vitamin C acidifies the urine, making the environment less friendly to bacteria. Vitamins designed for children are generally safe, but always ask your child's doctor before increasing the dose beyond the currently recommended daily allowance.

No Bubble Bath

Your child should avoid bubble baths and perfumed soaps because they can irritate the urethra.

Frequent Diaper Changes

If your child is in diapers, change him or her frequently to prevent stool from having prolonged contact with the genital area, which can increase the chance that bacteria will move up the urethra and into the bladder.

Proper Wiping Technique

In females, wiping from front to back after using the toilet will reduce exposure of the urethra to UTI-causing bacteria in the stool.

Cotton Underwear

Breathable cotton underwear is less likely to encourage bacterial growth near the urethra than nylon or other fabrics.

Frequent Bathroom Visits

Some children may object to using the school bathroom or may become so engrossed in a project that they delay urination. Children who experience UTIs should urinate at least every 3 to 4 hours to help flush bacteria from the urinary tract.

Follow-Up Visits

Your child's doctor may advise performing another urine culture after treatment of a UTI is completed to be sure that the infection has cleared.

Chapter 9

Urinary Tract Infections in Adults

Urinary tract infections (UTIs) are a serious health problem affecting millions of people each year.

Infections of the urinary tract are common—only respiratory infections occur more often. Women are especially prone to UTIs for reasons that are poorly understood. One woman in five develops a UTI during her lifetime. UTIs in men are not so common, but they can be very serious when they do occur.

What are the causes of UTI?

Normal urine is sterile. It contains fluids, salts, and waste products, but it is free of bacteria, viruses, and fungi. An infection occurs when microorganisms, usually bacteria from the digestive tract, cling to the opening of the urethra and begin to multiply. Most infections arise from one type of bacteria, *Escherichia coli (E. coli)*, which normally lives in the colon.

In most cases, bacteria first begin growing in the urethra. An infection limited to the urethra is called urethritis. From there bacteria often move on to the bladder, causing a bladder infection (cystitis). If the infection is not treated promptly, bacteria may then go up the ureters to infect the kidneys (pyelonephritis).

National Kidney and Urologic Diseases Information Clearinghouse (NKUDIC), a service of the National Institute of Diabetes and Digestive and Kidney Diseases (NIDDK), National Institutes of Health (NIH), Pub. No. 04-2097, November 2003.

Microorganisms called *Chlamydia* and *Mycoplasma* may also cause UTIs in both men and women, but these infections tend to remain limited to the urethra and reproductive system. Unlike *E. coli*, *Chlamydia* and *Mycoplasma* may be sexually transmitted, and infections require treatment of both partners.

The urinary system is structured in a way that helps ward off infection. The ureters and bladder normally prevent urine from backing up toward the kidneys, and the flow of urine from the bladder helps wash bacteria out of the body. In men, the prostate gland produces secretions that slow bacterial growth. In both sexes, immune defenses also prevent infection. But despite these safeguards, infections still occur.

Who is at risk?

Some people are more prone to getting a UTI than others. Any abnormality of the urinary tract that obstructs the flow of urine (a kidney stone, for example) sets the stage for an infection. An enlarged prostate gland also can slow the flow of urine, thus raising the risk of infection.

A common source of infection is catheters, or tubes, placed in the bladder. A person who cannot void or who is unconscious or critically ill often needs a catheter that stays in place for a long time. Some people, especially the elderly or those with nervous system disorders who lose bladder control, may need a catheter for life. Bacteria on the catheter can infect the bladder, so hospital staff take special care to keep the catheter sterile and remove it as soon as possible.

People with diabetes have a higher risk of a UTI because of changes in the immune system. Any disorder that suppresses the immune system raises the risk of a urinary infection.

UTIs may occur in infants who are born with abnormalities of the urinary tract, which sometimes need to be corrected with surgery. UTIs are rarely seen in boys and young men. In women, though, the rate of UTIs gradually increases with age. Scientists are not sure why women have more urinary infections than men. One factor may be that a woman's urethra is short, allowing bacteria quick access to the bladder. Also, a woman's urethral opening is near sources of bacteria from the anus and vagina. For many women, sexual intercourse seems to trigger an infection, although the reasons for this linkage are unclear.

According to several studies, women who use a diaphragm are more likely to develop a UTI than women who use other forms of birth control.

Recently, researchers found that women whose partners use a condom with spermicidal foam also tend to have growth of *E. coli* bacteria in the vagina.

Recurrent infections: Many women suffer from frequent UTIs. Nearly 20 percent of women who have a UTI will have another, and 30 percent of those will have yet another. Of the last group, 80 percent will have recurrences.

Usually, the latest infection stems from a strain or type of bacteria that is different from the infection before it, indicating a separate infection. (Even when several UTIs in a row are due to *E. coli*, slight differences in the bacteria indicate distinct infections.)

Research funded by the National Institutes of Health (NIH) suggests that one factor behind recurrent UTIs may be the ability of bacteria to attach to cells lining the urinary tract. A recent NIH-funded study found that bacteria formed a protective film on the inner lining of the bladder in mice. If a similar process can be demonstrated in humans, the discovery may lead to new treatments to prevent recurrent UTIs. Another line of research has indicated that women who are "non-secretors" of certain blood group antigens may be more prone to recurrent UTIs because the cells lining the vagina and urethra may allow bacteria to attach more easily. Further research will show whether this association is sound and proves useful in identifying women at high risk for UTIs.

Infections in pregnancy: According to some reports, about two to four percent of pregnant women develop a urinary infection. Scientists think that hormonal changes and shifts in the position of the urinary tract during pregnancy make it easier for bacteria to travel up the ureters to the kidneys. For this reason, many doctors recommend periodic testing of urine.

What are the symptoms of UTI?

Not everyone with a UTI has symptoms, but most people get at least some. These may include a frequent urge to urinate and a painful, burning feeling in the area of the bladder or urethra during urination. It is not unusual to feel bad all over—tired, shaky, washed out—and to feel pain even when not urinating. Often women feel an uncomfortable pressure above the pubic bone, and some men experience a fullness in the rectum. It is common for a person with a urinary infection to complain that, despite the urge to urinate, only a small amount of urine is passed. The urine itself may look milky or cloudy, even reddish if blood is present. A fever may mean that the infection has reached the kidneys. Other symptoms of a kidney infection include pain in the back or side below the ribs, nausea, or vomiting.

In children, symptoms of a urinary infection may be overlooked or attributed to another disorder. A UTI should be considered when a child or infant seems irritable, is not eating normally, has an unexplained fever that does not go away, has incontinence or loose bowels, or is not thriving. The child should be seen by a doctor if there are any questions about these symptoms, especially a change in the child's urinary pattern.

How is UTI diagnosed?

To find out whether you have a UTI, your doctor will test a sample of urine for pus and bacteria. You will be asked to give a "clean catch" urine sample by washing the genital area and collecting a "midstream" sample of urine in a sterile container. (This method of collecting urine helps prevent bacteria around the genital area from getting into the sample and confusing the test results.) Usually, the sample is sent to a laboratory, although some doctors' offices are equipped to do the testing.

In the urinalysis test, the urine is examined for white and red blood cells and bacteria. Then the bacteria are grown in a culture and tested against different antibiotics to see which drug best destroys the bacteria. This last step is called a sensitivity test.

Some microbes, like *Chlamydia* and *Mycoplasma*, can be detected only with special bacterial cultures. A doctor suspects one of these infections when a person has symptoms of a UTI and pus in the urine, but a standard culture fails to grow any bacteria.

When an infection does not clear up with treatment and is traced to the same strain of bacteria, the doctor will order a test that makes images of the urinary tract. One of these tests is an intravenous pyelogram (IVP), which gives x-ray images of the bladder, kidneys, and ureters. An opaque dye visible on x-ray film is injected into a vein, and a series of x rays is taken. The film shows an outline of the urinary tract, revealing even small changes in the structure of the tract.

If you have recurrent infections, your doctor also may recommend an ultrasound exam, which gives pictures from the echo patterns of sound waves bounced back from internal organs. Another useful test is cystoscopy. A cystoscope is an instrument made of a hollow tube with several lenses and a light source, which allows the doctor to see inside the bladder from the urethra.

How is UTI treated?

UTIs are treated with antibacterial drugs. The choice of drug and length of treatment depend on the patient's history and the urine tests that identify the offending bacteria. The sensitivity test is especially useful in helping the doctor select the most effective drug. The drugs most often used to treat routine, uncomplicated UTIs are trimethoprim (Trimpex), trimethoprim/sulfamethoxazole (Bactrim, Septra, Cotrim), amoxicillin (Amoxil, Trimox, Wymox), nitrofurantoin (Macrodantin, Furadantin), and ampicillin. A class of drugs called quinolones includes four drugs approved in recent years for treating UTI. These drugs include ofloxacin (Floxin), norfloxacin (Noroxin), ciprofloxacin (Cipro), and trovafloxacin (Trovan).

Often, a UTI can be cured with one or two days of treatment if the infection is not complicated by an obstruction or nervous system disorder. Still, many doctors ask their patients to take antibiotics for a week or two to ensure that the infection has been cured. Single-dose treatment is not recommended for some groups of patients, for example, those who have delayed treatment or have signs of a kidney infection, patients with diabetes or structural abnormalities, or men who have prostate infections. Longer treatment is also needed by patients with infections caused by *Mycoplasma* or *Chlamydia*, which are usually treated with tetracycline, trimethoprim/sulfamethoxazole (TMP/SMZ), or doxycycline. A follow-up urinalysis helps to confirm that the urinary tract is infection-free. It is important to take the full course of treatment because symptoms may disappear before the infection is fully cleared.

Severely ill patients with kidney infections may be hospitalized until they can take fluids and needed drugs on their own. Kidney infections generally require several weeks of antibiotic treatment. Researchers at the University of Washington found that two-week therapy with TMP/SMZ was as effective as six weeks of treatment with the same drug in women with kidney infections that did not involve an obstruction or nervous system disorder. In such cases, kidney infections rarely lead to kidney damage or kidney failure unless they go untreated.

Various drugs are available to relieve the pain of a UTI. A heating pad may also help. Most doctors suggest that drinking plenty of water helps cleanse the urinary tract of bacteria. During treatment, it is best to avoid coffee, alcohol, and spicy foods. And one of the best things a smoker can do for his or her bladder is to quit smoking. Smoking is the major known cause of bladder cancer.

Recurrent infections in women: Women who have had three UTIs are likely to continue having them. Four out of five such women get another within 18 months of the last UTI. Many women have them even more often. A woman who has frequent recurrences (three or more a year) should ask her doctor about one of the following treatment options:

- Take low doses of an antibiotic such as TMP/SMZ or nitrofurantoin daily for six months or longer. (If taken at bedtime, the drug remains in the bladder longer and may be more effective.) NIH-supported research at the University of Washington has shown this therapy to be effective without causing serious side effects.
- Take a single dose of an antibiotic after sexual intercourse.
- Take a short course (one or two days) of antibiotics when symptoms appear.

Dipsticks that change color when an infection is present are now available without a prescription. The strips detect nitrite, which is formed when bacteria change nitrate in the urine to nitrite. The test can detect about 90 percent of UTIs when used with the first morning urine specimen and may be useful for women who have recurrent infections.

Doctors suggest some additional steps that a woman can take on her own to avoid an infection:

- Drink plenty of water every day.
- Urinate when you feel the need; don't resist the urge to urinate.
- Wipe from front to back to prevent bacteria around the anus from entering the vagina or urethra.
- Take showers instead of tub baths.
- Cleanse the genital area before sexual intercourse.
- Avoid using feminine hygiene sprays and scented douches, which may irritate the urethra.

Some doctors suggest drinking cranberry juice. [See Chapter 11 for information on alternative treatments for urinary tract infections.]

Infections in pregnancy: A pregnant woman who develops a UTI should be treated promptly to avoid premature delivery of her baby and other risks such as high blood pressure. Some antibiotics are not safe to take during pregnancy. In selecting the best treatments, doctors consider various factors such as the drug's effectiveness, the stage of pregnancy, the mother's health, and potential effects on the fetus.

Complicated infections: Curing infections that stem from a urinary obstruction or nervous system disorder depends on finding and correcting the underlying problem, sometimes with surgery. If the root cause goes untreated, this group of patients is at risk of kidney damage. Also, such infections tend to arise from a wider range of bacteria, and sometimes from more than one type of bacteria at a time.

Infections in men: UTIs in men usually stem from an obstruction—for example, a urinary stone or enlarged prostate—or from a medical procedure involving a catheter. The first step is to identify the infecting organism and the drugs to which it is sensitive. Usually, doctors recommend lengthier therapy in men than in women, in part to prevent infections of the prostate gland.

Prostate infections (chronic bacterial prostatitis) are harder to cure because antibiotics are unable to penetrate infected prostate tissue effectively. For this reason, men with prostatitis often need long-term treatment with a carefully selected antibiotic. UTIs in older men are frequently associated with acute bacterial prostatitis, which can be fatal if not treated immediately.

Is there a vaccine to prevent recurrent UTIs?

In the future, scientists may develop a vaccine that can prevent UTIs from coming back. Researchers in different studies have found that children and women who tend to get UTIs repeatedly are likely to lack proteins called immunoglobulins, which fight infection. Children and women who do not get UTIs are more likely to have normal levels of immunoglobulins in their genital and urinary tracts.

Early tests indicate that a vaccine helps patients build up their own natural infection-fighting powers. The dead bacteria in the vaccine do not spread like an infection; instead, they prompt the body to produce antibodies that can later fight against live organisms. Researchers are testing injected and oral vaccines to see which works best. Another method being considered for women is to apply the vaccine directly as a suppository in the vagina.

Chapter 10

Urinary Tract Infection during Pregnancy

A urinary tract infection (UTI), also called bladder infection, is a bacterial inflammation in the urinary tract. Pregnant women are at increased risk for UTIs starting in week 6 through week 24.

Why are UTIs more common during pregnancy?

UTIs are more common during pregnancy because of changes in the urinary tract. The uterus sits directly on top of the bladder. As the uterus grows, its increased weight can block the drainage of urine from the bladder, causing an infection.

What are the signs and symptoms of UTIs?

If you have a urinary tract infection, you may experience one or more of the following symptoms:

- Pain or burning (discomfort) when urinating
- The need to urinate more often than usual
- A feeling of urgency when you urinate
- Blood or mucus in the urine
- Cramps or pain in the lower abdomen
- Pain during sexual intercourse

- Chills, fever, sweats, leaking of urine (incontinence)
- Waking up from sleep to urinate
- Change in amount of urine, either more or less
- Urine that looks cloudy, smells foul or unusually strong
- Pain, pressure, or tenderness in the area of the bladder
- When bacteria spreads to the kidneys you may experience: back pain, chills, fever, nausea, and vomiting.

How will the UTI affect my baby?

If the UTI goes untreated, it may lead to a kidney infection. Kidney infections may cause early labor and low birth weight. If your doctor treats a urinary tract infection early and properly, the UTI will not cause harm to your baby.

How do I know if I have a UTI?

A urinalysis and a urine culture can detect a UTI throughout pregnancy.

How is a UTI treated?

UTIs can be safely treated with antibiotics during pregnancy. Urinary tract infections are most commonly treated by antibiotics. Doctors usually prescribe a three to seven day course of antibiotics that is safe for you and the baby.

Call your doctor if you have fever, chills, lower stomach pains, nausea, vomiting, contractions, or if after taking medicine for three days, you still have a burning feeling when you urinate.

How can I prevent a UTI?

You may do everything right and still experience a urinary tract infection, but you can reduce the likelihood by doing the following:

- Drink six to eight glasses of water each day and unsweetened cranberry juice regularly.
- Eliminate refined foods, fruit juices, caffeine, alcohol, and sugar.
- Take vitamin C (250 to 500 mg), Beta-carotene (25,000 to 50,000 IU per day), and zinc (30 to 50 mg per day) to help fight infection.

- Develop a habit of urinating as soon as the need is felt and empty your bladder completely when you urinate.

- Urinate before and after intercourse.

- Avoid intercourse while you are being treated for an UTI.

- After urinating, blot dry (do not rub), and keep your genital area clean. Make sure you wipe from the front toward the back.

- Avoid using strong soaps, douches, antiseptic creams, feminine hygiene sprays, and powders.

- Change underwear and pantyhose every day.

- Avoid wearing tight-fitting pants.

- Wear all cotton or cotton-crotch underwear and pantyhose.

- Don't soak in the bathtub longer than 30 minutes or more than twice a day.

Chapter 11

Alternative Treatments for Urinary Tract Infections

Chapter Contents

Section 11.1

The Role of Cranberry in the Prevention and Treatment of Urinary Tract Infections

Excerpted from "Cranberry (*Vaccinium macrocarpon*) and Urinary Tract Infection," National Center for Complimentary and Alternative Medicine (NCCAM), National Institutes of Health (NIH), February 4, 2004.

Urinary tract infections (UTIs) are a serious health problem affecting millions of people each year. Nearly 20 percent of women who have a UTI will have another and 30 percent of those will have yet another.

Most infections arise from one type of bacteria, *Escherichia coli* (*E. coli*), which normally live in the colon. Usually, the latest infection stems from a strain or type of bacteria that is different from the infection before it, indicating a separate infection. (Even when several UTIs in a row are due to *E. coli*, slight differences in the bacterial strains indicate distinct infections.)

Research funded by the National Institutes of Health (NIH) suggests that one factor behind recurrent UTIs may be the ability of bacteria to attach to cells lining the urinary tract.

Cranberry Use

Traditionally UTIs are treated with antibacterial drugs, but these are expensive, can have side effects, and may lead to resistance. Therefore, physicians suggest additional steps that patients can take on their own to avoid infection, including drinking cranberry juice [see Chapter 9, "Urinary Tract Infections in Adults"]. Although cranberry juice is the form of cranberries most widely used, other cranberry products include cranberry powder in hard or soft gelatin capsules.

The use of cranberry among individuals to prevent or treat UTI is a common practice. The accumulating evidence from small, non-controlled and controlled clinical trials suggests that cranberry may relieve symptoms associated with UTI and may reduce the need for antibiotics. The findings from the preliminary research provide convincing reasons to support the conduct of small-scale, focused clinical studies.

Safety

Cranberry taken orally in food amounts appears safe, although ingesting large amounts may result in diarrhea and other gastrointestinal symptoms. Safety of amounts greater than that consumed in foods is unknown. One study of cranberry tablets suggests caution for patients at risk for nephrolithiasis until safety of cranberry is confirmed. Currently, there is insufficient reliable information available to assess the interaction of cranberry with dietary supplements, medications, foods, or laboratory tests.

Cranberry Product

The appropriate cranberry product, dose, and duration of intervention for prevention or treatment of UTI are unknown. While cranberry juice cocktail is the most studied product, concentrates and encapsulated powders have also been used. Some sources suggest six capsules of dried cranberry powder are equivalent to two ounces cranberry juice cocktail. The chemical composition of the study agents, in general, has not been described in the published literature, nor has the equivalence of the active constituents or markers among cocktails, concentrates, and capsules/tablets been described. Therefore, comparison among study agents or trial results has not been possible.

The single-strength juice is highly acidic and astringent which makes the juice unpalatable at full strength. Accordingly, the juice drink, i.e., cranberry juice cocktail, is a mixture of single-strength cranberry juice, sweetener, water, and vitamin C. Cocktails have been sweetened with fructose or artificially sweetened. The percent concentrate used in the cocktails has ranged, although cocktail with 33 percent pure juice is common.

Cranberries contain about 88 percent water. Among the other organic constituents are flavonoids, anthocyanins, catechin, triterpenoids, B-hydroxybutyric acid, citric, malic, glucuronic, quinic, and benzoic acids, ellagic acid, and vitamin C. Quinic acid and the ratio of quinic acid to malic acid are reasonably constant and are used to calculate percentage of cranberry juice content in juice drinks and to assess cranberry juice authenticity. Although anthocyanins change and degrade with processing and storage, the anthocyanin profile is unique to cranberry, and its qualitative pattern is characteristic.

Doses of the cocktails have ranged from 160 to 750 ml a day, usually in divided doses at meals. Intervention duration has also ranged, from five days to six months (longer trials for prevention). The rationale behind the amount and concentrate of cranberry juice given to participants and the duration of intervention is usually not provided.

Suggested Research Needs

Conclusions from the published literature suggest the following research directions:

- Study the effect of cranberry in prevention of UTI and as adjunct to antibiotics in the treatment of UTI.

- Demonstrate whether cranberry reduces symptomatic UTI (primary endpoint being UTI; secondary endpoints being bacteriuria, bacteria in the urine, or pyuria, pus in the urine).

- Conduct randomized controlled trials (RCTs) of longer duration in a broad array of patient types, especially younger women with symptomatic cystitis, as well as other patient groups with recurrent UTI.

- Determine the optimum amount of cranberry (dose-response), timing of ingestion, peak times to effect (temporal effect), and variations in response.

- Assess adherence to protocol and retention.

- Assess the contribution of cranberry juice to increased fluid intake (concentrate vs. juice vs. other beverage) and the effect on UTI.

- Collect data on adverse effects systematically.

- Assess interactions with medications (such as antibiotics and H_2 blockers), dietary supplements, foods, and laboratory tests.

- Evaluate relationship of cranberry to bacterial adherence.

- Evaluate relationship of cranberry and bacterial adherence to urinary pH.

- Conduct in vivo feeding studies to establish that proanthocyanidins are able to cross into the blood and urine to provide the antiadherence effect.

- Investigate the antiadhesive property on different strains of bacteria, as well as on various cellular substrates.

- Confirm/identify active agent(s) and/or other biochemical properties.

- Assess the equivalence of different cranberry products, e.g., juice cocktails, concentrates, encapsulated powders.

Section 11.2

Naturopathic Treatment for Urinary Tract Infections

"Urinary Tract Infections: Naturopathic Treatment," reprinted with permission. © 2005 Healthcommunities.com, Inc. All rights reserved.

Naturopathic Treatment

The natural therapeutics outlined in this section may help patients get through an existing urinary tract infection (UTI) without antibiotics. Some doctors believe that antibiotics contribute to recurrent infections from increasingly resistant bacteria. Lifestyle precautions and supportive natural measures can help reduce recurrent urinary tract infections.

Alkalinize the Urine

Although some controversy remains concerning what pH level is most conducive to bacteria growth in the urinary tract, most evidence indicates that UTIs benefit from an alkaline pH. The easiest way to alkalinize the urine is with minerals, specifically potassium citrate and sodium citrate. All citrates encourage an alkaline shift; so patients already taking a calcium/magnesium supplement should switch to a calcium citrate/magnesium citrate preparation. Mineral supplements should be taken before bedtime, as urine that remains in the bladder during sleep may irritate the tissue and promote an infection.

Disinfect the Urinary Tract

Some herbs have been clinically shown to have antiseptic properties. Drinking these herbs in beverage form throughout the day may be beneficial.

Drinking at least 16 ounces a day of cranberry or blueberry juice (not the sugar-sweetened variety) can have a preventative and therapeutic effect. These juices have antibiotic properties that interfere with the ability of bacteria to adhere to the bladder or urethral tissue. Choose a juice sweetened with apple or grape juice.

Herbal Therapeutics

The following herbal remedies usually do not cause side effects when used regularly at the suggested doses. Rarely, an herb at the prescribed dose causes stomach upset or headache. This may reflect the purity of the preparation or added ingredients such as synthetic binders or fillers. For this reason, only high quality, standardized extract formulas are recommended.

If possible, consult with a natural health practitioner such as a holistic medical doctor or licensed naturopathic physician before beginning any alternative treatment plan. As with all medications, more is not better and overdosing can lead to serious illness and, in rare cases, death.

A naturopathic physician may prescribe that one of these herbal preparations be used three to four times per day during a urinary tract infection:

- **Goldenseal root:** This herb has a long and well-documented history as a powerful antimicrobial agent. Use as a tea made from one teaspoon of dried herb per cup of hot water; in capsule form (1,000 mg); or as a tincture (one to two teaspoons in warm water).

- **Uva ursi:** Clinical research proves traditional use as an antiseptic with soothing and strengthening properties. Use as a tea made from two teaspoons of herb per cup of hot water; or as a tincture (one to two teaspoons in warm water).

Other herbs to consider as tea include:

- **Cleavers (*Galium aparine*):** Has a long history of use in treatment of urinary infections.

- **Marshmallow root (*Althea officinalis*):** Has very soothing demulcent properties. Best used in "cold infusion." Soak herb in cold water several hours, then strain and drink.

- **Buchu:** Is a soothing diuretic and antiseptic for the urinary system.

- **Cornsilk (*Zea mays*):** Is a soothing diuretic.

- **Horsetail (*Equisetum arvense*):** Is an astringent and mild diuretic with tissue-healing properties.

- **Usnea lichen:** Is very soothing and antiseptic.

Also be sure to drink two to three liters of water daily.

Homeopathic Remedies

A trained homeopathic practitioner is required to diagnose and prescribe a deep acting, constitutional remedy. The following remedies may help to relieve some of the acute symptoms associated with urinary tract infections.

The standard dosage for acute symptom relief is 12c to 30c [c is a measure of potency in homeopathic remedies], 3 to 5 pellets, 3 or 4 times a day until symptoms resolve. If the chosen remedy is correct, symptoms should improve shortly after the first or second dose. Do not take any remedy longer than a day or two without consulting a homeopathic practitioner (naturopathic physician or medical doctor).

Warning: Most homeopathic remedies are delivered in a small pellet form that has a lactose sugar base. Patients who are lactose intolerant should be advised that a homeopathic liquid may be a better choice.

- ***Cantharis:*** For intolerable urging with burning, "scalding" urination

- ***Apis mellifica:*** For stinging pain that is worse with heat

- ***Staphysagria:*** For a UTI that is the result of sexual intercourse

- ***Sarsaparilla:*** For pain that burns after urination has stopped

Physical Medicine

Castor oil packs can be applied for UTIs that have associated bladder cramping or pelvic discomfort. Apply castor oil directly to the skin and cover with a soft piece of flannel and heat (hot water bottle) for 30 minutes to one hour. The anti-inflammatory action of castor oil aids in pain relief.

Sitz baths can be helpful if there is swelling or burning of the urethral opening. An infusion of golden seal is anti-microbial and soothing. The other herbs indicated will also be helpful.

Chapter 12

Interstitial Cystitis

Understanding Interstitial Cystitis

Interstitial cystitis (IC), one of the chronic pelvic pain disorders, is a condition resulting in recurring discomfort or pain in the bladder and the surrounding pelvic region. The symptoms of IC vary from case to case and even in the same individual. People may experience mild discomfort, pressure, tenderness, or intense pain in the bladder and pelvic area. Symptoms may include an urgent need to urinate (urgency), frequent need to urinate (frequency), or a combination of these symptoms. Pain may change in intensity as the bladder fills with urine or as it empties. Women's symptoms often get worse during menstruation.

In IC, the bladder wall may be irritated and become scarred or stiff. Glomerulations (pinpoint bleeding caused by recurrent irritation) may appear on the bladder wall. Some people with IC find that their bladders cannot hold much urine, which increases the frequency of urination. Frequency, however, is not always specifically related to bladder size; many people with severe frequency have normal bladder capacity. People with severe cases of IC may urinate as many as 60 times a day.

National Kidney and Urologic Diseases Information Clearinghouse (NKUDIC), a service of the National Institute of Diabetes and Digestive and Kidney Diseases (NIDDK), National Institutes of Health (NIH), Pub. No. 03-3220, July 2003.

Also, people with IC often experience pain during sexual intercourse. IC is far more common in women than in men. Of the more than 700,000 Americans estimated to have IC, 90 percent are women.

IC Causes

Some of the symptoms of IC resemble those of bacterial infection, but medical tests reveal no organisms in the urine of patients with IC. Furthermore, patients with IC do not respond to antibiotic therapy. Researchers are working to understand the causes of IC and to find effective treatments.

One theory being studied is that IC is an autoimmune response following a bladder infection. Another theory is that a bacterium may be present in bladder cells but not detectable through routine urine tests. Some scientists have suggested that certain substances in urine may be irritating to people with IC, but no substance unique to people with IC has as yet been isolated. Researchers are beginning to explore the possibility that heredity may play a part in some forms of IC. In a few cases, IC has affected a mother and a daughter or two sisters, but it does not commonly run in families. No gene has yet been implicated as a cause.

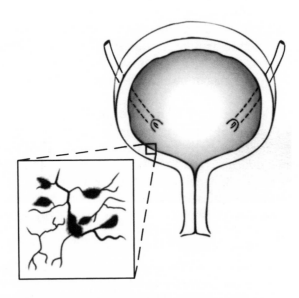

Figure 12.1. *Pinpoint bleeding on the bladder wall.*

Different Types of IC

Because IC varies so much in symptoms and severity, most researchers believe that it is not one, but several, diseases. In the past, cases were mainly categorized as ulcerative IC or nonulcerative IC, based on whether ulcers had formed on the bladder wall. But many researchers and clinicians have questioned the usefulness of this classification, since the vast majority of cases do not involve ulcers, and their presence or absence does not influence treatment options as much as other factors do.

Factors that influence treatment options include whether bladder capacity under anesthesia is great or small, and whether mast cells are present in the tissue of the bladder wall, which may be a sign of an allergic or autoimmune reaction. In some cases, the success or failure of a treatment helps characterize the type of IC. For example, some cases respond to changes in diet while others do not.

Diagnosing IC

Because symptoms are similar to those of other disorders of the urinary system and because there is no definitive test to identify IC, doctors must rule out other conditions before considering a diagnosis of IC. Among these disorders are urinary tract or vaginal infections, bladder cancer, bladder inflammation or infection caused by radiation to the pelvic area, eosinophilic and tuberculous cystitis, kidney stones, endometriosis, neurological disorders, sexually transmitted diseases, low-count bacteria in the urine, and, in men, chronic bacterial and nonbacterial prostatitis.

The diagnosis of IC in the general population is based on the presence of urgency, frequency, or pelvic/bladder pain; cystoscopic evidence (under anesthesia) of bladder wall inflammation, including Hunner ulcers or glomerulations (present in 90 percent of patients with IC); and the absence of other diseases that could cause the symptoms.

Diagnostic tests that help identify other conditions include urinalysis, urine culture, cystoscopy, biopsy of the bladder wall, distention of the bladder under anesthesia, urine cytology, and, in men, laboratory examination of prostate secretions.

Urinalysis and Urine Culture

These tests can detect and identify the most common organisms that infect the urine and that may cause symptoms similar to IC.

However, organisms such as *Chlamydia* cannot be detected with these tests, so a negative culture does not rule out all types of infection. A urine sample is obtained either by catheterization or by the "clean catch" method. For a clean catch, the patient washes the genital area before collecting urine "midstream" in a sterile container. White and red blood cells and bacteria in the urine may indicate an infection of the urinary tract, which can be treated with an antibiotic. If urine is sterile for weeks or months while symptoms persist, the doctor may consider a diagnosis of IC.

Culture of Prostate Secretions

In men, the doctor might obtain prostatic fluid and examine it for signs of an infection, which can then be treated with antibiotics.

Cystoscopy under Anesthesia with Bladder Distention

During cystoscopy, the doctor uses a cystoscope—an instrument made of a hollow tube about the diameter of a drinking straw with several lenses and a light—to see inside the bladder and urethra. The doctor will also distend or stretch the bladder to its capacity by filling it with a liquid or gas. Because bladder distention is painful in patients with IC, they must be given some form of anesthesia for the procedure. These tests can detect bladder wall inflammation; a thick, stiff bladder wall; and Hunner ulcers. Glomerulations are usually seen only after the bladder has been stretched to capacity.

The doctor may also test the patient's maximum bladder capacity—the maximum amount of liquid or gas the bladder can hold. This must be done under anesthesia since the bladder capacity is limited

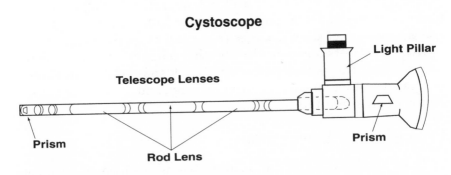

Cystoscope

Figure 12.2. Cystoscope.

by either pain or a severe urge to urinate. A small bladder capacity under anesthesia helps support the diagnosis of IC.

Biopsy

A biopsy is a tissue sample that is then examined under a microscope. Samples of the bladder and urethra may be removed during a cystoscopy and later examined with a microscope. A biopsy helps rule out bladder cancer.

Future Diagnostic Tools

As researchers learn more about the causes of IC, more accurate and less invasive diagnostic procedures are likely to emerge. For example, some researchers are studying the possibility that urine samples from people with IC contain substances not found in normal urine. If an IC marker in the urine can be found, patients may not have to undergo a cystoscopic examination or biopsy to receive a diagnosis.

IC Treatments

Scientists have not yet found a cure for IC, nor can they predict who will respond best to which treatment. Symptoms may disappear without explanation or coincide with an event such as a change in diet or treatment. Even when symptoms disappear, they may return after days, weeks, months, or years. Scientists do not know why.

Because the causes of IC are unknown, current treatments are aimed at relieving symptoms. Most people are helped for variable periods by one or a combination of treatments. As researchers learn more about IC, the list of potential treatments will change, so patients should discuss their options with a doctor.

Bladder Distention

Because many patients have noted an improvement in symptoms after a bladder distention has been done to diagnose IC, the procedure is often thought of as one of the first treatment attempts.

Researchers are not sure why distention helps, but some believe that it may increase capacity and interfere with pain signals transmitted by nerves in the bladder. Symptoms may temporarily worsen 24 to 48 hours after distention, but should return to predistention levels or improve after two to four weeks.

Bladder Instillation

During a bladder instillation, also called a bladder wash or bath, the bladder is filled with a solution that is held for varying periods of time, averaging 10 to 15 minutes, before being emptied.

The only drug approved by the U.S. Food and Drug Administration (FDA) for bladder instillation is dimethyl sulfoxide (DMSO, Rimso-50). DMSO treatment involves guiding a narrow tube called a catheter up the urethra into the bladder. A measured amount of DMSO is passed through the catheter into the bladder, where it is retained for about 15 minutes before being expelled. Treatments are given every week or two for six to eight weeks and repeated as needed. Most people who respond to DMSO notice improvement three or four weeks after the first six- to eight-week cycle of treatments. Highly motivated patients who are willing to catheterize themselves may, after consultation with their doctor, be able to have DMSO treatments at home. Self-administration is less expensive and more convenient than going to the doctor's office.

Doctors think DMSO works in several ways. Because it passes into the bladder wall, it may reach tissue more effectively to reduce inflammation and block pain. It may also prevent muscle contractions that cause pain, frequency, and urgency.

A bothersome but relatively insignificant side effect of DMSO treatments is a garlic-like taste and odor on the breath and skin that may last up to 72 hours after treatment. Long-term treatment has caused cataracts in animal studies, but this side effect has not appeared in humans. Blood tests, including a complete blood count and kidney and liver function tests, should be done about every six months.

Oral Drugs

Pentosan polysulfate sodium (Elmiron): This first oral drug developed for IC was approved by the FDA in 1996. In clinical trials, the drug improved symptoms in 38 percent of patients treated. Doctors do not know exactly how it works, but one theory is that it may repair defects that might have developed in the lining of the bladder.

The FDA-recommended oral dosage of Elmiron is 100 mg, three times a day. Patients may not feel relief from IC pain for the first two to four months. A decrease in urinary frequency may take up to six months. Patients are urged to continue with therapy for at least six months to give the drug an adequate chance to relieve symptoms.

Elmiron's side effects are limited primarily to minor gastrointestinal discomfort. A small minority of patients experienced some hair loss, but hair grew back when they stopped taking the drug. Researchers have found no negative interactions between Elmiron and other medications.

Elmiron may affect liver function, which should therefore be monitored by the doctor.

Because Elmiron has not been tested in pregnant women, the manufacturer recommends that it not be used during pregnancy, except in the most severe cases.

Other oral medications: Aspirin and ibuprofen are easy to obtain and may be a first line of defense against mild discomfort. Doctors may recommend other drugs to relieve pain.

Some patients have experienced improvement in their urinary symptoms by taking antidepressants or antihistamines. Antidepressants help reduce pain and may also help patients deal with the psychological stress that accompanies living with chronic pain. In patients with severe pain, narcotic analgesics such as acetaminophen (Tylenol) with codeine or longer acting narcotics may be necessary.

All drugs—even those sold over the counter—have side effects. Patients should always consult a doctor before using any drug for an extended time.

Transcutaneous Electrical Nerve Stimulation

With transcutaneous electrical nerve stimulation (TENS), mild electric pulses enter the body for minutes to hours two or more times a day either through wires placed on the lower back or just above the pubic area, between the navel and the pubic hair, or through special devices inserted into the vagina in women or into the rectum in men. Although scientists do not know exactly how TENS relieves IC pain, it has been suggested that the electrical pulses may increase blood flow to the bladder, strengthen pelvic muscles that help control the bladder, or trigger the release of substances that block pain.

TENS is relatively inexpensive and allows the patient to take an active part in treatment. Within some guidelines, the patient decides when, how long, and at what intensity TENS will be used. It has been most helpful in relieving pain and decreasing frequency in patients with Hunner ulcers. Smokers do not respond as well as nonsmokers. If TENS is going to help, improvement is usually apparent in three to four months.

Diet

There is no scientific evidence linking diet to IC, but many doctors and patients find that alcohol, tomatoes, spices, chocolate, caffeinated and citrus beverages, and high-acid foods may contribute to bladder irritation and inflammation. Some patients also note that their symptoms worsen after eating or drinking products containing artificial sweeteners. Patients may try eliminating various items from their diet and reintroducing them one at a time to determine which, if any, affect their symptoms. It is important, however, to maintain a varied, well-balanced diet.

Smoking

Many patients feel that smoking makes their symptoms worse. Because smoking is the major known cause of bladder cancer, one of the best things smokers can do for their bladder is to quit.

Exercise

Many patients feel that gentle stretching exercises help relieve IC symptoms.

Bladder Training

People who have found adequate relief from pain may be able to reduce frequency by using bladder training techniques. Methods vary, but basically patients decide to void (empty their bladder) at designated times and use relaxation techniques and distractions to keep to the schedule. Gradually, patients try to lengthen the time between scheduled voids. A diary in which to record voiding times is usually helpful in keeping track of progress.

Surgery

Many approaches and techniques are used, each of which has its own advantages and complications that should be discussed with a surgeon. Surgery should be considered only if all available treatments have failed and the pain is disabling. Most doctors are reluctant to operate because the outcome is unpredictable—some people still have symptoms after surgery.

Those considering surgery should discuss the potential risks and benefits, side effects, and long- and short-term complications with a

Your Daily Bladder Diary

This diary will help you and your health care team. Bladder diaries help show the causes of bladder control trouble. The "sample" line (below) will show you how to use the diary.

Your name: _____

Date: _____

Time	Drinks		Urine		ACCIDENTS		
	What kind?	How much?	How many times?	How much? (circle one)	Accidental leaks How much? (circle one)	Did you feel a strong urge to go? Circle one	What were you doing at the time? Sneezing, exercising, having sex, lifting, etc.
sample	Coffee	2 cps	4	sm ◑ med ● lg	sm ◑ med ● lg	yes (no)	Running
6–7 AM				○ sm ◐ med ● lg	○ sm ◐ med ● lg	yes no	
7–8 AM				○ sm ◐ med ● lg	○ sm ◐ med ● lg	yes no	
8–9 AM				○ sm ◐ med ● lg	○ sm ◐ med ● lg	yes no	
9–10 AM				○ sm ◐ med ● lg	○ sm ◐ med ● lg	yes no	
10–11 AM				○ sm ◐ med ● lg	○ sm ◐ med ● lg	yes no	
11–12 PM				○ sm ◐ med ● lg	○ sm ◐ med ● lg	yes no	
12–1 PM				○ sm ◐ med ● lg	○ sm ◐ med ● lg	yes no	
1–2 PM				○ sm ◐ med ● lg	○ sm ◐ med ● lg	yes no	
2–3 PM				○ sm ◐ med ● lg	○ sm ◐ med ● lg	yes no	
3–4 PM				○ sm ◐ med ● lg	○ sm ◐ med ● lg	yes no	
4–5 PM				○ sm ◐ med ● lg	○ sm ◐ med ● lg	yes no	
5–6 PM				○ sm ◐ med ● lg	○ sm ◐ med ● lg	yes no	
6–7 PM				○ sm ◐ med ● lg	○ sm ◐ med ● lg	yes no	

Figure 12.3. Voiding diary.

surgeon and with their family, as well as with people who have already had the procedure. Surgery requires anesthesia, hospitalization, and weeks or months of recovery, and as the complexity of the procedure increases, so do the chances for complications and for failure.

To locate a surgeon experienced in performing specific procedures, check with your doctor.

Two procedures—fulguration and resection of ulcers—can be done with instruments inserted through the urethra. Fulguration involves burning Hunner ulcers with electricity or a laser. When the area heals, the dead tissue and the ulcer fall off, leaving new, healthy tissue behind. Resection involves cutting around and removing the ulcers. Both treatments are done under anesthesia and use special instruments inserted into the bladder through a cystoscope. Laser surgery in the urinary tract should be reserved for patients with Hunner ulcers and should be done only by doctors who have had special training and have the expertise needed to perform the procedure.

Another surgical treatment is augmentation, which makes the bladder larger. In most of these procedures, scarred, ulcerated, and inflamed sections of the patient's bladder are removed, leaving only the base of the bladder and healthy tissue. A piece of the patient's colon (large intestine) is then removed, reshaped, and attached to what remains of the bladder. After the incisions heal, the patient may void less frequently. The effect on pain varies greatly; IC can sometimes recur on the segment of colon used to enlarge the bladder.

Even in carefully selected patients—those with small, contracted bladders—pain, frequency, and urgency may remain or return after surgery, and the patient may have additional problems with infections in the new bladder and difficulty absorbing nutrients from the shortened colon. Some patients are incontinent, while others cannot void at all and must insert a catheter into the urethra to empty the bladder.

A surgical variation of TENS, called sacral nerve root stimulation, involves permanent implantation of electrodes and a unit emitting continuous electrical pulses. Studies of this experimental procedure are now under way.

Bladder removal, called a cystectomy, is another surgical option. Once the bladder has been removed, different methods can be used to reroute the urine. In most cases, ureters are attached to a piece of colon that opens onto the skin of the abdomen; this procedure is called a urostomy, and the opening is called a stoma. Urine empties through the stoma into a bag outside the body. Some urologists are using a second technique that also requires a stoma but allows urine to be stored in a pouch inside the abdomen. At intervals throughout the day, the patient puts a catheter into the stoma and empties the pouch. Patients with either type of urostomy must be very careful to keep the area in and around the stoma clean to prevent infection. Serious potential complications may include kidney infection and small bowel obstruction.

A third method to reroute urine involves making a new bladder from a piece of the patient's colon and attaching it to the urethra. After healing, the patient may be able to empty the newly formed bladder by voiding at scheduled times or by inserting a catheter into the urethra. Only a few surgeons have the special training and expertise needed to perform this procedure.

Even after total bladder removal, some patients still experience variable IC symptoms in the form of phantom pain. Therefore, the decision to undergo a cystectomy should be made only after testing all alternative methods and after seriously considering the potential outcome.

Special Concerns

Cancer: There is no evidence that IC increases the risk of bladder cancer.

Pregnancy: Researchers have little information on pregnancy and IC but believe that the disorder does not affect fertility or the health of the fetus. Some women find that their IC goes into remission during pregnancy, while others experience a worsening of their symptoms.

Coping: The emotional support of family, friends, and other people with IC is very important in helping patients cope. Studies have found that patients who learn about the disorder and become involved in their own care do better than patients who do not. [The Interstitial Cystitis Association of America, Inc. has information on support groups. To find a group near you, go to their website at http://www.ichelp.org or contact them by telephone at 800-HELP-ICA (435-7422) or 301-610-5300.]

Chapter 13

Bladder Stones

Alternative names: Urinary tract stones; bladder calculi

Definition: Bladder stones are hard buildups of mineral that form in the urinary bladder.

Causes, Incidence, and Risk Factors

Bladder stones are usually the result of another urologic problem such as urinary tract infection, bladder diverticulum, neurogenic bladder, or an enlarged prostate. Approximately 95 percent of all bladder stones occur in men. Stones originating in the bladder are much less common than kidney stones.

Bladder stones may occur when urine in the bladder is concentrated and materials crystallize. The patient feels symptoms when the lining of the bladder is irritated by the stone or when the stone obstructs the flow of urine from the bladder.

Symptoms

* Frequent urge to urinate
* Interruption of the urine stream

- Difficulty urinating
- Inability to urinate except in certain positions
- Blood in the urine
- Abdominal pain, pressure
- Pain, discomfort in the penis
- Abnormally colored or dark-colored urine
- Urinary tract infection
  - Dysuria (painful urination)
  - Urinary urgency
  - Fever

Incontinence may also be associated with bladder stones.

Signs and Tests

- Physical examination, including rectal examination, may reveal enlarged prostate or other urologic conditions.
- Urinalysis may show blood or may indicate infection.
- Urine culture (clean catch) may reveal infection.
- Bladder or pelvic x-ray may show the presence of stones.

Treatment

Drinking six to eight glasses of water or more per day, enough to increase urinary output, may help the stones pass.

Stones that are not excreted spontaneously may be removed by your healthcare provider using a cystoscope or a lithotripter (a small tube that passes through the urethra to the bladder). Some stones may need to be removed using open surgery.

Extracorporeal shock wave lithotripsy (ESWL) may be an alternative to surgery. In this treatment, ultrasonic waves break up stones so that they may be expelled in the urine.

Medications are rarely used to try to dissolve the stones.

Underlying causes of bladder stones should be treated. Most commonly bladder stones are seen in conjunction with benign prostatic hyperplasia (BPH) or bladder outlet obstruction.

For patients with BPH and bladder stones, transurethral resection of the prostate (TURP) can be performed with ESWL.

Expectations (Prognosis)

Most bladder stones are expelled or can be removed without permanent damage to the bladder. They may recur if the underlying cause is not corrected.

If the stones are left untreated they may cause permanent damage to the bladder or kidneys.

Complications

- Recurrence of stones
- Urinary tract infection, chronic or recurrent
- Obstruction of the urethra
- Reflux nephropathy
- Acute bilateral obstructive uropathy
- Chronic bladder dysfunction (incontinence or urinary retention)
- Calling your healthcare provider

Call your healthcare provider if symptoms indicate that you may have bladder stones.

Prevention

Prompt treatment of urinary tract infections or other urologic conditions may help prevent bladder stones.

Chapter 14

Other Bladder Disorders

Chapter Contents

Section 14.1

Neurogenic Bladder

The normal function of the bladder is to store and expel urine in a coordinated, controlled fashion. This coordinated activity is regulated by the central and peripheral nervous systems. But what happens when the bladder malfunctions as a result of dysfunction, trauma, disease or injury? The information below should help you recognize this problem before it causes serious damage.

What happens under normal conditions?

The urinary bladder, a spherical organ, has a soft inner lining (similar to the inner cheek) and an outer muscle layer. In addition to the bladder, the bladder neck (funnel-like outlet of the bladder which leads to the urethra), the urethra (tube-like structure which serves as a channel to carry urine from the bladder to the external surface), and the external urethral sphincter muscle (group of muscles which surround the urinary passage below the bladder neck) complete the lower urinary tract.

The muscles and nerves of the urinary system must function in a coordinated fashion with the bladder in order to perform its two major functions of storage and elimination of urine. Nerves carry messages from the bladder to the brain and then from the brain to the muscles of the bladder telling them to either tighten or release, allowing the bladder to empty during urination.

What is neurogenic bladder?

Neurogenic bladder is the loss of normal bladder function caused by damage to part of the nervous system. The damage can cause the bladder to be underactive, in which it is unable to contract and unable to empty completely, or it can be overactive, in which it contracts too quickly or frequently.

What are some risk factors for neurogenic bladder?

Risk factors for neurogenic bladder include various birth defects, which adversely affect the spinal cord and function of the bladder, including spina bifida and other spinal cord abnormalities. Tumors within the spinal cord or pelvis may also disrupt normal nervous tissue function and place an individual at risk. Traumatic spinal cord injury is also a major risk factor for development of neurogenic bladder.

What are the symptoms of neurogenic bladder?

Inability to control urination, also known as urinary incontinence, is perhaps the most common symptom associated with the neurogenic bladder. This may be caused by abnormalities in bladder capacity or malfunction of control mechanisms such as the bladder neck and/or external urethral sphincter muscle that are important for the bladder's storage function.

Symptoms including a dribbling urinary stream, straining during urination or inability to urinate may also be associated with neurogenic bladder. Urinary retention may result either from loss of bladder muscle contracting performance or loss of appropriate coordination between the bladder muscle and the external urethral sphincter muscle.

Irritating symptoms, such as urinary frequency and urgency, may be evidence of bladder hyperactivity. Other irritating symptoms may include painful urination (dysuria), which may be a result of a urinary tract infection (UTI) caused by urine being held too long in the bladder. UTI with fever is a sign of potential severe kidney infection (pyelonephritis) and is a more worrisome situation as it may result in permanent damage of the kidney(s).

Stones may also form in the urinary tract of individuals with a neurogenic bladder caused by the stoppage of urine flow and/or infection.

Abnormal backup of urine from the bladder to the kidney(s), also known as vesicoureteral reflux (VUR), may develop as a means of releasing high pressure within the bladder. A UTI is of particular concern as VUR may place the patient at significant risk for a severe kidney infection by transporting infected bladder urine directly to the kidney(s).

How is neurogenic bladder diagnosed?

When neurogenic bladder is suspected, both the nervous system (including the brain) and the bladder itself are tested. In addition to complete medical history and physical examination, diagnostic procedures may include the following:

- x-rays of the skull and spine
- an electroencephalogram (EEG) to identify brain dysfunction
- imaging tests of the bladder and ureters
- function tests that involve filling the bladder to see how much it can hold and if it empties completely

How is neurogenic bladder treated?

Medication for treatment of overactive bladder may improve or relieve irritating symptoms and/or incontinence. Antibiotics are important for treatment and prevention of urinary tract infections (UTIs), especially in patients with vesicoureteral reflux. Other medications may improve bladder control by increasing outlet resistance at the bladder neck.

Clean intermittent bladder catheterization (CIC) was developed by Dr. Jack Lapides in the early 1970s as a means of emptying the bladder in the case of a bladder muscle that is unable to contract or in patients with loss of appropriate coordination between the bladder muscle and the external urethral sphincter muscle.

Surgical cutting of the external urethral sphincter with the use of an endoscope passed through the urethra may allow free flow of urine into an appropriate receptacle and eliminate the need for CIC in order to empty the bladder. Also, endoscopic injection of paralytic agents directly into the external urethral sphincter muscle is another technique that provides temporary relief.

Permanent stents can also be used in the bladder neck for effective urinary transportation.

At times, however, damage to bladder anatomy and function is so severe that capacity needs to be improved with bladder augmentation (increasing bladder size with various tissues), vesicoureteral reflux needs to be corrected and/or an alternate tube for emptying the bladder may need to be surgically constructed.

What can be expected after treatment for neurogenic bladder?

A person can expect extensive follow-up evaluation of bladder and kidney function. This may involve repeated x-rays, ultrasound, blood tests, and bladder function tests.

Although some characteristics of the neurogenic bladder may improve or resolve, most issues typically require constant attention and reevaluation.

Proactive management of patients with a neurogenic bladder may decrease the risk of damage to the bladder and kidney(s) and, therefore, potentially limit the need for future intervention. This has been shown in management of neurogenic bladder patients with spina bifida.

Frequently Asked Questions

What is the likelihood that my child with spina bifida will develop neurogenic bladder?

The risk of neurogenic bladder is significant in this population and, therefore, careful and frequent evaluation of bladder function is recommended.

What are expected limitations for a patient with neurogenic bladder?

Limits are typically a function of the cause of neurogenic bladder (such as spinal cord injury, for example), rather than the neurogenic bladder itself.

Can the effects of a neurogenic bladder be prevented?

Some effects of neurogenic bladder are preventable with aggressive management with medication and at times appropriate surgical reconstruction.

Section 14.2

Cystocele (Fallen Bladder)

National Kidney and Urologic Diseases Information Clearinghouse (NKUDIC), a service of the National Institute of Diabetes and Digestive and Kidney Diseases (NIDDK), National Institutes of Health (NIH), Pub. No. 05-4557, November 2004.

A cystocele (SIS-tuh-seal) occurs when the wall between a woman's bladder and her vagina weakens and allows the bladder to droop into the vagina. This condition may cause discomfort and problems with emptying the bladder.

A bladder that has dropped from its normal position may cause two kinds of problems—unwanted urine leakage and incomplete emptying of the bladder. In some women, a fallen bladder stretches the opening into the urethra, causing urine leakage when the woman coughs, sneezes, laughs, or moves in any way that puts pressure on the bladder.

A cystocele is mild (grade 1) when the bladder droops only a short way into the vagina. With more severe (grade 2) cystocele, the bladder sinks far enough to reach the opening of the vagina. The most advanced (grade 3) cystocele occurs when the bladder bulges out through the opening of the vagina.

A cystocele may result from muscle straining while giving birth. Other kinds of straining—such as heavy lifting or repeated straining during bowel movements—may also cause the bladder to fall. The hormone estrogen helps keep the muscles around the vagina strong. When women go through menopause (when they stop having periods), their bodies stop making estrogen, so the muscles around the vagina and bladder may grow weak.

A doctor may be able to diagnose a grade 2 or grade 3 cystocele from a description of symptoms and from physical examination of the vagina because the fallen part of the bladder will be visible. A voiding cystourethrogram (sis-toe-yoo-REETH-roe-gram) is a test that involves taking x-rays of the bladder during urination. This x-ray shows the shape of the bladder and lets the doctor see any problems that might block the normal flow of urine. Other tests may be needed to find or rule out problems in other parts of the urinary system.

Treatment options range from no treatment for a mild cystocele to surgery for a serious cystocele. If a cystocele is not bothersome, the doctor may only recommend avoiding heavy lifting or straining that could cause the cystocele to worsen. If symptoms are moderately bothersome, the doctor may recommend a pessary—a device placed in the vagina to hold the bladder in place. Pessaries come in a variety of shapes and sizes to allow the doctor to find the most comfortable fit for the patient. Pessaries must be removed regularly to avoid infection or ulcers. [For more information on pessaries, see Chapter 20, "Treatments for Urinary Incontinence in Women."]

Large cystoceles may require surgery to move the bladder back into a more normal position and keep it there. This operation may be performed by a gynecologist, a urologist, or a urogynecologist. The patient should be prepared to stay in the hospital for several days and take four to six weeks to recover fully.

Section 14.3

Bladder Diverticulum

Many people may have small, bulging pouches in their bladder and never know it. These pouches are usually harmless, but read on to learn more about what problems they can cause.

What is bladder diverticulum?

They are pouches in the bladder wall that a person is born with (congenital) or later acquires. A congenital bladder diverticulum represents an area of weakness in the bladder wall through which some of the lining of the bladder is forced out. (A small balloon squeezed in a fist will create a diverticular-like effect between the fingers.) Bladder diverticula may be multiple and they often occur at the entrance of the upper urinary system into the bladder (ureterovesical junction).

Acquired diverticula are usually related to bladder obstruction, most commonly as a result of benign prostatic hyperplasia (BPH).

What are the symptoms of bladder diverticulum?

Under normal conditions a diverticulum is of no significance. But sometimes it causes special problems if a bladder tumor happens to be in one, or if one is next to a ureter that allows urine to go from the bladder back up to the kidney (vesicoureteral reflux). Under most situations however, diverticula are without symptoms and not clinically significant. A diverticulum usually becomes significant if it becomes very large and causes incomplete bladder emptying and stagnation of urine. If the urine within the diverticulum becomes infected, that infection may not be able to clear because of the stagnation. Under such circumstances, treatment may be indicated. If a diverticulum is related to bladder outlet obstruction, the obstruction must also be treated.

How is bladder diverticulum diagnosed?

Diverticulum is not visible and will be detected only if it causes trouble. Usually it is found during an examination for the cause of recurring urinary tract infections. X-rays or a cystoscopy are used to identify it.

How is bladder diverticulum treated?

Surgical removal is the treatment of a symptomatic bladder diverticulum. This may be done from entirely within the bladder in certain situations, but often requires dissection both inside and outside of the bladder. This surgery may be somewhat difficult because of the inflammation of a chronically infected diverticulum.

What can be expected after treatment for bladder diverticulum?

Treatment will usually have good results. Postoperatively, catheter drainage of the bladder is indicated for one to two weeks. Bladder diverticula are either congenital (you are born with them) or acquired. Acquired diverticula are usually related to bladder obstruction, most commonly as a result of benign prostatic hypertrophy. Those that become symptomatic usually are large singular diverticula.

Under normal conditions a diverticulum is of no significance. They sometimes present special problems if a bladder tumor happens to be in one, or if one is next to a ureter that allows vesicoureteral reflux (urine can go from the bladder back up to the kidney). Under most situations however, they are asymptomatic and not clinically significant. A diverticulum usually becomes significant if it becomes very large and therefore is a cause of incomplete bladder emptying and stagnation of urine. If the urine within the diverticulum becomes infected, that infection may not be able to clear because of the stagnation. Under such circumstances, treatment may be indicated. If a diverticulum is related to bladder outlet obstruction, the obstruction must also be treated.

Treatment of a symptomatic bladder diverticulum is surgical excision. This may be done from entirely within the bladder in certain situations, but often requires dissection both inside and outside of the bladder. This surgery may be somewhat difficult because of the inflammation of a chronically infected diverticulum. Nevertheless treatment will usually have good results. Postoperatively catheter drainage of the bladder is indicated for one to two weeks.

Section 14.4

Bladder Fistula

What happens when the bladder has abnormal connections with other organs? The information below should help you recognize this problem before it causes serious damage.

What is bladder fistula?

Bladder fistula refers to an abnormal connection between the bladder and another organ or the skin. Most commonly this involves the bowel (enterovesical fistula) or the vagina (vesicovaginal fistula). Although relatively rare, fistulization to the skin can result from an injury or previous surgery in the face of bladder outlet obstruction.

Vesicovaginal fistulas are seen after a urologic or gynecological surgery or in relation to gynecological cancers. Fistulas to the bowel are most commonly seen as a result of inflammatory bowel disease such as Crohn disease or diverticulitis. About 20 percent of bowel fistulas are caused by bowel cancer. Fistulas are rarely caused by bladder pathology. Fistulas to both the vagina and the bowel may also develop as a result of previous radiation therapy.

What are the symptoms of bladder fistula?

Symptoms are frequent urinary tract infections or the passage of gas from the urethra during urination.

How is bladder fistula diagnosed?

Bladder fistula is diagnosed by the use of an excretory urogram, which is an x-ray examination of the bladder. An excretory urogram study uses a contrast dye to enhance the x-ray images. The dye is injected into the patient's system, and its progress through the urinary tract is then recorded on a series of quickly captured images. The examination enables the radiologist to review the anatomy and the function of the bladder and urinary tract.

How is bladder fistula treated?

Treatment of bladder fistula usually requires partial surgical removal. If it is caused by a disease such as colon cancer or inflammatory disease, surgical removal is usually done in conjunction with removal of the primary disease.

What can be expected after treatment for bladder fistula?

The success of surgery is directly related to the ability to remove the primary disease and the presence of healthy tissue with which the fistula is closed. Ideally, healthy tissue with good blood supply is brought between the bladder and the other organ. The presence of unremovable cancer or tissue exposed to radiation and having a bad blood supply make a good result more difficult to obtain. The patient can expect to have a catheter in their bladder for a few weeks postoperatively.

Section 14.5

Bladder Trauma

Fortunately traumatic injury to the bladder is uncommon. The bladder is located within the bony structures of the pelvis and is protected from most external forces. But injuries can occur as a result of blunt or penetrating trauma. The following information should help explain why timely evaluation and proper management are critical for the best outcomes.

What happens under normal conditions?

The bladder is a hollow, balloon-shaped organ that is located within the pelvis. The bladder stores urine—the liquid waste made by the kidneys when they clean the blood. Muscular tissue within the bladder wall allows it to enlarge or shrink as urine is held or emptied.

How does bladder trauma happen?

When the bladder is empty, it is protected from injury from a blow to the lower abdomen by the bones of the pelvis. As it fills, the top of the bladder rises into the abdomen and makes it more vulnerable to be ruptured. In the child, the pelvic bones are not fully developed and so it is more easily injured than in the adult. If the force of the impact is great enough to fracture the bones of the pelvis, the bladder may be injured even if it is empty. Bullets or knives can also injure the bladder despite its level of fullness.

What are causes of injury to the bladder?

The most common way the bladder is injured is in motor vehicle accidents, falls from a high place or having a heavy object fall on the lower abdomen of a person. Automobile passengers that have a full bladder and are wearing a seat belt around the lower abdomen may

167

have the force of the collision focus on the lower abdomen and thus the full bladder. To prevent this, wear your seat belt properly as a lap belt and always empty your bladder when planning a long car ride.

What are the symptoms of bladder trauma?

Virtually everyone who has a blunt injury to the bladder will see blood in the urine. Those with penetrating injury many not actually see bleeding. There may be pain below the belly button but many times the pain from other injuries makes the discomfort from the bladder hardly noticeable. If there is a large hole in the bladder and all of the urine leaks into the abdomen, it is impossible to pass urine. In women, if the injury is severe enough, the vagina may be torn open as well as the bladder. If this happens, urine may leak from the bladder through the vagina. Blood may also come out of the vagina in this instance. Other symptoms may include: difficulty beginning to urinate, weak urinary stream, painful urination, fever, and severe back pain.

How is bladder trauma diagnosed?

The diagnosis of injury to the bladder is done by placing a catheter into the bladder and performing a series of x-rays. If the doctor is worried that the urethra is injured an x-ray of this organ may be done before a catheter is inserted. Before the x-rays are taken, the bladder is filled with a liquid that will make it visible on the x-rays.

What are the different types of bladder injuries and how are they treated?

Contusion: Most of the time the bladder wall does not rupture but is only bruised. If this happens, merely leaving a large diameter catheter in the bladder so clots may pass is all that is necessary. Once the urine has become clear and the doctor does not need the catheter in the bladder for other reasons (accurate measurement of urine made during the day or in patients too sick to urinate on their own), it can be removed.

Intraperitoneal rupture: If the tear is on the top of the bladder, the hole will usually communicate with the abdominal cavity that holds all of the vital organs (liver, spleen, and bowel). This injury should be surgically repaired. Urine that leaks into the abdomen is a serious problem. The repair is performed by making an abdominal incision and sewing the tear closed. A catheter is left in the bladder for a few days to rest the bladder after the surgery, either through the urethra or coming directly out the abdominal wall, below the belly button.

Extraperitoneal rupture: If the tear is at the bottom or sides of the bladder, the urine will not leak into the abdominal cavity but into the tissues around the bladder. Many urologists think these patients should all have surgical repair of the injury, but in some circumstances these injuries can be treated by simply placing a large diameter catheter into the bladder to keep it empty and allow the urine and blood to drain out into a collection bag. If the catheter does not drain properly, surgical repair is required. Allowing the bladder to repair itself in this fashion usually takes at least ten days and the catheter is not removed until an x-ray is done as described above to prove the leak has sealed.

Penetrating injuries: Patients who have injury to the bladder from a penetrating object are usually operated upon and the hole(s) is surgically repaired. Most of the time other organs in the area will be injured and need repair as well. A catheter is left in the bladder to drain the urine and blood as described above.

What can be expected after treatment for injuries to the bladder?

After the catheter is removed, urination should return to normal in a few weeks. Antibiotics are commonly given to the patient for a few days to eliminate any infection in the bladder from the injury or the catheter. In some patients, the bladder remains overactive for many weeks or months due to the irritation of the injury. Medication to calm this bladder overactivity may be given to help the symptoms of having to pass urine frequently or the feeling that when you get the first sensation to pass urine, you think you have to get to the bathroom immediately or you might wet yourself (urgency).

Part Three

Urinary Incontinence

Chapter 15

What Is Urinary Incontinence?

What is urinary incontinence and what causes it?

When you are not able to hold your urine until you can get to a bathroom, you have what's called urinary incontinence (also called loss of bladder control). In contrast, bladder control means you urinate only when you want to. Incontinence can often be temporary, and it is always caused by an underlying medical condition. Incontinence can often be temporary, and it is always caused by an underlying medical condition.

More than 13 million Americans experience loss of bladder control. However, women suffer from incontinence twice as often as men do. Both women and men can have trouble with bladder control from neurological (nerve) injury, birth defects, strokes, multiple sclerosis (MS), and physical problems associated with aging.

Older women have more bladder control problems than younger women do. The loss of bladder control, however, is not something that has to happen as you grow older. It can be treated and often cured, whatever your age. Don't let any embarrassment about incontinence prevent you from talking to your healthcare provider about your condition. Find out if you have a medical condition that needs treatment.

"Frequently Asked Questions about Urinary Incontinence," The National Women's Health Information Center, a project of U.S. Department of Health and Human Services, Office on Women's Health, October 2002.

What does the bladder system look like and how does it work?

Bladder control means more than just telling yourself to wait to urinate until you get to the bathroom. It is not that simple. It takes teamwork from many organs, muscles, and nerves in your body.

Most of the bladder control system is inside your pelvis, the area of your abdomen between your hips and below the belly button. Your bladder is a muscle shaped like a balloon. When the bladder stores urine, the bladder muscle relaxes. When you urinate, the bladder muscle tightens to squeeze urine out of the bladder.

More muscles help with bladder control. Two sphincter muscles surround the tube that carries urine from your bladder down to an opening in the front of the vagina. The tube is called the urethra. Urine leaves your body through this tube. The sphincter muscles keep the urethra closed by squeezing like rubber bands.

Pelvic floor muscles support the uterus, or womb, and rectum and bladder. They also help keep the urethra closed.

When the bladder is full, nerves in your bladder signal the brain. That's when you get the urge to urinate. Once you reach the toilet, your brain sends a message down to the sphincter muscles and the pelvic floor muscles. The brain tells them to relax. The brain also tells the bladder muscles to tighten up to squeeze urine out of the bladder.

Loss of bladder control in women most often happens because of problems with the muscles that help to hold or release urine: the bladder muscle, the sphincter muscles, and the pelvic floor muscles. Incontinence occurs if your bladder muscles suddenly contract (or squeeze) or if the muscles around the urethra suddenly relax.

Are there different types of urinary incontinence?

Yes, there are different types of incontinence. They include:

- **Stress incontinence:** Leaking small amounts of urine during physical movement (coughing, sneezing, or exercising). Stress incontinence is the most common form of incontinence in women. It is treatable.

- **Urge incontinence:** Leaking large amounts of urine at unexpected times, including during sleep, after drinking a small amount of water, or when you touch water or hear it running (as when washing dishes).

- **Functional incontinence:** Not being able to reach a toilet in time because of physical disability, obstacles, or problems in thinking or communicating that prevent a person from reaching a toilet. For example, a person with Alzheimer disease may not think well enough to plan a trip to the bathroom in time to urinate or a person in a wheelchair may be blocked from getting to a toilet in time.

- **Overflow incontinence:** Leaking small amounts of urine because the bladder is always full. With this condition, the bladder never empties completely. Overflow incontinence is rare in women.

- **Mixed incontinence:** A combination of incontinence, most often when stress and urge incontinence occur together.

- **Transient incontinence:** Leaking urine on a temporary basis due to a medical condition or infection that will go away once the condition or infection is treated. It can be triggered by medications, urinary tract infections, mental impairment, restricted mobility, and stool impaction (severe constipation).

Do pregnancy, childbirth, and menopause affect urinary incontinence?

Yes. During pregnancy, the added weight and pressure of the unborn baby can weaken pelvic floor muscles, which affects your ability to control your bladder. Sometimes the position of your bladder and urethra can change because of the position of the baby, which can cause problems. Vaginal delivery and an episiotomy (the cut in the muscle that makes it easier for the baby to come out) can weaken bladder control muscles. Pregnancy and childbirth can cause damage to bladder control nerves.

After delivery, the problem of urinary incontinence often goes away by itself. But if you are still having problems six weeks after delivery, talk to your healthcare provider. Bladder control problems don't always show up right after childbirth. Some women do not have problems with incontinence until they reach their 40s.

Menopause (when your periods stop completely) can cause bladder control problems for some women. During menopause, the amount of the female hormone estrogen in your body starts decreasing. The lack of estrogen causes the bladder control muscles to weaken. Estrogen controls how your body matures, your monthly periods, and body changes during pregnancy and breastfeeding. Estrogen also helps keep the lining of the bladder and urethra plump and healthy.

Talk with your healthcare provider about whether taking estrogen to prevent further bladder control problems is best for you. Tell him or her if you or your family has a history of cancer. If you face a high risk of breast cancer or uterine cancer, your healthcare provider may not prescribe estrogen for you.

How is urinary incontinence diagnosed?

If you are having a problem with incontinence, the first step is to see your healthcare provider. She or he can refer you to a urologist, a doctor who specializes in treating the urinary tract. Some urologists further specialize in the female urinary tract. Gynecologists and obstetricians specialize in the female reproductive tract and childbirth. A urogynecologist focuses on urological problems in women. Family practitioners and internists treat patients for all kinds of complaints. Any of these doctors may be able to help you.

To diagnose the problem, your healthcare provider will first ask you about your symptoms and for a complete medical history. Your provider should ask you about your overall health, any problems you are having, medications you are taking, surgeries you have had, pregnancy history, and past illnesses. You will also be asked about your bladder habits: how often you empty your bladder, how and when you leak urine, or when you have accidents.

Your provider will then do a physical exam to look for signs of any medical conditions that can cause incontinence, such as tumors that block the urinary tract, impacted stool, and poor reflexes that may be nerve-related.

A test may be done to figure out how much your bladder can hold and how well your bladder muscles function. For this test, you will be asked to drink plenty of fluids and urinate into a measuring pan, after which your provider will measure any urine that remains in the bladder. Your provider may also recommend other tests, including the following:

- **Stress test:** You relax, then cough hard as the provider watches for loss of urine.

- **Urinalysis:** You give a urine sample that is then tested for signs of infection or other causes of incontinence.

- **Blood tests:** You give a blood sample, which is sent to a laboratory to test for substances related to the causes of incontinence.

- **Ultrasound:** Sound waves are used to take a picture of the kidneys, bladder, and urethra, so any problems in these areas that could cause incontinence can be seen.

- **Cystoscopy:** A thin tube with a tiny camera is placed inside the urethra to view the inside of the urethra and bladder.

- **Urodynamics:** Pressure in the bladder and the flow of urine are measured using special techniques.

You may be asked to keep a diary for a day or a week in order to record when you empty your bladder. This diary should include the times you urinate and the amounts of urine you produce. To measure your urine, you can use a special pan that fits over the toilet rim. These pans are available at drug stores or surgical supply stores.

How is urinary incontinence treated?

There are a number of ways to treat incontinence. Your healthcare provider will work with you to figure out which way(s) is best for you. Don't give up or be embarrassed! Remember, many women have incontinence and all types of incontinence can be treated, no matter what your age. Treatments include the following:

- **Pelvic muscle exercises:** Simple exercises to strengthen the muscles near the urethra, also called Kegel exercises. Taking a few minutes each day to do these exercises can help to reduce or cure stress leakage. A healthcare provider can teach you these exercises, most of which require no special equipment. One exercise, however, does use cones of different weights. You stand and hold a cone-shaped object inside your vagina. You then substitute cones of increasing weight to strength the muscles that keep the urethra closed.

- **Electrical stimulation:** Brief doses of electrical stimulation can strengthen muscles in the lower pelvis in a way similar to exercising the muscles. Special devices called electrodes are temporarily placed inside the vagina or rectum to stimulate nearby muscles. This treatment can be used to reduce both stress incontinence and urge incontinence.

- **Biofeedback:** Biofeedback uses measuring devices to help you become aware of your body's functioning. A therapist trained in biofeedback places an electrical patch over your bladder and urethral muscles. A wire connected to the patch is linked to a TV screen. You and your therapist watch the screen to track when these muscles contract, so you can learn to gain control over these muscles. Biofeedback can be used with pelvic muscle exercises and electrical stimulation to relieve stress incontinence and urge incontinence.

- **Timed voiding or bladder training:** Two techniques that help you to train your bladder to hold urine better. In timed voiding (urinating), you fill in a chart of when you urinate and when you leak urine. From the patterns that appear in your chart, you can plan to empty your bladder before you would otherwise leak. Bladder training—biofeedback and muscle conditioning—can change your bladder's schedule for storing and emptying urine. These techniques are effective for urge incontinence and overflow incontinence.

- **Weight loss:** Extra weight can cause bladder control problems. If you are overweight, talk with your healthcare provider about a diet and exercise program to help you lose weight.

- **Dietary changes:** Certain foods and drinks can cause incontinence, such as caffeine (in coffee, soda, chocolate), tea, and alcohol. You can often reduce incontinence by restricting these liquids in your diet.

- **Medicines:** Medications can reduce many types of leakage. They can also help tighten or strengthen pelvic floor muscles and muscles around the urethra. Some drugs can also calm overactive bladder muscles. Some drugs, especially hormones such as estrogen, are believed to cause muscles involved in urination to function normally.

  Be aware that some drugs can produce harmful side effects if used for long periods of time. In particular, estrogen therapy can increase a person's risk for cancers of the breast and endometrium (lining of the uterus). Talk to your provider about the risks and benefits of medications.

- **Implants:** Substances are injected (through a needle) into tissues around the urethra. The implant adds bulk and helps the urethra to stay closed. This treatment reduces stress incontinence. Collagen (a natural fibrous tissue from cows) and fat from a person's body have been used. This procedure takes about 30 minutes and can be done in a provider's office using local anesthesia.

The success rate of implants varies. Injections must be repeated after a time because the body slowly gets rids of the substances. Before getting a collagen injection, you need to have a skin test to make sure you are not allergic to this substance.

- **Surgery:** This treatment is primarily used only after other treatments have been tried. Different types of surgery can be done, depending on what kind of incontinence problem you have. Some surgeries raise, or lift, the bladder up to a more normal position. Other surgeries use implants to help the bladder function better.

- **Catheterization:** A catheter is a small tube that you can learn to insert yourself through the urethra into the bladder to drain urine. Catheters can be used once in while or all the time. If used all the time, the tube connects to a bag that you can attach to your leg. If you use a long-term (or indwelling) catheter, you need to watch for signs of urinary tract infection.

- **Pessary:** A pessary is a stiff ring that is inserted by a health-care provider into the vagina, where it presses against the wall of the vagina and the nearby urethra. The pressure helps to hold up the bladder and reduce stress leakage. If you use a pessary, watch for signs of vaginal and urinary tract infections. Visit your provider right away if you think you have an infection. Have your provider check the pessary on a regular basis.

- **Urethral inserts:** A urethral insert is a small device that you place inside the urethra, a technique that you can learn to do yourself. You remove the device when you go to the bathroom and then put it back into your urethra until you need to urinate again.

- **Urine seals:** Urine seals are small foam pads that you place over the urethra opening. The pad seals itself against your body, keeping you from leaking. You remove and throw it away after urinating. You then place a new seal over the urethra.

- **Dryness aids:** Absorbent pads or diapers help many women, but they do not cure bladder control problems. They can also cause low self-esteem (how you feel about yourself) and irritate the skin. Some women use urinals (pans) beside their beds when they sleep if they suffer from urge incontinence.

Chapter 16

Some Medications Can Cause Incontinence

Do you have a bladder control problem?

If so, one cause of your problem may be sitting in your medicine cabinet. Medicines (drugs) can cause people to lose bladder control.

Do not stop taking any medicine without talking to your doctor. If your medicine is causing your bladder problem, your doctor may find another medicine. If you need to keep taking the same medicine, your doctor can help you find another way to regain bladder control.

How does bladder control work?

Your bladder is a muscle shaped like a balloon. While the bladder stores urine, the muscle relaxes. When you go to the bathroom, the bladder muscle tightens to squeeze urine out of the bladder.

Two sphincter (SFINK-tur) muscles surround a tube called the urethra (yoo-REE-thrah). Urine leaves your body through this tube.

The sphincters keep the urethra closed by squeezing like rubber bands. Pelvic floor muscles under the bladder also help keep the urethra closed.

When the bladder is full, nerves in your bladder signal the brain. That's when you get the urge to go to the bathroom.

"Your Medicines and Bladder Control," National Kidney and Urologic Diseases Information Clearinghouse (NKUDIC), a service of the National Institute of Diabetes and Digestive and Kidney Diseases (NIDDK), National Institutes of Health (NIH), Pub. No. 02-4185, April 2002.

Once you reach the toilet, your brain tells the sphincter and pelvic floor muscles to relax. This allows urine to pass through the urethra. The brain signal also tells the bladder to tighten up. This squeezes urine out of the bladder.

Bladder control means you urinate only when you want to. For good bladder control, all parts of your system must work together. Pelvic muscles must hold up the bladder and urethra. Sphincter muscles must open and shut the urethra. Nerves must control the muscles of the bladder and pelvic floor.

How can medicines cause leaking?

Leaking can happen when medicines affect any of these muscles or nerves. For instance, medicines to treat high blood pressure may make the sphincter muscles too tight or too loose. Medicines to treat colds can have the same effect.

You may take medicine to calm your nerves so that you can sleep or relax. This medicine may dull the nerves in the bladder and keep them from signaling the brain when the bladder is full. Without the message and urge, the bladder overflows. Drinking alcohol can also cause these nerves to fail.

Water pills (diuretics) take fluid from swollen areas of your body and send it to the bladder. This may cause the bladder to leak because it fills more quickly than usual. Caffeine drinks such as coffee and cola have the same effect. Some foods such as chocolate also can cause bladder problems.

What can you do about your bladder control problem?

Before your next doctor visit, make a list of all the prescription medicines you take. Also list medicines you buy without a prescription. Or you can bring all your medicines with you to show the doctor. Ask your doctor if any of the medicines could cause your bladder problem. Your pharmacist can also give you information about your medicines.

You may have to continue taking a medicine that causes a bladder control problem. Ask your doctor to help you find another way to control your bladder. Other ways might include exercises for the muscles that close the bladder, devices to stimulate the muscles, or training the bladder to hold more urine.

Chapter 17

Urinary Incontinence in Children

Parents or guardians of children who experience bed-wetting at night or "accidents" during the day should treat this problem with understanding and patience. This loss of urinary control is called "urinary incontinence" or just "incontinence." Although it affects many young people, it usually disappears naturally over time, which suggests that incontinence, for some people, may be a normal part of growing up. Incontinence at the normal age of toilet training may cause great distress. Daytime or nighttime incontinence can be embarrassing. It is important to understand that many children experience occasional incontinence and that treatment is available for most children who have difficulty controlling their bladders.

How does the urinary system work?

Urination, or voiding, is a complex activity. The bladder is a balloon-like organ that lies in the lowest part of the abdomen. The bladder stores urine, then releases it through the urethra, the canal that carries urine to the outside of the body. Controlling this activity involves nerves, muscles, the spinal cord, and the brain.

The bladder is composed of two types of muscles: the detrusor, a muscular sac that stores urine and squeezes to empty, and the sphincter,

National Kidney and Urologic Diseases Information Clearinghouse (NKUDIC), a service of the National Institute of Diabetes and Digestive and Kidney Diseases (NIDDK), National Institutes of Health (NIH), Pub. No. 04-4095, April 2004.

a circular group of muscles at the bottom or neck of the bladder that automatically stay contracted to hold the urine in and automatically relax when the detrusor contracts to let the urine into the urethra. A third group of muscles below the bladder (pelvic floor muscles) can contract to keep urine back.

A baby's bladder fills to a set point, then automatically contracts and empties. As the child gets older, the nervous system matures. The child's brain begins to get messages from the filling bladder and begins to send messages to the bladder to keep it from automatically emptying until the child decides it is the time and place to void.

Failures in this control mechanism result in incontinence. Reasons for this failure range from the simple to the complex.

Incontinence happens less often after age five. About ten percent of five-year-olds, five percent of ten-year-olds, and one percent of eighteen-year-olds experience episodes of incontinence. It is twice as common in boys as in girls.

What causes nighttime incontinence?

After age five, wetting at night—often called bed-wetting or sleep-wetting—is more common than daytime wetting in boys. Experts do not know what causes nighttime incontinence. Young people who experience nighttime wetting are usually physically and emotionally normal. Most cases probably result from a mix of factors including slower physical development, an overproduction of urine at night, a lack of ability to recognize bladder filling when asleep, and, infrequently, anxiety. For many, there is a strong family history of bed-wetting, suggesting an inherited factor.

Slower physical development: Between the ages of five and ten, nocturnal incontinence may be the result of a small bladder capacity, long sleeping periods, and underdevelopment of the body's alarms that signal a full or emptying bladder. This form of incontinence will fade away as the bladder grows and the natural alarms become operational.

Excessive output of urine during sleep: Normally, the body produces a hormone that can slow the making of urine. This hormone is called antidiuretic hormone, or ADH. The body normally produces more ADH at night so that the need to urinate is lower. If the body doesn't produce enough ADH at night, the making of urine may not be slowed down, leading to bladder overfilling. If a child does not sense the bladder filling and awaken to urinate, then wetting will occur.

Anxiety: Experts suggest that anxiety-causing events occurring in the lives of children ages two to four might lead to incontinence before the child achieves total bladder control. Anxiety experienced after age four might lead to wetting after the child has been dry for a period of six months or more. Such events include angry parents, unfamiliar social situations, and overwhelming family events such as the birth of a brother or sister.

Incontinence itself is an anxiety-causing event. Strong bladder contractions leading to leakage in the daytime can cause embarrassment and anxiety that lead to wetting at night.

Genetics: Certain inherited genes appear to contribute to incontinence. In 1995, Danish researchers announced they had found a site on human chromosome 13 that is responsible, at least in part, for nighttime wetting. If both parents were bed wetters, a child has an 80 percent chance of being a bed wetter also. Experts believe that other, undetermined genes also may be involved in incontinence.

Obstructive sleep apnea: Nighttime incontinence may be one sign of another condition called obstructive sleep apnea, in which the child's breathing is interrupted during sleep, often because of inflamed or enlarged tonsils or adenoids. Other symptoms of this condition include snoring, mouth breathing, frequent ear and sinus infections, sore throat, choking, and daytime drowsiness. In some cases, successful treatment of this breathing disorder may also resolve the associated nighttime incontinence.

Structural problems: Finally, a small number of cases of incontinence are caused by physical problems in the urinary system in children. Rarely, a blocked bladder or urethra may cause the bladder to overfill and leak. Nerve damage associated with the birth defect spina bifida can cause incontinence. In these cases, the incontinence can appear as a constant dribbling of urine.

What causes daytime incontinence?

Daytime incontinence that is not associated with urinary infection or anatomic abnormalities is less common than nighttime incontinence and tends to disappear much earlier than the nighttime versions. One possible cause of daytime incontinence is an overactive bladder. Many children with daytime incontinence have abnormal elimination habits, the most common being infrequent voiding and constipation.

185

An overactive bladder: Muscles surrounding the urethra (the tube that takes urine away from the bladder) have the job of keeping the passage closed, preventing urine from passing out of the body. If the bladder contracts strongly and without warning, the muscles surrounding the urethra may not be able to keep urine from passing. This often happens as a consequence of urinary tract infection and is more common in girls.

Infrequent voiding: Infrequent voiding refers to a child's voluntarily holding urine for prolonged intervals. For example, a child may not want to use the toilets at school or may not want to interrupt enjoyable activities, so he or she ignores the body's signal of a full bladder. In these cases, the bladder can overfill and leak urine. Additionally, these children often develop urinary tract infections (UTIs), leading to an irritable or overactive bladder.

Other causes: Some of the same factors that contribute to nighttime incontinence may act together with infrequent voiding to produce daytime incontinence. These factors include the following:

- small bladder capacity
- structural problems
- anxiety-causing events
- pressure from a hard bowel movement (constipation)
- drinks or foods that contain caffeine, which increases urine output and may also cause spasms of the bladder muscle, or other ingredients to which the child may have an allergic reaction, such as chocolate or artificial coloring

Sometimes overly strenuous toilet training may make the child unable to relax the sphincter and the pelvic floor to completely empty the bladder. Retaining urine (incomplete emptying) sets the stage for urinary tract infections.

What treats or cures incontinence?

Growth and development: Most urinary incontinence fades away naturally. Here are examples of what can happen over time:

- Bladder capacity increases.
- Natural body alarms become activated.
- An overactive bladder settles down.

- Production of ADH becomes normal.
- The child learns to respond to the body's signal that it is time to void.
- Stressful events or periods pass.

Many children overcome incontinence naturally (without treatment) as they grow older. The number of cases of incontinence goes down by 15 percent for each year after the age of five.

Medications: Nighttime incontinence may be treated by increasing ADH levels. The hormone can be boosted by a synthetic version known as desmopressin, or DDAVP, which recently became available in pill form. Patients can also spray a mist containing desmopressin into their nostrils. Desmopressin is approved for use by children.

Another medication, called imipramine, is also used to treat sleepwetting. It acts on both the brain and the urinary bladder. Researchers estimate that these medications may help as many as 70 percent of patients achieve short-term success. Many patients, however, relapse once the medication is withdrawn.

If a young person experiences incontinence resulting from an overactive bladder, a doctor might prescribe a medicine that helps to calm the bladder muscle. This medicine controls muscle spasms and belongs to a class of medications called anticholinergics.

Bladder training and related strategies: Bladder training consists of exercises for strengthening and coordinating muscles of the bladder and urethra, and may help the control of urination. These techniques teach the child to anticipate the need to urinate and prevent urination when away from a toilet.

Techniques that may help nighttime incontinence include determining bladder capacity, drinking less fluid before sleeping, and developing routines for waking up. Unfortunately, none of these techniques guarantees success.

Techniques that may help daytime incontinence include urinating on a schedule, such as every two hours (timed voiding), avoiding caffeine or other foods or drinks that you suspect may contribute to your child's incontinence, and following suggestions for healthy urination, such as relaxing muscles and taking your time.

Moisture alarms: At night, moisture alarms can awaken a person when he or she begins to urinate. These devices include a water-sensitive pad worn in pajamas, a wire connecting to a battery-driven control, and an alarm that sounds when moisture is first detected. For the alarm to be effective, the child must awaken as soon as the alarm goes off, go to the bathroom, and change the bedding. This may require having another person sleep in the same room to awaken the bed wetter.

Is incontinence also called enuresis?

Yes. Incontinence is also called enuresis.

- **Primary enuresis** is wetting in a person who has never been dry for at least six months.

- **Secondary enuresis** is wetting that begins after at least six months of dryness.

- **Nocturnal enuresis** is wetting that usually occurs during sleep (nighttime incontinence).

- **Diurnal enuresis** is wetting when awake (daytime incontinence).

Chapter 18

Urinary Incontinence in Men

Urinary incontinence (UI) is the accidental leakage of urine. Over a lifespan, there are gender differences in the frequency of UI. In childhood, girls usually develop bladder control at an earlier age than boys, and bedwetting (nocturnal enuresis) is less common in girls than in boys. However, adult women are far more likely to experience UI because of the anatomy of their urinary tract and the stresses caused by pregnancy and childbirth. Nevertheless, men may experience UI as a result of prostate problems, and both men and women can experience nerve damage that leads to UI. Its prevalence increases with age, but it is not an inevitable part of aging.

UI is a medical problem. To find a treatment that addresses the root of the problem, you need to talk to your healthcare provider. The four forms of UI are as follows:

- **Temporary or reversible incontinence** related to urinary tract infection, constipation, or delirium

- **Stress incontinence** caused by weak pelvic and sphincter muscles

- **Urge incontinence** caused by damaged or irritable nerves

- **Overflow incontinence** that results when an individual is unable to empty the bladder

National Kidney and Urologic Diseases Information Clearinghouse (NKUDIC), a service of the National Institute of Diabetes and Digestive and Kidney Diseases (NIDDK), National Institutes of Health (NIH), Pub. No. 04-5280, March 2004.

Causes of UI in Men

For the urinary system to do its job, muscles and nerves must work together to hold urine in the bladder and then release it at the right time. Babies are not born with the ability to control urination. As children grow, they learn to interpret nerve signals and develop the muscle control required to stay dry. In children between the ages of five and ten, some incontinence may result from limited bladder capacity or delayed development of the nerve pathways that signal a full or emptying bladder. This form of incontinence fades away as the bladder grows and nerves become mature. Other types of nerve problems, however, can cause urination problems that are more difficult to overcome.

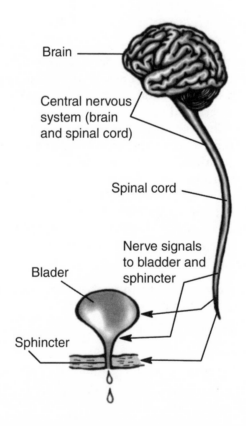

Brain

Central nervous system (brain and spinal cord)

Spinal cord

Nerve signals to bladder and sphincter

Blader

Sphincter

Figure 18.1. Nerves carry signals from the brain to the bladder and sphincter. Any disease, condition, or injury that damages nerves can lead to urination problems.

Nerve Problems

Any disease, condition, or injury that damages nerves can lead to urination problems. Nerve problems can occur at any age.

- Men who have had diabetes for many years may develop nerve damage that affects their bladder control as well as their sexual function.

- Stroke, Parkinson disease, and multiple sclerosis all affect the brain and nervous system, so they can also cause incontinence.

- Overactive bladder is a condition in which the bladder squeezes at the wrong time. The condition may be caused by nerve problems, or it may occur without any clear cause. A person with overactive bladder may have any two or all three of the following symptoms:

  - Urinary frequency (urination eight or more times a day or two or more times at night)

  - Urinary urgency (the sudden, strong need to urinate immediately)

  - Urge incontinence (urine leakage that follows a sudden, strong urge)

- Spinal cord injury can cause incontinence by interrupting the nerve signals required for bladder control.

- In neural birth defects such as spina bifida or myelomeningocele, the backbone and spinal canal do not close before birth. In severe cases, nerve damage can result in many problems, including lack of control over urination.

Prostate Problems

The prostate is a male gland about the size and shape of a walnut. It surrounds the urethra just below the bladder, where it adds fluid to semen before ejaculation.

BPH: The prostate gland commonly becomes enlarged as a man ages. This condition is called benign prostatic hyperplasia (BPH) or benign prostatic hypertrophy. As the prostate enlarges, it may squeeze the urethra. The bladder wall thickens and becomes irritable, and the bladder begins to contract even when it contains only small amounts of urine. This results in more frequent urination. BPH rarely causes symptoms before age 40, but more than half of men in their sixties and up to 90 percent in their seventies and eighties have some symptoms of BPH. The symptoms vary, but the most common ones involve changes or problems with urination, such as a hesitant, interrupted, weak stream; urgency and leaking or dribbling; more frequent urination, especially at night; and urge incontinence. Problems with urination do not necessarily signal blockage caused by an enlarged prostate. Other changes associated with aging can cause urination problems experienced by both men and women.

Radical prostatectomy: The surgical removal of the entire prostate gland—called radical prostatectomy—may be recommended to treat prostate cancer. The surgeon may approach the prostate through the abdomen or through the perineal area (between the scrotum and the anus). The surgery may lead to erection problems and UI, although nerve-sparing procedures in the abdominal approach may make these side effects less likely.

External beam radiation: This therapy uses an x-ray machine to deliver radiation to the prostate gland. The treatment is not painful, but can cause loss of bladder control as well as fatigue, skin redness and irritation, rectal burning or injury, diarrhea, inflammation of the bladder wall (cystitis), blood in the urine, loss of sexual function, and loss of appetite.

Prostate Symptom Scores

If your prostate could be involved in your incontinence, you may be asked a series of standardized questions, either the International Prostate Symptom Score or the American Urological Association (AUA) Symptom Scale. Some of the questions you will be asked for the AUA Symptom Scale are as follows:

- Over the past month or so, how often have you had to urinate again in less than two hours?

- Over the past month or so, from the time you went to bed at night until the time you got up in the morning, how many times did you typically get up to urinate?

- Over the past month or so, how often have you had a sensation of not emptying your bladder completely after you finished urinating?

- Over the past month or so, how often have you had a weak urinary stream?

- Over the past month or so, how often have you had to push or strain to begin urinating?

Your answers to these questions may help identify the problem or determine which tests are needed. Your symptom score evaluation can be used as a baseline to see how effective later treatments are at relieving those symptoms.

How UI Is Diagnosed

Medical history: The first step in solving a urinary problem is talking to your healthcare provider. Your general medical history, including any major illnesses or surgeries, and details about your continence problem and when it started will help your doctor determine the cause. You should talk about how much fluid you drink a day and whether you use alcohol or caffeine. You should also talk about the medicines you take, both prescription and nonprescription, because they might be part of the problem.

Voiding diary: You may be asked to keep a voiding diary, which is a record of fluid intake and trips to the bathroom, plus any episodes of leakage. Studying the diary will give your healthcare provider a better idea of your problem and help direct additional tests.

Physical examination: A physical exam will check for prostate enlargement or nerve damage. In a digital rectal exam, the doctor inserts a gloved finger into the rectum and feels the part of the prostate next to it. This exam gives the doctor a general idea of the size and condition of the gland. To check for nerve damage, the doctor may ask about tingling sensations or feelings of numbness and may check for changes in sensation, muscle tone, and reflexes.

EEG and EMG: An electroencephalogram (EEG), a test where wires are taped to the forehead, can sense dysfunction in the brain. An electromyogram (EMG) measures nerve activity in muscles and muscular activity that may be related to loss of bladder control.

Ultrasound: For an ultrasound, or sonography, a technician holds a device, called a transducer, that sends harmless sound waves into the body and catches them as they bounce back off the organs inside to create a picture on a monitor. In abdominal ultrasound, the technician slides the transducer over the surface of your abdomen for images of the bladder and kidneys. In transrectal ultrasound, the technician uses a wand inserted in the rectum for images of the prostate. Depending on your symptoms, your doctor may recommend one of these tests.

Urodynamics: Urodynamic testing focuses on the bladder's ability to store urine and empty steadily and completely, and on your sphincter control mechanism. It can also show whether the bladder is having abnormal contractions that cause leakage. The testing involves measuring pressure in the bladder as it is filled with fluid through a small catheter. This test can help identify limited bladder capacity, bladder overactivity or underactivity, weak sphincter muscles, or urinary obstruction. If the test is performed with EMG surface pads, it can also detect abnormal nerve signals and uncontrolled bladder contractions.

How UI Is Treated

No single treatment works for everyone. Your treatment will depend on the type and severity of your problem, your lifestyle, and your preferences, starting with the simpler treatment options. Many men regain urinary control by changing a few habits and doing exercises to strengthen the muscles that hold urine in the bladder. If these behavioral treatments do not work, you may choose to try medicines or a continence device—either an artificial sphincter or a catheter. Finally, for some men, surgery is the best choice.

Behavioral Treatments

For some men, avoiding incontinence is as simple as limiting fluids at certain times of the day or planning regular trips to the bathroom—a therapy called timed voiding or bladder training. As you gain control, you can extend the time between trips. Bladder training also includes Kegel exercises to strengthen the pelvic muscles, which help hold urine in the bladder. Extensive studies have not yet shown that Kegel exercises are effective in reducing incontinence in men, but many clinicians find them to be an important element in therapy for men.

Some people with nerve damage cannot tell whether they are doing Kegel exercises correctly or not. If you are not sure, you may still be able to learn proper Kegel exercises by doing special training with biofeedback, electrical stimulation, or both. Biofeedback uses sensors to detect muscle activity and create a visual or audio signal when the appropriate muscles are being used. A small probe, about the size of a pen, is inserted in the anus to record muscle contractions during the exercises. If you squeeze the right muscle, you will see a change on a television screen or hear a tone from a speaker.

Mild electrical pulses delivered to the pelvic muscles cause them to contract and grow stronger. This technique can also help you locate the right muscles to use during Kegel exercises.

Performing Kegel Exercises

The first step is to find the right muscles. Imagine that you are trying to stop yourself from passing gas. Squeeze the muscles you would use. If you sense a "pulling" feeling, those are the right muscles for pelvic exercises.

It is important not to squeeze other muscles at the same time and not to hold your breath. Also, be careful not to tighten your stomach, leg, or buttock muscles. Squeezing the wrong muscles can put more pressure on your bladder control muscles. Squeeze just the pelvic muscles.

Repeat, but do not overdo it. Pull in the pelvic muscles and hold for a count of three. Then relax for a count of three. Work up to three sets of ten repeats. Start doing your pelvic muscle exercises lying down. This is the easiest because the muscles then do not need to work against gravity. When your muscles get stronger, do your exercises sitting or standing. Working against gravity is like adding more weight.

Be patient. Do not give up. It takes just five minutes, three times a day. Your bladder control may not improve for three to six weeks, although most people notice an improvement after a few weeks.

Medications

Medicines can affect bladder control in different ways. Some medicines help prevent incontinence by blocking abnormal nerve signals that make the bladder contract at the wrong time, while others slow the production of urine. Still others relax the bladder or shrink the prostate. Before prescribing a medicine to treat incontinence, your doctor may consider changing a prescription you already take. For example, diuretics are often prescribed to treat high blood pressure because they reduce fluid in the body by increasing urine production. Some men may find that switching from a diuretic to another kind of blood pressure medicine takes care of their incontinence.

If changing medicines is not an option, your doctor may choose from the following types of drugs for incontinence:

- **Alpha-blockers:** Terazosin (Hytrin), doxazosin (Cardura), tamsulosin (Flomax), and alfuzosin (Uroxatral) are used to treat problems caused by prostate enlargement and bladder outlet obstruction. They act by relaxing the smooth muscle of the prostate and bladder neck, allowing normal urine flow and preventing abnormal bladder contractions that can lead to urge incontinence.

- **5-alpha reductase inhibitors:** Finasteride (Proscar) and dutasteride (Avodart) work by inhibiting the production of the male hormone DHT [dihydrotestosterone], which is thought to be responsible for prostate enlargement. These 5-alpha reductase inhibitors relieve voiding problems by shrinking an enlarged prostate.

  The National Institute of Diabetes and Digestive and Kidney Diseases (NIDDK) sponsored the Medical Therapy of Prostate Symptoms (MTOPS) trial, a multicenter study that found that doxazosin and finasteride taken together reduced the risk of BPH progression by 67 percent compared with placebo. The risk of progression was reduced by 39 percent with doxazosin alone and by 34 percent with finasteride alone.

- **Imipramine:** Marketed as Tofranil, this drug belongs to a class of drugs called tricyclic antidepressants. It relaxes muscles and blocks nerve signals that might cause bladder spasms. Imipramine is also used to treat bedwetting in children.

- **Antispasmodics:** Propantheline (Pro-Banthine), tolterodine (Detrol LA), and oxybutynin (Ditropan XL) belong to a class of drugs that work by relaxing the bladder muscle and relieving spasms. Their most common side effect is dry mouth, although larger doses may cause blurred vision, constipation, a faster heartbeat, headache, and flushing.

Catheters

If all other methods fail or are found unacceptable, you may consider controlling incontinence by using a catheter, a thin tube inserted through the urethra to drain the bladder. Catheters must be managed with great care to avoid infection and stone formation.

- **Clean intermittent bladder catheterization:** If you have problems emptying your bladder because of an enlarged prostate or because of nerve damage, you may use a catheter at regular times, or as needed, to drain urine and prevent overflow incontinence. Depending on your situation, the catheterization may be done for you, or you may learn to do it yourself. You will need to learn sterile technique to avoid urinary tract infections.

- **Condom catheter:** Some men may prefer a drainage system that fits over the penis like a condom. You must take the same care to avoid infection as you do with other catheters. Condom catheters can also carry a risk of skin breakdown.

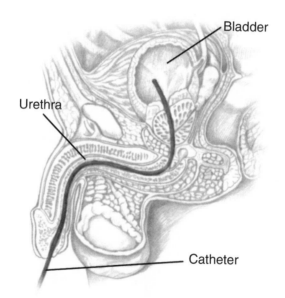

Bladder

Urethra

Catheter

Figure 18.2. Clean intermittent bladder catheterization.

Urethral Injections

Another method to help keep the urethra closed is to inject a fat-like substance into the area that surrounds the opening of the bladder into the urethra. A variety of bulking agents are available for injection. Your doctor will discuss which one may be best for you. Collagen, for example, is a natural tissue from cows. After using local anesthesia or sedation, a doctor can inject the material in about half an hour. Over time, the body slowly eliminates the collagen, so you may need repeat injections. Before you receive collagen, a doctor will perform a skin test to determine whether you could have an allergic reaction to the material.

Artificial Sphincter

Some men may eliminate urine leakage with an artificial sphincter, an implanted device that keeps the urethra closed until you are ready to urinate. This device can help people who have incontinence because of weak sphincter muscles or because of nerve damage that

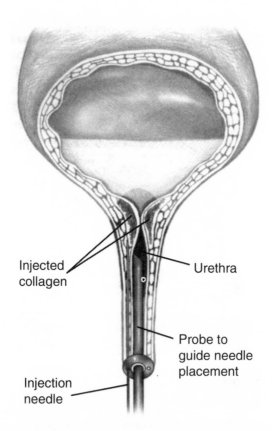

Injected collagen

Urethra

Probe to guide needle placement

Injection needle

Figure 18.3. *Urethral injections. Adding bulk to the tissue around the bladder opening helps keep the urethra closed.*

interferes with sphincter muscle function. It does not solve incontinence caused by uncontrolled bladder contractions.

Surgery to place the artificial sphincter requires general or spinal anesthesia. The device has three parts: a cuff that fits around the urethra, a small balloon reservoir placed in the abdomen, and a pump placed in the scrotum. The cuff is filled with liquid that makes it fit tightly around the urethra to prevent urine from leaking. When it is time to urinate, you squeeze the pump with your fingers to deflate the cuff so that the liquid moves to the balloon reservoir and urine can flow through the urethra. When your bladder is empty, the cuff automatically refills in the next two to five minutes to keep the urethra tightly closed.

Male Sling

Surgery can improve some types of urinary incontinence in men. In a sling procedure, the surgeon creates a support for the urethra by wrapping a strip of material around the urethra and attaching the ends of the strip to the pelvic bone. The sling keeps constant pressure on the urethra so that it does not open until the patient consciously releases the urine.

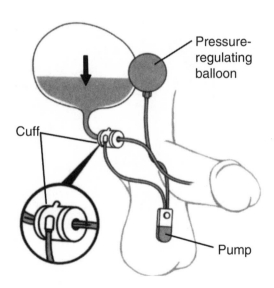

Figure 18.4. Artificial sphincter.

Urinary Diversion

If the bladder must be removed or all bladder function is lost because of nerve damage, you may consider surgery to create a urinary diversion. In this procedure, the surgeon creates a reservoir by removing a piece of the small intestine and directing the ureters to the reservoir. The surgeon also creates a stoma, an opening on the lower abdomen where the urine can be drained through a catheter or into a bag.

Social Support

UI should not cause embarrassment. It is a medical problem like arthritis or diabetes. Your healthcare provider can help you find a solution. You may also find it helpful to join a support group. In many areas, men dealing with the aftereffects of prostate cancer treatment have organized support groups.

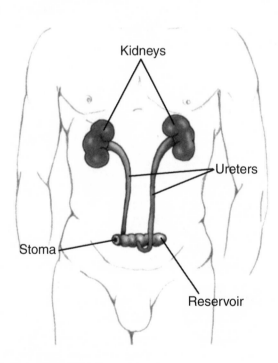

Figure 18.5. Urinary diversion.

Hope through Research

NIDDK has many research programs aimed at finding treatments for urinary disorders, including UI in men. In addition to the MTOPS trial, which focused on drug therapies to treat BPH, the NIDDK is forming a consortium of seven collaborative Prostate Evaluation Treatment Centers and a Biostatistical Coordinating Center to develop and conduct randomized, controlled clinical trials of new surgical treatments to achieve the same long-term outcomes as traditional transurethral resection of the prostate (TURP) but with less morbidity, lower costs, a shorter hospital stay, and more rapid recovery. The first trial will evaluate the safety and effectiveness of transurethral needle ablation (TUNA), transurethral microwave therapy (TUMT), and medical therapy with an alpha-blocker and finasteride combined. The results of this first trial will provide the knowledge needed by both physicians and patients to make the most appropriate choices for long-term management of BPH.

Chapter 19

Urinary Incontinence in Women

Chapter Contents

Section 19.1

Facts about Urinary Incontinence in Women

"Urinary Incontinence in Women," National Kidney and Urologic Diseases Information Clearinghouse (NKUDIC), a service of the National Institute of Diabetes and Digestive and Kidney Diseases (NIDDK), National Institutes of Health (NIH), Pub. No. 04-4132, September 2004.

Women experience incontinence twice as often as men. Pregnancy and childbirth, menopause, and the structure of the female urinary tract account for this difference. But both women and men can become incontinent from neurologic injury, birth defects, strokes, multiple sclerosis, and physical problems associated with aging.

Older women, more often than younger women, experience incontinence. But incontinence is not inevitable with age. Incontinence is treatable and often curable at all ages. If you experience incontinence, you may feel embarrassed. It may help you to remember that loss of

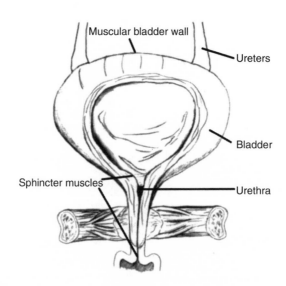

Figure 19.1. *Front view of bladder and sphincter muscles.*

bladder control can be treated. You will need to overcome your embarrassment and see a doctor to learn if you need treatment for an underlying medical condition.

Incontinence in women usually occurs because of problems with muscles that help to hold or release urine. The body stores urine—water and wastes removed by the kidneys—in the bladder, a balloon-like organ. The bladder connects to the urethra, the tube through which urine leaves the body.

During urination, muscles in the wall of the bladder contract, forcing urine out of the bladder and into the urethra. At the same time, sphincter muscles surrounding the urethra relax, letting urine pass out of the body (see Figure 19.1). Incontinence will occur if your bladder muscles suddenly contract or muscles surrounding the urethra suddenly relax.

What are the types of incontinence?

Stress incontinence: If coughing, laughing, sneezing, or other movements that put pressure on the bladder cause you to leak urine, you may have stress incontinence. Physical changes resulting from pregnancy, childbirth, and menopause often cause stress incontinence. It is the most common form of incontinence in women and is treatable.

Pelvic floor muscles support your bladder (see Figure 19.2). If these muscles weaken, your bladder can move downward, pushing slightly

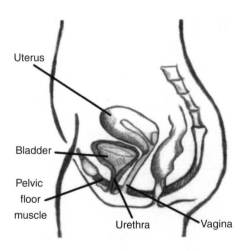

Figure 19.2. Side view of female pelvic muscles.

out of the bottom of the pelvis toward the vagina. This prevents muscles that ordinarily force the urethra shut from squeezing as tightly as they should. As a result, urine can leak into the urethra during moments of physical stress. Stress incontinence also occurs if the muscles that do the squeezing weaken.

Stress incontinence can worsen during the week before your menstrual period. At that time, lowered estrogen levels might lead to lower muscular pressure around the urethra, increasing chances of leakage. The incidence of stress incontinence increases following menopause.

Urge incontinence: If you lose urine for no apparent reason while suddenly feeling the need or urge to urinate, you may have urge incontinence. The most common cause of urge incontinence is inappropriate bladder contractions.

Medical professionals describe such a bladder as "unstable," "spastic," or "overactive." Your doctor might call your condition "reflex incontinence" if it results from overactive nerves controlling the bladder.

Urge incontinence can mean that your bladder empties during sleep, after drinking a small amount of water, or when you touch water or hear it running (as when washing dishes or hearing someone else taking a shower).

Involuntary actions of bladder muscles can occur because of damage to the nerves of the bladder, to the nervous system (spinal cord and brain), or to the muscles themselves. Multiple sclerosis, Parkinson disease, Alzheimer disease, stroke, and injury—including injury that occurs during surgery—all can harm bladder nerves or muscles.

Functional incontinence: People with functional incontinence may have problems thinking, moving, or communicating that prevent them from reaching a toilet. A person with Alzheimer disease, for example, may not think well enough to plan a timely trip to a restroom. A person in a wheelchair may be blocked from getting to a toilet in time. Conditions such as these are often associated with age and account for some of the incontinence of elderly women in nursing homes.

Overflow incontinence: If your bladder is always full so that it frequently leaks urine, you have overflow incontinence. Weak bladder muscles or a blocked urethra can cause this type of incontinence. Nerve damage from diabetes or other diseases can lead to weak bladder muscles; tumors and urinary stones can block the urethra. Overflow incontinence is rare in women.

Other types of incontinence: Stress and urge incontinence often occur together in women. Combinations of incontinence—and this combination in particular—are sometimes referred to as "mixed incontinence."

"Transient incontinence" is a temporary version of incontinence. It can be triggered by medications, urinary tract infections, mental impairment, restricted mobility, and stool impaction (severe constipation), which can push against the urinary tract and obstruct outflow.

How is incontinence evaluated?

The first step toward relief is to see a doctor who is well acquainted with incontinence to learn what type you have. A urologist specializes in the urinary tract, and some urologists further specialize in the female urinary tract. Gynecologists and obstetricians specialize in the female reproductive tract and childbirth. A urogynecologist focuses on urological problems in women. Family practitioners and internists see patients for all kinds of complaints. Any of these doctors may be able to help you. [Other medical professionals who may be involved in your care include a nurse, nurse practitioner, or physical therapist.]

To diagnose the problem, your doctor will first ask about symptoms and medical history. Your pattern of voiding and urine leakage may suggest the type of incontinence. Other obvious factors that can help define the problem include straining and discomfort, use of drugs, recent surgery, and illness. If your medical history does not define the problem, it will at least suggest which tests are needed.

Your doctor will physically examine you for signs of medical conditions causing incontinence, such as tumors that block the urinary tract, stool impaction, and poor reflexes or sensations, which may be evidence of a nerve-related cause.

Your doctor will measure your bladder capacity and residual urine for evidence of poorly functioning bladder muscles. To do this, you will drink plenty of fluids and urinate into a measuring pan, after which the doctor will measure any urine remaining in the bladder. Your doctor may also recommend the following procedures:

- **Stress test:** You relax, then cough vigorously as the doctor watches for loss of urine.

- **Urinalysis:** Urine is tested for evidence of infection, urinary stones, or other contributing causes.

- **Blood tests:** Blood is taken, sent to a laboratory, and examined for substances related to causes of incontinence.

- **Ultrasound:** Sound waves are used to "see" the kidneys, ureters, bladder, and urethra.

- **Cystoscopy:** A thin tube with a tiny camera is inserted in the urethra and used to see the inside of the urethra and bladder.

- **Urodynamics:** Various techniques measure pressure in the bladder and the flow of urine.

Your doctor may ask you to keep a diary for a day or more, up to a week, to record when you void. This diary should note the times you urinate and the amounts of urine you produce. To measure your urine, you can use a special pan that fits over the toilet rim.

How is incontinence treated?

Exercises: Kegel exercises to strengthen or retrain pelvic floor muscles and sphincter muscles can reduce or cure stress leakage. Women of all ages can learn and practice these exercises, which are taught by a healthcare professional.

Most Kegel exercises do not require equipment. However, one technique involves the use of weighted cones. For this exercise, you stand and hold a cone-shaped object within your vagina. You then substitute cones of increasing weight to strengthen the muscles that help keep the urethra closed.

Electrical stimulation: Brief doses of electrical stimulation can strengthen muscles in the lower pelvis in a way similar to exercising the muscles. Electrodes are temporarily placed in the vagina or rectum to stimulate nearby muscles. This will stabilize overactive muscles and stimulate contraction of urethral muscles. Electrical stimulation can be used to reduce both stress incontinence and urge incontinence.

Biofeedback: Biofeedback uses measuring devices to help you become aware of your body's functioning. By using electronic devices or diaries to track when your bladder and urethral muscles contract, you can gain control over these muscles. Biofeedback can be used with pelvic muscle exercises and electrical stimulation to relieve stress and urge incontinence.

Timed voiding or bladder training: Timed voiding (urinating) and bladder training are techniques that use biofeedback. In timed voiding, you fill in a chart of voiding and leaking. From the patterns that appear in your chart, you can plan to empty your bladder before you would otherwise leak. Biofeedback and muscle conditioning—known as bladder training—can alter the bladder's schedule for storing and emptying urine. These techniques are effective for urge and overflow incontinence.

Medications: Medications can reduce many types of leakage. Some drugs inhibit contractions of an overactive bladder. Others relax muscles, leading to more complete bladder emptying during urination. Some drugs tighten muscles at the bladder neck and urethra, preventing leakage. And some are believed to cause muscles involved in urination to function normally.

Some of these medications can produce harmful side effects if used for long periods. In particular, estrogen therapy has been associated with an increased risk for cancers of the breast and endometrium (lining of the uterus). Talk to your doctor about the risks and benefits of long-term use of medications.

Pessaries: A pessary is a stiff ring that is inserted by a doctor or nurse into the vagina, where it presses against the wall of the vagina and the nearby urethra. The pressure helps reposition the urethra, leading to less stress leakage. If you use a pessary, you should watch for possible vaginal and urinary tract infections and see your doctor regularly.

Implants: Implants are substances injected into tissues around the urethra. The implant adds bulk and helps to close the urethra to reduce stress incontinence. Collagen (a fibrous natural tissue from cows) and fat from the patient's body have been used. Implants can be injected by a doctor in about half an hour using local anesthesia.

Implants have a partial success rate. Injections must be repeated after a time because the body slowly eliminates the substances. Before you receive collagen, a doctor must perform a skin test to determine whether you would have an allergic reaction to the material.

Surgery: Doctors usually suggest surgery to alleviate incontinence only after other treatments have been tried. Many surgical options have high rates of success.

Most stress incontinence results from the bladder dropping down toward the vagina. Therefore, common surgery for stress incontinence involves pulling the bladder up to a more normal position. Working through an incision in the vagina or abdomen, the surgeon raises the bladder and secures it with a string attached to muscle, ligament, or bone.

For severe cases of stress incontinence, the surgeon may secure the bladder with a wide sling. This not only holds up the bladder but also compresses the bottom of the bladder and the top of the urethra, further preventing leakage.

In rare cases, a surgeon implants an artificial sphincter, a doughnut-shaped sac that circles the urethra. A fluid fills and expands the sac, which squeezes the urethra closed. By pressing a valve implanted under the skin, you can cause the artificial sphincter to deflate. This removes pressure from the urethra, allowing urine from the bladder to pass.

Catheterization: If you are incontinent because your bladder never empties completely (overflow incontinence) or your bladder cannot empty because of poor muscle tone, past surgery, or spinal cord injury, you might use a catheter to empty your bladder. A catheter is a tube that you can learn to insert through the urethra into the bladder to drain urine. Catheters may be used once in a while or on a constant basis, in which case the tube connects to a bag that you can attach to your leg. If you use a long-term (or indwelling) catheter, you should watch for possible urinary tract infections.

Other procedures: Many women manage urinary incontinence with pads that catch slight leakage during activities such as exercising. Also, you often can reduce incontinence by restricting certain liquids, such as coffee, tea, and alcohol.

Finally, many women who could be treated resort instead to wearing absorbent undergarments, or diapers—especially elderly women in nursing homes. This is unfortunate, because diapering can lead to diminished self-esteem, as well as skin irritation and sores. If you are an elderly woman, you and your family should discuss with your doctor the possible effectiveness of treatments such as timed voiding, pelvic muscle exercises, and electrical stimulation before resorting to absorbent pads or undergarments.

Section 19.2

Pregnancy, Childbirth, and Bladder Control

National Kidney and Urologic Diseases Information Clearinghouse (NKUDIC), a service of the National Institute of Diabetes and Digestive and Kidney Diseases (NIDDK), National Institutes of Health (NIH), Pub. No. 02-4189, May 2002.

Do pregnancy and childbirth affect bladder control?

Yes. But don't panic. If you lose bladder control after childbirth, the problem often goes away by itself. Your muscles may just need time to recover.

When do you need medical help?

If you still have a problem after six weeks, talk to your doctor. Without treatment, lost bladder control can become a long-term problem. Accidental leaking can also signal that something else is wrong in your body.

Bladder control problems do not always show up right after childbirth. Some women do not begin to have problems until later, often in their 40s.

You and your healthcare team must first find out why you have lost bladder control. Then you can discuss treatment.

After treatment, most women regain or improve their bladder control. Regaining control helps you enjoy a healthier and happier life.

Can you prevent bladder problems?

Yes. Women who exercise certain pelvic muscles have fewer bladder problems later on. These muscles are called pelvic floor muscles. If you plan to have a baby, talk to your doctor. Ask if you should do pelvic floor exercises. Exercises after childbirth also help prevent bladder problems in middle age. Ask your healthcare team how to do pelvic exercises.

211

What do pregnancy and childbirth have to do with bladder control?

The added weight and pressure of pregnancy can weaken pelvic floor muscles. Other aspects of pregnancy and childbirth can also cause problems:

- changed position of bladder and urethra

- vaginal delivery

- episiotomy (the cut in the muscle that makes it easier for the baby to come out)

- damage to bladder control nerves

Section 19.3

Menopause and Bladder Control

National Kidney and Urologic Diseases Information Clearinghouse (NKUDIC), a service of the National Institute of Diabetes and Digestive and Kidney Diseases (NIDDK), National Institutes of Health (NIH), Pub. No. 04-4186, April 2004.

Does menopause affect bladder control?

Yes. Some women have bladder control problems after they stop having periods (menopause or change of life). If you are going through menopause, talk to your healthcare team.

After your periods end, your body stops making the female hormone estrogen. Estrogen controls how your body matures, your monthly periods, and body changes during pregnancy and breast-feeding.

Some scientists believe estrogen may help keep the lining of the bladder and urethra plump and healthy. They think that lack of estrogen could contribute to weakness of the bladder control muscles.

Pressure from coughing, sneezing, or lifting can push urine through the weakened muscle. This kind of leakage is called stress incontinence. It is one of the most common kinds of bladder control problems in older women.

Recent studies have raised doubts about the benefits of taking estrogen after menopause. The studies also point to added risks from taking estrogen for many years. No studies have shown that taking estrogen improves bladder control in women who have gone through menopause. Your doctor can suggest many other possible treatments to improve bladder control. [See Section 19.4, "Hormone Therapy and Bladder Control," for more information.]

What else causes bladder control problems in older women?

Sometimes bladder control problems are caused by other medical conditions. These problems include the following:

- infections
- nerve damage from diabetes or stroke
- heart problems
- medicines
- feeling depressed
- difficulty walking or moving

A very common kind of bladder control problem for older women is urge incontinence. This means the bladder muscles squeeze at the wrong time—or all the time—and cause leaks. If you have this problem, your healthcare team can help you retrain yourself to go to the toilet on a schedule.

What should you do about bladder control after menopause?

Talk to your healthcare team. You may have stress or urge incontinence, but other things could also be happening. Medicines and exercises can restore bladder control in many cases. Your doctor will give you a checkup first.

What treatments can help you regain bladder control?

It depends on what kind of bladder control problem you have. Your healthcare team may also recommend some of the following:

- limiting caffeine
- exercising pelvic muscles
- training the bladder to hold more urine

If these simple treatments do not work, your healthcare team may have you try something different. These treatments might include the following:

- biofeedback
- electrical stimulation of pelvic muscles
- a device inserted in the vagina to hold up the bladder
- a device inserted directly into the urethra to block leakage
- surgery to lift a sagging bladder into a better position

Section 19.4

Hormone Therapy and Bladder Control

Hormone therapy, which doctors have often prescribed to post-menopausal women to prevent urinary incontinence, may actually increase its incidence and severity, a new study finds.

Data from the Women's Health Initiative (WHI)—the major study of hormonal therapy—found that risks for developing one kind or another of urinary incontinence were significantly greater for women who got the therapy than for those who didn't.

Many experts are now reluctant to recommend hormone replacement therapy (HRT) to incontinent patients, and these findings may support that trend.

"Would I prescribe hormonal treatment for urinary incontinence? No, never," said Dr. Jean Fourcroy, a trustee of the National Association for Continence.

The findings appear in the February 23, [2005], issue of the *Journal of the American Medical Association.*

Researchers led by Dr. Susan Hendrix of Wayne State University School of Medicine, in Detroit, looked over data on nearly 23,300 women aged 50 to 79. They focused on symptoms of urinary incontinence occurring within one year of initiating HRT.

The team reported that the incidence of developing stress incontinence (urinary incontinence triggered by stressors such as heavy lifting or even coughing) more than doubled for women prescribed estrogen alone as a hormone therapy, compared to women given a placebo.

Urge incontinence, caused by an involuntary contraction of bladder muscles, was 32 percent more likely in women taking estrogen-only HRT, while the incidence of mixed incontinence, which has a multitude of causes, was increased by 79 percent.

Hormone-related increases in risk for stress or mixed incontinence were somewhat lower in women getting a combination of hormones, such as estrogen plus progestin, the researchers note. And in the case of urge incontinence, mixed hormonal therapy appeared to confer no increase in risk over a placebo.

Women already diagnosed with urinary incontinence at the start of the study reported an increase in the frequency and degree of the problem after being prescribed hormonal therapy, the researchers add.

The report on urinary incontinence and hormonal therapy couldn't have been made earlier because the complete Women's Health Initiative trial didn't end until February 2004 and "it takes a long time to be sure the records are complete and to get the information together," explained Hendrix, a professor of obstetrics and gynecology.

The finding that hormonal therapy worsened the outlook was "quite surprising," Hendrix said, and the treatment probably is still being prescribed for incontinence by many physicians.

"We have to educate patients and physicians about the effects of the medication so we can treat patients better," she said.

The report is yet another blow for HRT from data arising from the Women's Health Initiative. In July 2002, one arm of the study was unexpectedly halted after results found combined therapy increased women's risks for heart attack, stroke, blood clots, and breast cancer. Sales of HRT have fallen sharply since that time.

This finding of an increased risk of urinary incontinence "is something of a surprise, because smaller trials have shown a benefit," said Dr. Catherine E. DuBeau, an associate professor of medicine at the University of Chicago, who wrote an accompanying editorial in the journal.

Her editorial advises that "clinicians should no longer prescribe long-term oral conjugated estrogens for treatment of urge, stress or mixed urinary incontinence in postmenopausal women aged 50 years or older."

However, the finding "is not the final word on using estrogens to treat urinary incontinence," DuBeau said. "There is still a lot we don't know about [the effectiveness of] topical estrogens," such as lotions or creams.

The most important result of the study "will be to get the word out to women that they don't have to suffer from urinary incontinence," DuBeau said. Many women find the issue so embarrassing that they never tell their doctors about it, she said, even though a variety of helpful treatments are available, starting with behavioral therapy and moving on to drug treatment, if necessary. An implantable device has also been approved for use in extreme cases, she said.

Fourcroy said the study does have some weaknesses that could benefit from further analysis.

"One of the biggest things is that relief of urinary incontinence is associated with weight loss," Fourcroy said, and the new report has no information on participants' body-mass index, a measure of obesity. "We might see some subset differences if we looked at body-mass index information," she said.

But the bottom line, she said, is that hormonal therapy "is not the way to go."

More Information

The various forms of urinary incontinence, their causes and treatment, are outlined by the National Association for Continence on their website at http://www.nafc.org/about_incontinence.

Sources

Susan Hendrix, M.D., professor, obstetrics and gynecology, Wayne State University, Detroit; Catherine E. DuBeau, M.D., associate professor, medicine, University of Chicago; Jean Fourcroy, M.D., trustee, National Association for Continence, and consultant, urology and endocrinology, Bethesda, Maryland; February 23, 2005, *Journal of the American Medical Association*.

—by Ed Edelson, HealthDay *reporter*

Chapter 20

Treatments for Urinary Incontinence in Women

Chapter Contents

Section 20.1

Urinary Incontinence Treatment Tips for Women

"Treatments for Urinary Incontinence in Women," National Kidney and Urologic Diseases Information Clearinghouse (NKUDIC), a service of the National Institute of Diabetes and Digestive and Kidney Diseases (NIDDK), National Institutes of Health (NIH), Pub. No. 03-5104, June 2003.

Urinary incontinence (UI) is a medical problem. Your doctor or nurse can help you find a solution. No single treatment works for everyone, but most women can be treated without surgery. The treatment you select depends on your lifestyle and your preferences. Many women try the simpler treatment options first, such as changing a few habits and doing exercises to strengthen the muscles that hold urine in the bladder. If these behavioral treatments do not work, you may choose to try medicines or vaginal devices. Sometimes mild electrical stimulation to the pelvic nerves may help. And for some women, surgery is the best solution.

Behavioral Remedies: Bladder Retraining and Kegel Exercises

Your doctor or nurse may ask you to keep a bladder diary—a record of your fluid intake, trips to the bathroom, episodes of urine leakage, and an estimate of the amount of leakage. By looking at this record, the doctor may see a pattern and suggest making it a point to use the bathroom at regular timed intervals, a habit called timed voiding. As you gain control, you can extend the time between scheduled trips to the bathroom. Behavioral treatment also includes Kegel exercises to strengthen the muscles that help hold in urine.

How to Do Kegel Exercises

The first step is to find the right muscles. Imagine that you are sitting on a marble and want to pick up the marble with your vagina. Imagine "sucking" the marble into your vagina.

Try not to squeeze other muscles at the same time. Be careful not to tighten your stomach, legs, or buttocks. Squeezing the wrong muscles can put more pressure on your bladder control muscles. Just squeeze the pelvic muscles. Don't hold your breath. Do not practice while urinating.

Repeat, but don't overdo it. At first, find a quiet spot to practice—your bathroom or bedroom—so you can concentrate. Pull in the pelvic muscles and hold for a count of three. Then relax for a count of three. Work up to three sets of ten repeats. Start doing your pelvic muscle exercises lying down. This is the easiest position to do them because the muscles do not need to work against gravity. When your muscles get stronger, do your exercises sitting or standing. Working against gravity is like adding more weight.

Be patient. Don't give up. It takes just five minutes a day. You may not feel your bladder control improve for three to six weeks. Still, most people do notice an improvement after a few weeks.

Some people with nerve damage cannot tell whether they are doing Kegel exercises correctly or not. If you are not sure, ask your doctor or nurse to examine you while you try to do them. If it turns out that you are not squeezing the right muscles, you may still be able to learn proper Kegel exercises by doing special training with biofeedback, electrical stimulation, or both.

Medicines for Overactive Bladder

Overactive bladder occurs when abnormal nerves send signals to the bladder at the wrong time, causing its muscles to squeeze without warning. Normal women may void up to 12 times a day, but women with overactive bladder may find that they must urinate more frequently. Specifically, the symptoms of overactive bladder include the following:

- **Urinary frequency:** urination 13 or more times a day or two or more times at night

- **Urinary urgency:** the sudden, strong need to urinate immediately

- **Urge incontinence:** leakage or gushing of urine that follows a sudden, strong urge

If you have an overactive bladder, your doctor may prescribe a medicine to block the nerve signals that cause frequent urination and urgency.

Drugs that relax muscles and prevent bladder spasms include oxybutynin chloride (Ditropan) and tolterodine tartrate (Detrol), which belong to the class of drugs called bladder relaxants. Their most common side effect is dry mouth, although larger doses may cause blurred vision, constipation, a faster heartbeat, and flushing. Ditropan XL and Detrol LA are long-acting drugs that can be taken once a day.

Imipramine hydrochloride (Tofranil), a tricyclic antidepressant that relaxes bladder muscles and tightens urethral muscles, may be used instead of or in combination with Ditropan XL or Detrol LA. Side effects may include fatigue, dry mouth, dizziness, blurred vision, nausea, and insomnia.

If you take medicine to treat an overactive bladder, you should take several precautions.

- Wear sunglasses if your eyes become more sensitive to light.

- Take care not to become overheated.

- Chew gum or suck on sugarless hard candy to avoid dry mouth.

Different medicines can affect the nerves and muscles of the urinary tract in different ways. Pills to treat swelling (edema) or high blood pressure may increase your urine output and contribute to bladder control problems. Talk with your doctor; you may find that taking an alternative to a medicine you already take may solve the problem without adding another prescription.

Electrical Stimulation for Nerve Problems

Mild electrical pulses can be used to stimulate the nerves that control the bladder and sphincter muscles. Depending on which nerves the doctor plans to treat, these pulses can be given through the vagina or by using patches on the skin. Other forms of electrical stimulation or neuromodulation are also available.

Vaginal Devices for Stress Incontinence

Stress incontinence is urine leakage that occurs when an action puts pressure on the bladder. Laughing, sneezing, coughing, rising from a chair, lifting an object, and running can all cause the stomach muscles to press down on the bladder and force urine out. Stress incontinence usually results from weak pelvic muscles, the muscles that hold the bladder in place and keep urine inside.

A pessary is a stiff ring that is inserted by a doctor or nurse into the vagina, where it presses against the wall of the vagina and the nearby urethra. The pressure helps reposition the urethra, leading to less stress leakage. If you use a pessary, you should watch for possible vaginal and urinary tract infections and see your doctor regularly.

Injections for Stress Incontinence

Collagen, one of the bulking agents used for injections, is a natural tissue from cows. It is injected into tissues around the bladder neck and urethra to add bulk and close the bladder opening to reduce stress incontinence. After using local anesthesia or sedation, a doctor can inject the material in about half an hour. Over time, the body slowly eliminates the collagen, so you may need repeat injections. Before you receive collagen, a doctor will perform a skin test to determine whether you could have an allergic reaction to the material. A variety of bulking agents are available for injection. Your doctor will discuss which one may be best for you.

Surgery for Stress Incontinence

In some women, the bladder can move out of its normal position, especially following childbirth. Surgeons have developed different techniques for supporting the bladder in its normal position. The two main types of surgery are retropubic suspension and the sling procedure.

Retropubic suspension uses sutures (surgical threads) to support the bladder neck. The threads are secured to the pubic bone and other structures within the pelvis to form a cradle for the bladder. To place the sutures, the surgeon makes an incision in the abdomen a few inches below the navel.

Sling procedures are performed through a vaginal incision. The conventional sling procedure uses a strip of material to support the bladder neck. The sling may be made of natural tissue or synthetic (man-made) material. Both ends of the sling are attached to the pubic bone or tied in front of the abdomen just above the pubic bone. Another sling method uses a synthetic tape, but the ends are not tied but rather pulled up above the pubic bone.

Surgeons report that the retropubic suspension and sling procedures cure stress incontinence for at least four years in more than 80 percent of their cases. Possible side effects include persistent stress incontinence, bladder overactivity, and voiding changes.

Talk with your doctor about whether surgery will help your condition and what type of surgery is best for you. The procedure you choose may depend on your own preferences or on your surgeon's experience. Ask what you should expect after the procedure. You may also wish to talk to someone who has recently had the procedure.

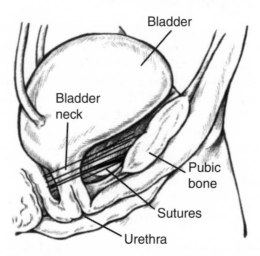

Figure 20.1. *Side view. Supporting sutures in place following retropubic or transvaginal suspension.*

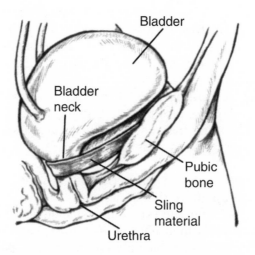

Figure 20.2. *Sling in place, secured to the pubic bone.*

Hope through Research

The National Institute of Diabetes and Digestive and Kidney Diseases (NIDDK) has many research programs aimed at finding treatments for urinary disorders, including urinary incontinence. The NIDDK is sponsoring the Urinary Incontinence Treatment Network, a multicenter study that will evaluate and compare treatment methods for stress and mixed incontinence in women. The researchers have established criteria for selecting patients and measuring results. The goal of the study is to learn which treatment methods have the best short- and long-term outcomes for treating stress urinary incontinence in women.

Section 20.2

Exercising Your Pelvic Muscles

National Kidney and Urologic Diseases Information Clearinghouse (NKUDIC), a service of the National Institute of Diabetes and Digestive and Kidney Diseases (NIDDK), National Institutes of Health (NIH), Pub. No. 02-4188, April 2002.

Why You Should Exercise Your Pelvic Muscles

Life's events can weaken pelvic muscles. Pregnancy, childbirth, and being overweight can do it. Luckily, when these muscles get weak, you can help make them strong again.

Pelvic floor muscles are just like other muscles. Exercise can make them stronger. Women with bladder control problems can regain control through pelvic muscle exercises, also called Kegel exercises.

Pelvic Fitness in Minutes a Day

Exercising your pelvic floor muscles for just five minutes, three times a day can make a big difference to your bladder control. Exercise strengthens muscles that hold the bladder and many other organs in place.

223

The part of your body including your hip bones is the pelvic area. At the bottom of the pelvis, several layers of muscle stretch between your legs. The muscles attach to the front, back, and sides of the pelvis bone.

Two pelvic muscles do most of the work. The biggest one stretches like a hammock. The other is shaped like a triangle. These muscles prevent leaking of urine and stool.

How to Exercise Your Pelvic Muscles

Find the right muscles. This is very important. Your doctor, nurse, or physical therapist will help make sure you are doing the exercises the right way.

You should tighten the two major muscles that stretch across your pelvic floor. They are the "hammock" muscle and the "triangle" muscle. Here are three methods to check for the correct muscles.

1. Try to stop the flow of urine when you are sitting on the toilet. If you can do it, you are using the right muscles.

2. Imagine that you are trying to stop passing gas. Squeeze the muscles you would use. If you sense a "pulling" feeling, those are the right muscles for pelvic exercises.

3. Lie down and put your finger inside your vagina. Squeeze as if you were trying to stop urine from coming out. If you feel tightness on your finger, you are squeezing the right pelvic muscle.

Don't squeeze other muscles at the same time. Be careful not to tighten your stomach, legs, or other muscles. Squeezing the wrong muscles can put more pressure on your bladder control muscles. Just squeeze the pelvic muscle. Don't hold your breath.

Repeat, but don't overdo it. At first, find a quiet spot to practice—your bathroom or bedroom—so you can concentrate. Lie on the floor. Pull in the pelvic muscles and hold for a count of three. Then relax for a count of three. Work up to ten to fifteen repeats each time you exercise.

Do your pelvic exercises at least three times a day. Every day, use three positions: lying down, sitting, and standing. You can exercise while lying on the floor, sitting at a desk, or standing in the kitchen. Using all three positions makes the muscles strongest.

Be patient. Don't give up. It's just five minutes, three times a day. You may not feel your bladder control improve until after three to six weeks. Still, most women do notice an improvement after a few weeks.

Exercise aids. You can also exercise by using special weights or biofeedback. Ask your healthcare team about these exercise aids.

Hold the Squeeze 'til after the Sneeze

You can protect your pelvic muscles from more damage by bracing yourself.

Think ahead, just before sneezing, lifting, or jumping. Sudden pressure from such actions can hurt those pelvic muscles. Squeeze your pelvic muscles tightly and hold on until after you sneeze, lift, or jump.

After you train yourself to tighten the pelvic muscles for these moments, you will have fewer accidents.

Section 20.3

Using a Pessary

This section contains text reproduced with permission from "Pessary: What It Is and How to Use One," May 1, 2000, http://familydoctor.org/ 578.xml. Copyright © 2000 American Academy of Family Physicians. All rights reserved. It also includes text reproduced with permission from "Practical Use of the Pessary," May 1, 2000, *American Family Physician.* Copyright © 2000 American Academy of Family Physicians. All rights reserved.

Pessary: What It Is and How to Use One

What is a pessary?

A pessary is a plastic device that fits into your vagina to help support your uterus (womb), vagina, bladder or rectum.

The pessary is most often used for "prolapse" of the uterus. Prolapse means that your uterus droops or tends to "fall out" because it loses support after you give birth or have pelvic surgery. This problem is usually fixed with surgery, but you can also use a pessary to help keep the uterus in place.

A pessary can help if you have a "cystocele" (when your bladder droops down into your vagina) or if you have a "rectocele" (when your rectum sticks up into the bottom of your vagina).

A pessary can also help many women with stress urinary incontinence (the leaking of urine when you cough, strain or exercise). Pregnant women with incontinence can also use a pessary.

What kind of pessary will I use?

Your doctor will decide which type of pessary you should use depending on the problem you have. The pessary has to be fit just right. There are no tools that can tell what the right size is. The pessary is fit by trial and error. It usually takes a few tries to get the right one.

After the first fitting, you'll need to go back to the doctor's office to have the pessary rechecked. Your doctor will probably check the pessary in a few days. After that you will probably be checked every few months. Sometimes the size or shape of the pessary will have to be changed.

How do I care for my pessary?

It's important that you follow your doctor's instructions about caring for your pessary. Most pessaries can be worn for many days to weeks at a time before they have to be taken out and cleaned with ordinary soap and water. You may be able to take out, clean, and reinsert your pessary yourself, or your doctor may want you to come into the office so he or she can do it. Be sure to keep your check-up appointments and clean the pessary as your doctor tells you.

Does the pessary cause any side effects?

You may notice more vaginal discharge than normal. Your vaginal discharge may also develop an odor. Certain vaginal gels can help with these side effects. Your doctor may or may not have you douche as well.

Vaginal irritation is another possible side effect. Women who are past menopause may need to use estrogen cream for the irritation.

Can the pessary get lost or fall out?

The vagina is a closed tube. The pessary can't go anywhere else inside the body. The pessary can fall out of the vagina if you strain or lift something. This usually means that your pessary is too small. Check with your doctor if your pessary keeps falling out.

What else should I know?

Many pessaries can be worn during intercourse—your doctor will tell you if you can't. Be sure to tell your doctor promptly if you have any discomfort with the pessary or if you have trouble urinating or having a bowel movement.

This text provides a general overview on this topic and may not apply to everyone. To find out if this text applies to you and to get more information on this subject, talk to your family doctor.

Practical Use of the Pessary

The pessary is an effective tool in the management of a number of gynecologic problems. The pessary is most commonly used in the management of pelvic support defects such as cystocele and rectocele. Pessaries can also be used in the treatment of stress urinary incontinence. The wide variety of pessary styles may cause confusion for physicians during the initial selection of the pessary. However, an understanding of the different styles and their uses will enable physicians to make an appropriate choice. Complications can be minimized with simple vaginal hygiene and regular follow-up visits.

The pessary is one of the oldest medical devices available. The type of pessary that is appropriate for each patient depends on the condition being treated. Although many physicians are unfamiliar with the

Table 20.1. Gynecologic Conditions that Can Be Managed with Pessaries

Stress urinary incontinence

Vaginal vault prolapse

Cystocele

Enterocele

Rectocele

Uterine prolapse

Preoperative preparation

Information from references 1 through 4.

pessary, it remains a useful device for the nonsurgical management of a number of gynecologic conditions (Table 20.1). Physicians who are familiar with the use of a pessary will be equipped to manage a variety of pelvic support defects, including genuine stress urinary incontinence.

How is the pessary used?

Pelvic support defects: The pessary is most commonly used in the nonsurgical management of pelvic support defects. Multiple vaginal deliveries can weaken the musculature of the pelvic floor. Hysterectomy or other pelvic surgery can predispose a woman to weakness of the pelvic floor, as can conditions that involve repetitive bearing down, such as chronic constipation, chronic coughing or repetitive heavy lifting.[1]

Although surgical repair of certain pelvic support defects offers a more permanent solution, some patients may elect to use a pessary as a temporary management option. As the geriatric population continues to increase, more patients are presenting with pelvic floor defects. While many of these patients are poor candidates for surgery, most of them can safely use a pessary.

Classification of uterine prolapse: Uterine prolapse is classified by degree. In first-degree uterine prolapse, the cervix is visible when the perineum is depressed. In second-degree prolapse, the cervix is visible outside of the vaginal introitus, while the uterine fundus remains inside. In third-degree prolapse, or procidentia, the entire uterus is outside of the vaginal introitus. Uterine prolapse is associated with incontinence, vaginitis, cystitis and, possibly, uterine malignancy.[5]

Types of vaginal prolapse: Variants of vaginal prolapse include rectocele, enterocele, cystocele, and vault prolapse. A rectocele occurs when the fascial layers between the rectum and the vagina become weak. This weakening allows the rectum to herniate, causing a bulging of the posterior vagina. The patient may report having to manually reduce the rectocele before defecation. An enterocele is the herniation of the sigmoid colon into the upper posterior vaginal wall. An enterocele differs from a rectocele in that it is a true hernia, lined by peritoneum and usually containing small bowel.

A cystocele occurs when the tissues between the bladder and the vagina weaken, leading to a herniation of the bladder. This herniation causes a bulge in the anterior vaginal wall. Other portions of the vaginal vault may prolapse as well. Such vault prolapse may or may not cause symptoms.

Treatment of uterine prolapse: First- and second-degree uterine prolapse are usually managed with a ring pessary. The doughnut and inflatable pessaries are also useful in the treatment of mild to moderate uterine prolapse. If the uterine prolapse is associated with a cystocele, a ring pessary with support is useful.

The cube pessary is designed to manage third-degree uterine prolapse. Because the cube is held in place by suction, removal can be somewhat difficult for some patients. This type of pessary can support the uterus even with a lack of vaginal tone. The cube pessary should be removed and cleaned daily, because it has no drainage capability.[5]

A doughnut, inflatable or Gellhorn pessary can also be used in patients with third-degree uterine prolapse. The Gellhorn pessary is designed to manage severe uterine or vaginal prolapse. While the Gellhorn offers strong support, it can also be difficult for the patient to remove. If a cystocele or rectocele accompanies the third-degree uterine prolapse, a Gehrung pessary may be the most helpful. However, the Gehrung can be difficult to insert.

Treatment of vaginal prolapse: In patients with a mild cystocele, treatment using a ring with support, a dish with support, a Hodge with support or a doughnut pessary will suffice. To manage a large prolapse of the anterior vaginal wall, the Gellhorn pessary may be the best choice, although insertion and removal can be difficult. Inflatable and cube pessaries are also useful in patients with a larger cystocele. In patients with rectoceles and enteroceles, the use of a Gellhorn, doughnut, inflatable or cube pessary is usually required to provide the necessary support.

Stress urinary incontinence: Stress urinary incontinence, which is the involuntary loss of urine during exertion, is a common problem that affects many women. In one survey of women older than 18 years, 22 percent complained of symptoms associated with stress urinary incontinence.[6]

Pessaries should be used by patients for whom conservative management is appropriate. Good candidates for a pessary trial might include a pregnant patient, an elderly woman in whom surgery would be risky and a woman whose previous operation for stress incontinence failed. A pessary can also be used by women who only have stress urinary incontinence with strenuous exercise. The prevalence of stress urinary incontinence with strenuous exercise may be as high as 27 percent.[2]

Incontinence pessaries: The pessary compresses the urethra against the upper posterior portion of the symphysis pubis and elevates the bladder neck. This causes an increase in outflow resistance and corrects the angle between the bladder and the urethra so that Valsalva maneuvers alone are not strong enough to cause leakage of urine. Any style of pessary that can accomplish this will help with the management of stress urinary incontinence.

The incontinence ring and incontinence dish pessaries are most commonly used in patients with stress urinary incontinence. A Hodge pessary with or without support, depending on the presence of a cystocele, can also be used. Introl, a bladder neck support prosthesis that is marketed by UroMed, is also available. The prosthesis has two prongs that support the urethrovesical junction and bladder neck. This device was found to be effective in 83 percent of adult women with stress urinary incontinence.[7]

For women who have urinary incontinence during strenuous activities such as jogging, aerobics or tennis, a cube pessary that is inserted before exercise may be all that is needed. A Hodge pessary with support is also effective in the prevention of exercise incontinence.[3]

The pessary can be used to differentiate between patients with stress urinary incontinence that is secondary to a correctable anatomic defect and those with bladder instability. A properly fitted pessary can simulate the result of surgical correction of incontinence, thereby yielding diagnostic and prognostic information.[8]

What are some management issues concerning the pessary?

Selection and fitting: Selection of an appropriate pessary depends primarily on the condition for which the patient is being treated. Pessaries are available from Milex, the largest manufacturer, at a cost of $31.00 to $51.50 each. [Editor's note: According to the Milex website, their products are not for sale to the general public. Patients are requested to contact their physician to obtain Milex products. For more information go to http://www.milexproducts.com.] Of the pessaries that are indicated for a particular condition (Table 20.2), the style that works the best for the particular patient should be chosen. For example, a Gellhorn pessary can offer excellent support for uterine prolapse as long as the perineal body is intact. If the perineal body is weak, a cube or doughnut pessary will be more effective.[4] An incontinence ring pessary usually helps with stress urinary incontinence, but if the patient has some degree of cystocele, a Hodge with support or a Gehrung pessary may be more effective.

Pessaries are fit by trial and error. In patients who use a diaphragm, the size of the diaphragm does not correlate with the size of the pessary. Proper fitting of the pessary often requires the patient to try several sizes and/or styles. A variety of styles and sizes should be made available during the patient's fitting session. The manufacturer of the pessary can provide pessaries in the most common sizes that will fit the majority of patients. The manufacturer can also provide detailed instructions on how to fit each particular style of pessary.

After a complete pelvic examination has been performed, the physician should start with an average-sized pessary in the simplest style. When the pessary has been put into place, the fit and effectiveness should be checked. The largest pessary that the patient can wear comfortably is generally the most effective. The examiner's finger should pass easily between the pessary and the vaginal wall. The physician should check the pessary to be sure that the intended function is met. When the indication of the pessary is for stress urinary incontinence, the patient should cough to test for any leakage of urine.

Finally, the examiner should ask the patient to stand, sit, squat and perform Valsalva maneuvers to be sure that the device will not become dislodged. It is also recommended that the patient void before leaving the office. If the patient is unable to void with the pessary in position, the device should be removed and the patient should be fitted with the next smaller size. The patient should be instructed to immediately report any discomfort or difficulty with urination or defecation while wearing the pessary.

Contraindications: There are few contraindications to the use of a pessary. Active infections of the pelvis or vagina, such as vaginitis or pelvic inflammatory disease, preclude the use of a pessary until the infection has been resolved. Patients who are noncompliant or unlikely to follow up should not be fitted for a pessary. Most pessaries are made of silicone; some are made of latex. An allergy to the product would also be a contraindication.

Follow up: After the initial fitting of the pessary, the patient should be followed up within a few days so that the physician can recheck the fit. The pessary should be removed so that the vagina can be examined for irritation, pressure sores or allergic reaction. Having to change the size of the pessary at least once after the initial fitting is not uncommon. The patient should then be instructed to follow-up within one to two weeks for another examination, after which time the examinations can be spaced to every two to three months. In the motivated patient who is able to demonstrate effective removal, insertion and care of the pessary, these examinations may be spaced further at the discretion of the physician.[9]

At each follow-up examination, the pessary should be removed and cleaned with soap and water while the vagina is inspected for erosions, pressure necrosis or allergic reaction. If inspection of the pessary reveals cracking or other defects, it should be replaced. The patient who is using a pessary should be considered to be under the

Table 20.2. Various Types of Pessaries and Their Uses

Type	Uses	Most common sizes	Ease of insertion and removal
Ring*	Mild uterine prolapse	3 to 5	Easy
Incontinence ring*	Stress urinary incontinence	2 to 7	Easy
Ring with support*	Mild uterine prolapse/ Mild cystocele	3 to 5	Easy
Incontinence dish*	Stress urinary incontinence/ Mild uterine prolapse	3 to 5	Medium
Dish with support*	Mild cystocele/ Stress urinary incontinence/ Mild uterine prolapse	3 to 5	Medium
Doughnut*	Moderate uterine prolapse/ Mild cystocele	2½ to 3 inches	Medium
Gellhorn*	Moderate uterine prolapse/ Mild cystocele	2¼ to 2¾ inches	Difficult
Inflatable*	Moderate uterine prolapse	Medium and large	Easy
Cube*	Moderate to severe uterine prolapse/Mild cystocele/ Mild rectocele/Other vaginal vault prolapse	2 to 4	Medium

care of the person who placed it for the duration of its use. Pessaries should never be placed in elderly, debilitated patients without excellent follow-up.

Complications: Although the pessary is an extremely safe device, it is still a foreign body in the vagina. Because of this, the most common side effect of the pessary is increased vaginal discharge and odor.[4] This side effect can be minimized with the use of an acidic vaginal gel such as Trimo-San, which also helps to relieve minor irritation and itching. Some physicians recommend that patients douche with dilute vinegar or hydrogen peroxide for relief.[4,10]

Postmenopausal women with thin vaginal mucosa are more susceptible to vaginal ulceration with use of a pessary. Treatment with

Table 20.2. Various Types of Pessaries and Their Uses (*continued*)

Type	Uses	Most common sizes	Ease of insertion and removal
Gehrung*	Moderate to severe cystocele/ Mild rectocele/Moderate to severe uterine prolapse	3 to 5	Difficult
Gehrung with knob*	Same uses as Gehrung/ Stress urinary incontinence	3 to 5	Difficult
Hodge*	Mild cystocele	2 to 4	Medium
Hodge with support*	Mild cystocele/ Stress urinary incontinence	2 to 4	Medium
Smith, Risser*	Mild cystocele/ Stress urinary incontinence	2 to 4	Medium
Introl†	Stress urinary incontinence	Call manufacturer	Easy

* Manufactured by Milex Products, Inc. (Chicago, IL, telephone: 800-621-1278, website: http://www.milexproducts.com).

† Manufactured by UroMed, Inc. (Norwood, MA, telephone: 800-403-9189, website: http://www.uromed.com).

Information from references 1 through 4, and 7.

estrogen cream can make the vaginal mucosa more resistant to erosion and should be used before or concurrently with the fitting of the pessary in such patients.[9,10]

A pessary that is neglected can become embedded in vaginal mucosa and may be difficult to remove. In some cases, the use of estrogen cream may enable easier removal of the pessary by decreasing inflammation and promoting epithelial maturation.[11] In extreme and rare cases, the pessary must be removed surgically.[4] Even with a neglected, embedded pessary, the development of a fistula is extremely rare.[4]

In the patient with an improperly fitted ring pessary, the cervix and lower uterus can herniate through the open center of the ring and become incarcerated. If not recognized, this incarceration could lead to strangulation and necrosis of the cervix and uterus.[4]

While vaginal cytology may reveal inflammatory changes, the presence of a pessary does not increase the patient's risk of developing vaginal cancer.[4]

Is the pessary really useful?

Although many physicians are unfamiliar with the pessary, this useful gynecologic device has stood the test of time. Currently, family practice and obstetrics gynecology residencies include little education and training on the use of the pessary.[11] Incorporating the use of the pessary into a physician's practice requires minimal investment; however, it may significantly improve the lifestyle of patients who have limited therapeutic alternatives. The pessary is clearly a safe and useful treatment alternative for a number of gynecologic conditions that are seen by family physicians every day.

—by Anthony J. Viera, LT, MC, USNR
and Margaret Larkins-Pettigrew, LCDR, MC, USNR

References

1. Davila, G.W. Vaginal prolapse: management with nonsurgical techniques. *Postgraduate Medicine* 1996;99: 171-6,181,184-5.

2. Nygaard, I., DeLancey, J.O., Arnsdorf, L., Murphy, E. Exercise and incontinence. *Obstetrics and Gynecology* 1990; 75:848-51.

3. Nygaard, I. Prevention of exercise incontinence with mechanical devices. *Journal of Reproductive Medicine* 1995;40:89-94.

4. Miller, D.S. Contemporary use of the pessary. In: Sciarra, J.J., ed. *Gynecology and Obstetrics*. Revised 1997 ed. Philadelphia: Lippincott-Raven, 1997:1-12.

5. Zeitlin, M.P., Lebherz, T.B. Pessaries in the geriatric patient. *The Journal of the American Geriatrics Society* 1992;40:635-9.

6. Yarnell, J.W., Voyle, G.J., Richards, C.J., Stephenson, T.P. The prevalence and severity of urinary incontinence in women. *Journal of Epidemiology and Community Health* 1981; 35:71-4.

7. Davila, G.W., Ostermann, K.V. The bladder neck support prosthesis: a nonsurgical approach to stress incontinence in adult women. *The American Journal of Obstetrics and Gynecology* 1994;171:206-11.

8. Bhatia, N.N., Bergman, A. Pessary test in women with urinary incontinence. *Obstetrics and Gynecology* 1985;65: 220-6.

9. Brubacker, L. The vaginal pessary. In Friedman, A.J., ed. *American Urogynecologic Society Quarterly Report* 1991;9(3).

10. Deger, R.B., Menzin, A.W., Mikuta, J.J. The vaginal pessary: past and present. *Postgraduate Obstetrics and Gynecology* 1993;13(18):1-8.

11. Poma, P.A. Management of incarcerated vaginal pessaries. *The Journal of the American Geriatrics Society* 1981;29:325-7.

Chapter 21

Minimally Invasive Management of Urinary Incontinence

Urinary incontinence is a very common problem affecting as many as 13 million people in the United States. Many of these people suffer in silence unnecessarily, since incontinence can be managed or treated. The following information should help you discuss this condition with your urologist and what treatments are available to you.

What happens under normal conditions?

Coordinated activity between the urinary tract and the brain controls urinary function. The bladder stores urine because the smooth muscle of the bladder (detrusor muscle) relaxes and the bladder neck and urethral sphincter mechanism are closed. The urethral sphincter is a circular muscle that wraps around the urethra. During urination, the bladder neck opens, the sphincter relaxes and the bladder muscle contracts. Incontinence occurs if closure of the bladder neck is inadequate (stress incontinence) or the bladder muscle is overactive and contracts involuntarily (urge incontinence).

What is urinary incontinence?

Urinary incontinence is the involuntary loss of urine and is not necessarily a part of aging. It is a common condition experienced by men and women of all ages.

What are the different types of urinary incontinence?

Stress urinary incontinence: Stress incontinence is leakage that occurs when there is an increase in abdominal pressure caused by physical activities like coughing, laughing, sneezing, lifting, straining, getting out of a chair or bending over. The major risk factor for stress incontinence is damage to pelvic muscles that may occur during pregnancy and childbirth.

Urge urinary incontinence: Also referred to as "overactive bladder," this type of incontinence is usually accompanied by a sudden, strong urge to urinate and an inability to get to the toilet fast enough. Frequently, some patients with urge incontinence may leak urine with no warning. Risk factors for urge incontinence include aging, obstruction of urine flow, inconsistent emptying of the bladder, and a diet high in bladder irritants (such as coffee, tea, colas, chocolate and acidic fruit juices).

Mixed urinary incontinence: Mixed incontinence is a combination of urge and stress incontinence.

Overflow urinary incontinence: Overflow incontinence occurs when the bladder does not empty properly and the amount of urine produced exceeds the capacity of the bladder. It is characterized by frequent urination and dribbling. Poor bladder emptying occurs if there is an obstruction to flow or if the bladder muscle cannot contract effectively.

What is minimally invasive management of urinary incontinence?

Some of the causes of incontinence are temporary and easily reversible. Reversible causes include urinary tract infection, vaginal infection or irritation, medication, constipation, and restricted mobility. However, in some cases, further medical intervention is necessary. Minimally invasive treatment options are those treatments that do not involve surgery and should be the first line of treatment for patients. However, they may also be used in conjunction with surgical therapy.

Fluid management: This option consists of instructing a patient to increase or reduce their fluid intake. Incontinent patients may need to reduce the amount of caffeine or other dietary irritants (such as acidic fruit juices, colas, coffee, and tea), while at the same time increase water intake to produce an adequate amount of non-irritating, non-concentrated urine. A recommended water intake is six to eight glasses per day.

Bladder training: A diary is the starting point for bladder training. Patients are instructed to record fluid intake, urination times, and when their urinary accidents occur. The diary allows the patient to see how often they actually urinate and when incontinence occurs. The diary is also used to set time intervals for urination. Patients who urinate infrequently are instructed to do "timed urination" where they urinate by the clock every one to two hours during waking hours. By achieving regular bladder emptying they should have fewer incontinent episodes. Timed urination may be effective in patients with both urge and stress incontinence.

Bladder retraining: Bladder retraining is used for patients with urinary frequency. The goal of retraining is to increase the amount of urine that the patient can hold within their bladder. Patients are instructed to keep a diary to determine their urination interval. Patients are then instructed to gradually increase their urination interval by 15 to 30 minutes per week. The goal is to have patients urinating every two to four hours while awake with less urgency and less incontinence.

Pelvic floor exercises: Also known as Kegel exercises, this type of minimally invasive treatment focuses on strengthening the external sphincter muscle and the pelvic muscles. Patients who are able to contract and relax their pelvic floor muscles can improve their strength by doing the exercises regularly. Other patients require help from a healthcare professional to learn how to contract those muscles. Biofeedback and electrical stimulation can be used to aid patients in doing pelvic floor exercises. During electrical stimulation, a small amount of stimulation from a sensor placed in the vagina or rectum is delivered to the muscles of the pelvic floor. Like any exercise program, the patient must continue to do the exercises to maintain the benefit. Patients with stress incontinence benefit from pelvic floor exercises by increasing resistance at the urethra and by increasing the strength of the voluntary pelvic floor muscles. Patients can also be taught to compensate by contracting the pelvic muscles with certain activities like coughing.

Pelvic floor muscle exercises are effective for urge incontinence, since a contraction of the pelvic floor can interrupt a contraction of the bladder smooth muscle and stop or delay an accident.

Medicinal treatment: Stress incontinence may be treated with drugs that tighten the bladder neck, such as pseudoephedrine or imipramine. Just as pseudoephedrine causes constriction of the blood vessels in the nose, it also causes the muscles at the bladder neck to contract. Because of its effect on the smooth muscle in blood vessels, it should not be used in patients with a history of hypertension. Imipramine is a tricyclic antidepressant. In addition to causing the bladder muscle to relax, it also causes the smooth muscles at the bladder neck to contract. Urge incontinence is also treated with drugs that have anticholinergic properties. Anticholinergics allow for relaxation of the bladder smooth muscle. A commonly used anticholinergic is oxybutynin chloride. This drug works well to treat urge incontinence but has side effects including dry mouth, confusion, constipation, blurred vision and an inability to urinate. New drugs or new formulations of older drugs have been developed in an effort to reduce side effects. Oxybutynin is now formulated in a slow-release tablet taken once daily. The slow release of this new drug allows for a steady level of the drug and fewer side effects. Tolterodine tartrate is another new anticholinergic that is different than the older ones in that it has less effect on the salivary glands and therefore causes less dry mouth. It is also available in a slow-release, one-a-day form. Postmenopausal women with incontinence may benefit from hormone treatment. Normally the bladder neck and the urethra are closed at rest. With loss of estrogen, the tissues become weakened or dried and normal closure is lost. Hormone replacement improves the health of these tissues and allows for closure to be regained through increased tone and improved blood supply. [Recent studies have raised questions about the use of hormone replacement therapy in treating incontinence in postmenopausal women. See Chapter 19, "Urinary Incontinence in Women," for more information.]

What can be expected from minimally invasive treatment for urinary incontinence?

Minimally invasive therapies can lead to improvement in incontinence but not necessarily a cure. Improvement generally does not occur overnight. Patients need time to adapt to behavioral changes. Results with pelvic floor exercises may take three to six months. Some patients may notice an immediate effect with medical therapy, whereas in others an effect may not be seen for approximately four weeks. Incontinence may also recur after treatment. Continuing behavioral techniques or continuing or resuming pharmacologic treatment as well as practicing preventive strategies may prevent such recurrence. Incontinence may also be prevented by good toileting habits including regular urination, pelvic floor exercises, avoidance of constipation, avoidance of bladder irritants, and adequate water intake.

Frequently Asked Questions

What should I do if I suffer from incontinence?

Talk to your healthcare provider. Incontinence can sometimes be treated by a primary care physician or it may be necessary for you to see a urologist who specializes in treating incontinence. You can help your doctor by bringing a list of your medications to your appointment. Prior to the appointment, you might want to record for two to four days the amount and type of liquids that you consume, the number of times you urinate and the number of accidents you have.

What can I do about my incontinence prior to being seen by a healthcare provider?

You can urinate every two to three hours during the day, drink six to eight glasses of water, avoid bladder irritants (e.g., coffee, tea, colas, chocolate and acidic fluid juices), avoid constipation, and do pelvic floor exercises.

What foods or drinks are irritating to the bladder?

Caffeine is a common bladder irritant but there are other substances that can also cause bladder irritation. Not all incontinent patients are bothered by certain foods or drinks. The only way to know if diet is a factor is to eliminate possible irritants and see if continence is improved. Some of the most common bladder irritants are: alcohol, carbonated beverages (with and without caffeine), coffee or tea (with and without caffeine), chocolate, citrus fruits, tomatoes, and acidic fruit juices.

How do I know if I am doing pelvic floor exercises properly?

When you do pelvic floor exercises only the pelvic floor should move. The pelvic floor muscles are tightened as if you wanted to stop urinating midstream or stop the passage of gas. The abdominal, buttock or leg muscles should not be tightened. By doing the exercises in front of a mirror or by placing a hand on the abdominal or buttock muscles you will be able to tell if you are contracting any of the wrong muscles. If the exercises are done properly, they can be done anywhere. There are written instructions available from support groups or from your healthcare provider.

Could any of my medications be causing my incontinence?

Certain types of medications can cause or exacerbate incontinence. These medications include diuretics, sedatives, narcotics, antidepressants, antihistamines, calcium channel-blockers, and alpha-blockers.

Will my incontinence get worse as I continue to get older?

Your urinary incontinence will not necessarily get worse, but it also will not improve without treatment.

I have a small amount of incontinence very infrequently that doesn't bother me. Is this abnormal and do I need to be treated?

Any leakage of urine is abnormal. You should consider treatment if your incontinence prevents you from doing the activities that you want to do. Although pads or diapers may prevent embarrassing accidents, there are other treatment options currently available that can eliminate your need to wear such protection.

Chapter 22

Surgical Techniques to Treat Incontinence

Chapter Contents

Section 22.1

Surgical Management of Urinary Incontinence

Bladder control is a common yet complex problem that can seriously affect a person's life. Fortunately, with today's high-tech procedures and powerful drugs, a diagnosis may simply mean the road to
bladder control is challenging, rather than impossible. So read below
to learn more about the available treatment options so you are better prepared when talking with your urologist.

What can be expected under normal conditions?

The urinary tract is similar to a plumbing system, with special
pipes that allow water and salts to flow through them. The urinary
tract includes the kidneys, two ureters, the bladder and the urethra.

The kidneys act as a filtration system for the blood, cleansing it of
poisonous materials and retaining valuable glucose, salts, and minerals. Urine, the waste product of the filtration, is produced in the kidney and flows through two 10- to 12-inch long tubes called the ureters,
which connect the kidneys to the bladder. The ureters are about one-
fourth of an inch in diameter and their muscular walls contract to
make waves of movement that force the urine into the bladder. The
bladder is expandable and stores the urine until it can be conveniently
disposed of. It also is a one-way flap valve that allows unimpeded urinary flow into the bladder but prevents urine from flowing backward
(vesicoureteral reflux) into the kidneys. It also closes passageways into
the ureters so that urine cannot flow back into the kidneys. The tube
through which the urine flows out of the body is called the urethra.

What is urinary incontinence?

Urinary incontinence is the involuntary loss of urine. It is not a
disease but rather a symptom that can be caused by a wide range of

conditions. Incontinence can be caused by diabetes, a stroke, multiple sclerosis, Parkinson disease, some surgeries or even childbirth. More than 15 million Americans, mostly women, suffer from incontinence. Although it is more common in women over 60, it can occur at any age. Most healthcare professionals classify incontinence by its symptoms or circumstances in which it occurs. In the normal population, the incidence of incontinence in the female over 65 is more than 25 percent and in the male it is about 15 percent.

What are the various types of urinary incontinence?

Stress incontinence: Stress urinary incontinence is the most common type of leakage. This occurs when urine is lost during activities such as walking, aerobics or even sneezing and coughing. The added abdominal pressure associated with these events can cause urine to leak. The pelvic floor muscles, which support the bladder and urethra, can be weakened, thus preventing the sphincter muscles from working properly. This can also occur if the sphincter muscles themselves are weakened or damaged from previous childbirth or surgical trauma. Menopausal women can also suffer from small amounts of leakage as a result of decreased estrogen levels. In men, the most common cause of incontinence is surgery on the prostate. This is more frequent after radical prostatectomy for cancer than after transurethral surgery for BPH.

Urge incontinence: Also referred to as "overactive bladder," urge incontinence is another form of leakage. This can happen when a person has an uncontrollable urge to urinate but cannot reach the bathroom in time and has an accident. At other times, running water or cold weather can cause such an event. Some people have no warning and experience leakage just by changing body position (e.g., getting out of bed). Overactive bladder is also associated with strokes, multiple sclerosis, and spinal cord injuries.

Overflow incontinence: This type of incontinence occurs when the bladder is full, is unable to empty and yet leaks. Frequent small urinations and constant dribbling are symptoms. This is rare in women and more common in men with a history of surgery or prostate problems.

Functional incontinence: This type of incontinence is the inability to access a proper facility or urinal container because of physical or mental disability.

Mixed incontinence: Mixed incontinence refers to a combination of types of incontinence, most commonly stress and urge incontinence.

How is the diagnosis made?

As with any medical problem, a good history and physical examination are critical. A urologist will first ask questions about the individual's habits and fluid intake as well as their family, medical and surgical history. A thorough pelvic examination looking for correctable reasons for leakage, including impacted stool, constipation, and hernias will be conducted. Usually a urinalysis and cough stress test will be conducted at the first evaluation. If some findings suggest further evaluation, other tests may be recommended—such as a cystoscopy or even urodynamic testing. This outpatient test is usually done with a tiny tube in the bladder inserted through the urethra and sometimes with a small rectal tube, as well.

What are some treatment options for each type of incontinence?

In most cases of incontinence, minimally invasive management (fluid management, bladder training, pelvic floor exercises, and medication) is prescribed. However, if that fails, surgical treatment can be necessary.

Stress incontinence: One of the surgical treatments for this condition in males is the use of urethral injections of bulking agents to improve the function of the sphincter. The injections are done under local anesthesia and can be repeated. Unfortunately, the cure rate is only 10 to 30 percent. Another alternative is to perform a urethral compression procedure with the use of a vascular graft or a segment of cadaveric tissue to compress the urethra in the area between the scrotum and the rectum. The results are very preliminary and at this time only experimental. The most effective treatment for male incontinence is implantation of an artificial sphincter. The device is inserted under the skin and consists of a cuff around the urethra, a fluid-filled, pressure-regulating balloon in the abdomen and a pump in the scrotum which is controlled by the patient. The fluid in the abdominal balloon is transferred to the urethra cuff, closing the urethra and preventing leakage of urine.

Stress incontinence in the female is treated at the beginning with behavior modification and pelvic exercise. Sometime techniques like biofeedback or electrical stimulation of the pelvic muscles can help. But when the symptoms are more severe and conservative measures are not helping the treatment is surgery. In selected cases bulking agents can be used to increase continence. The operation is done under local anesthesia and is minimally invasive but the cure rates are lower compared to open surgical procedures.

Anterior repair (Kelly plication) is a common option used by gynecologists but has not given good long-term results. Another option is abdominal surgery (Burch suspension) in which the vaginal tissues are affixed to the pubic bone. The long-term results are good but the surgery requires longer recuperation time and is generally only used when other abdominal surgeries are also required. The most common and most popular surgery for stress incontinence is the sling procedure. In this operation a strip of tissue is applied under the urethra to provide compression and improve urethral closure. The operation is minimally invasive and patients recuperate very quickly. The tissue used to create the sling can be a segment of the patient's abdominal wall, specially treated fascia, skin from a cadaver or a synthetic material.

Urge incontinence: For urge incontinence there is a large array of treatment options available. The first step should be behavior modification—drinking less fluids; avoiding caffeine, alcohol or spices; not drinking at bedtime and urinating around the clock and not at the last moment. Exercising the pelvic muscle (Kegel exercises) also helps. It is important to keep a log on the frequency of urination, number of accidents, the amount lost, the fluid intake and the number of pads used if required. The mainstay of treatment for overactive bladder is medication. This consists of the use of bladder relaxants that prevent the bladder from contracting without the patient's permission. The most common side effect of the medication is dryness of the mouth, constipation or changes in vision. Sometimes, reduction of medication takes care of the side effects.

Other alternatives can be considered in patients who fail to respond to behavior modification and/or medication. A new and exiting technology is the use of a bladder pacemaker to control bladder function. This technology consists of a small electrode that is inserted in the patient's back close to the nerve that controls bladder function. The electrode is connected to a pulse generator and the electrical impulses control bladder function. There is more than 60 to 75 percent cure or improvement with this technology. In more difficult cases, the bladder can be made bigger using a segment of small intestine. This operation, called augmentation cystoplasty, is very successful in curing incontinence but its main drawback is the need in 10 to 30 percent of the patients to perform self-catheterization to empty their bladder.

Overflow incontinence: For overflow incontinence, the treatment is to completely empty the bladder and prevent urine leakage. Patients with diabetic bladder or patients with prostatic obstruction often develop this type of incontinence. Overflow incontinence due to obstruction should be treated with medication or surgery to remove the blockage. If no blockage is found, the best treatment is to instruct the patient to perform self-catheterization a few times a day. By emptying the bladder regularly the incontinence disappears and the kidneys are protected.

What can be expected after treatment?

The goal of any treatment for incontinence is to improve quality of life for the patient. In most cases, great improvements and even cure of the symptoms are possible. Medical therapy is usually effective, but not if the patient sips fluids all day and does not time their urination. Similarly, large shifts in weight gain and activities that promote abdominal and pelvic straining put any repair to the test and cannot be expected to stand the test of time. Positive, long-term outcomes can almost be assured with common sense, proper body mechanics, and care.

Medical treatment of overactive bladder (urgency and urge incontinence) can be very successful, but factors like prior surgery, lack of hormones, neurological conditions, and age may make the treatment less effective. There are mild complications from medications, including constipation and dryness of the mouth that some patients cannot tolerate. Surgery, like the insertion of a bladder pacemaker, can result in 50 to 70 percent cure or great improvement of the symptoms. Enlargement of the bladder using a segment of intestine may cure the urgency incontinence in more than 80 percent of the cases but the main drawback is the need in 10 to 30 percent of the patients to perform self-catheterization for the rest of their life. It is sometimes the only choice when other treatments fail.

Surgery for urinary incontinence in the male like the artificial sphincter can cure or greatly improve more than 70 to 80 percent of the patients. Prior radiation, bladder malfunction, and/or scar tissue in the urethra may result in a deterioration of the results. Being a mechanical device, it may require modification over time.

Surgery for urinary incontinence (stress incontinence) in the female is in general very successful, but choosing the proper procedure is important. Many patients with stress incontinence also have other conditions like bladder prolapse, rectocele or uterine prolapse that must be treated at the same time. The combination of urgency incontinence symptoms requires medical treatment first to try to improve the symptoms. The procedure of choice will depend on multiple factors, like the need for abdominal surgery for other conditions, the degree of incontinence, the degree of mobility of the urethra and bladder and the surgeon's personal experience. For simple stress incontinence with mild to moderate urethral incontinence, a sling is the procedure of choice. The patient can expect more than 80 to 90 percent cure or great improvement. Injectables can cure 30 percent of patients but may require multiple applications.

Frequently Asked Questions

What is a bulking agent?

It is a substance used to inject under the urethra to improve urinary continence.

What is an artificial sphincter?

An artificial sphincter is a patient-controlled device made of silicone rubber that has:

- an inflatable cuff that fits around the tube through which urine leaves the body (urethra) close to the point where it joins the bladder.
- a balloon that regulates the pressure of the cuff.
- a bulb to control inflation and deflation of the cuff.

The balloon is placed within the pelvic space, and the control bulb is placed in the scrotum of a male or the external vaginal lips of a female.

The cuff is inflated to keep urine from leaking. When urination is desired, the cuff is deflated, allowing urine to drain out.

What are bladder relaxants?

They are medications used to improve the urgency and frequency of urination.

Section 22.2

Bladder Augmentation

The bladder is a balloon-like organ in the lower half of the abdomen, which stores urine and expels urine when it is full. If the bladder isn't large enough to hold the usual amount of urine made by the kidneys, a bladder augmentation may be necessary.

What happens under normal conditions?

The urinary tract is made up of two kidneys, two ureters, a bladder, and a urethra. The kidneys are located just below the ribs and filter blood, retaining valuable glucose, salts, minerals, and removing waste (urine) from the body. The urine flows from the kidneys through two long tubes called the ureters, and then collects in the bladder.

The bladder is expandable such that it can store urine until it can be conveniently emptied. When one urinates, the bladder empties, and the urine flows through the urethra out of the body.

What is bladder augmentation?

Bladder augmentation is an operation performed to increase the size of the bladder. This type of surgery is for patients whose bladder is not large enough to hold the usual amount of urine made by the kidneys. In some patients, the urine may leak from the bladder, causing wetting (incontinence).

For other patients, the bladder muscle may lose its ability to stretch (expand). If this happens, pressure within the bladder can become too high. This increased pressure may be harmful to the kidneys because urine may not drain properly. This may cause the urine to back up through the ureters all the way to the kidneys. This backup is called reflux.

The result of any of the scenarios listed above may be urinary tract infections and possible kidney damage.

How is bladder augmentation performed?

Bladder augmentation is performed to increase the size of the bladder and to improve its ability to stretch (expand). A section of the bowel or stomach is used. During the operation, the surgeon makes an incision in the abdomen (belly) and the top of the bladder is opened so that it can be made larger. A section is removed from the bowel or stomach, which is placed over the opening in the bladder as a patch, and then sewn into place.

What can be expected after bladder augmentation?

Following a bladder augmentation, the bladder may not be able to expel the stored urine by itself. As a result, many patients must learn to pass a tube backwards through the urethra into the bladder to catheterize themselves, so that they can empty the bladder if they cannot drain it by urinating alone. This is called clean intermittent catheterization (CIC). If the bladder cannot empty itself it is important to pass a tube (catheter) regularly so that the bladder does not over expand and rupture.

Before bladder augmentation surgery, routine tests are done to measure the function and structure of the bladder and kidneys. These tests may include blood tests, x-rays and bladder pressure studies (urodynamics). The same tests may be done after surgery to make sure that the bladder is healing.

Frequently Asked Questions

How does a patient get ready for surgery?

A few days before surgery, the patient may need to start a low fiber diet and begin taking antibiotics to prepare the bowel for surgery. The day before surgery the patient comes to the hospital and the doctor may recommend that the patient have clear liquids only.

What is a bowel prep, also known as a "clean out"?

A bowel prep, or "clean out," is cleansing of the bowel using a special liquid. The liquid comes in the form of a drink that can be swallowed or dripped into the stomach through a narrow tube called a nasogastric tube. During this cleansing, patients should expect to have several loose stools. The bowel prep may take four to six hours to complete. When the stools are clear and watery, the bowel prep is finished.

Why is a bowel prep needed?

A bowel prep may be necessary to prevent infection. It makes the bowel as clean and free of contamination as possible.

When will the patient be able to eat and drink after the surgery?

The patient will not be able to eat or drink for as long as one week after surgery. The patient will receive all fluids, "food" and medicines through an IV tube in the arm. The doctors and nurses will listen to the abdomen each day. Soon after the lower belly begins to make "gurgle" sounds again, the patient may be ready to start eating but this will be determined by the doctor. The patient will start with clear fluids, and soon afterwards, will be able to eat regular food again.

When will the patient be able to go back to school or work?

Most children and young adults are ready to return to school or work within a few weeks after leaving the hospital. However, each person is different, and some may not be ready to resume regular activities until three to four weeks after leaving the hospital.

Chapter 23

New Developments for Treating Incontinence

What is incontinence?

Incontinence is the inability to control the passage of urine or stool. Current figures indicate that 20 million Americans suffer with involuntary loss of bladder control (urinary incontinence) and that 10 percent of these people also have problems with bowel control (fecal incontinence).

Often, embarrassment and the stigma associated with incontinence prevent the person from seeking treatment, even when incontinence threatens his or her quality-of-life and that of his or her family.

Urinary and fecal incontinence can be cured or significantly improved once the underlying cause has been detected. However, it's important to recognize that incontinence is a symptom and not a disease. Its cause may be quite complex and involve many factors. Your physician should complete an in-depth evaluation before beginning treatment.

What can I do to address this problem?

Getting help means taking the first step. See your doctor. Diagnostic tests for incontinence can be completed in the outpatient setting and are not painful. Once these tests have confirmed the cause of your incontinence, your physician can make specific recommendations for treatment, many of which do not require surgery. No matter how serious the problem seems, incontinence is a condition that can be significantly helped and, in most cases, cured.

How can incontinence be treated?

Urinary incontinence can be caused by many different factors. Your physician will suggest a treatment plan after considering these factors and your specific symptoms. Common treatments for urge and stress incontinence, two common types of incontinence, are described below.

Urge incontinence is an urgent desire to void, which is followed by an involuntary loss of urine. This condition can be caused by an "overactive" bladder. Normally, strong muscles (sphincters) control the flow of urine from the bladder. The muscle of an "overactive" bladder spasms (contracts) with enough force to override the sphincter muscles of the urethra and allow urine to pass out of the bladder.

Medications: Medications can work very well to return normal function to the bladder. The type of medication used should also be chosen for your specific needs. Your physician may prescribe a low dose and then gradually increase the dose. In this way, he or she can evaluate how well the drug is working and reduce your risk of experiencing side effects. Your physician should discuss with you the risks and benefits of using medications. Common medications used include the following:

- Anticholinergic medications (these medications control muscle spasms in the bladder)
  - Oxybutynin (Ditropan), Oxybutynin XL (Ditropan XL), Oxybutynin TDDS [transdermal drug delivery system] (Oxytrol)
  - Propantheline (Pro-Banthine)
  - Dicyclomine (Antispas, Bentyl, Di-Spaz, Dibent, Or-Tyl, Spasmoject)
  - Tolterodine (Detrol)
- Antidepressant medication
  - Imipramine (Norfranil, Tipramine, Tofranil)

Self-help techniques include the following:

- Empty your bladder regularly, especially before physical activity.
- Avoid drinking caffeine or a lot of fluid before activities.
- Avoid lifting heavy objects.
- Practice Kegel exercises.
- Practice timed voidings. (Go to the bathroom on a regular schedule rather than waiting for the urge.)

The following aids are used with self-help techniques:

- **Perineometer:** This device is used to measure the force of the sphincter muscles.
- **Vaginal cones (for women):** The woman inserts a tampon-shaped cone into the vagina and holds it in place by contracting the pelvic muscles. As the muscles get stronger, the weight of the cone is increased.
- **Electrical stimulation:** Mild electrical impulses are used to stimulate contractions of the pelvic floor muscles. Devices for electrical stimulation can be implanted near the spine or activated by the urethra, vagina or rectum (non-implanted devices). Electrical stimulation can be used for incontinence that does or does not involve neurological problems.
- **Biofeedback:** In biofeedback devices are used to help you see the strength of your contractions. Biofeedback can help you learn how to perform Kegel exercises.

Surgery: Your physician may recommend surgery if other treatments fail to improve your symptoms. Surgical procedures for urge incontinence can be used to:

- Increase the storage capacity of the bladder (hydro-distention).
- Limit nerve impulses to the control muscles (denervation).
- Divert the flow of urine.
- Neuromodulation (modulate nerve to bladder/penis).

Stress incontinence occurs when an activity such as a cough or sneeze increases abdominal pressure on the bladder. Typically, a small amount of urine leaks from the urethra. This problem can result from a number of factors, including weak muscles of the pelvic floor, a weak sphincter muscle at the neck of the bladder, or a problem with the way the sphincter muscle opens and closes. Women who have given birth are more likely to have stress incontinence.

Treatments for stress incontinence: Self-help techniques and aids as previously described, can be used to treat mild stress incontinence.

Bulking agents: Bulking agents are substances that are injected into the lining of the urethra. They increase the size of the lining of the urethra, which creates resistance against the flow of urine. Collagen is one bulking agent commonly used.

Surgery: When these methods fail, surgery may be an option. Surgery is now minimally invasive and an outpatient procedure in the majority of the cases. Surgery can be used to:

- Increase resistance in the urethra.
- Implant an artificial sphincter.
- Tighten the pelvic floor muscles.
- Change pressure within the urethra using an implant device.

Kegel exercises: Kegel exercises, also called pelvic floor exercises, help strengthen the muscles that support the bladder, uterus and bowels. By strengthening these muscles, you can reduce or prevent problems such as leaking urine.

How to do Kegel exercises: Imagine you are trying to stop the flow of urine or trying not to pass gas. When you do this, you are contracting the muscles of the pelvic floor and are practicing Kegel exercises. While doing Kegel exercises, try not to move your leg, buttock or abdominal muscles. In fact, no one should be able to tell that you are doing Kegel exercises.

Kegel exercises should be done every day. We [The Cleveland Clinic] recommend doing five sets of Kegel exercises a day. Each time you contract the muscles of the pelvic floor, hold for a slow count of five and then relax. Repeat this ten times for one set of Kegels.

Part Four

Disorders of the Ureters, Urethra, and Genitals

Chapter 24

Congenital Defects of the Urinary Tract and Genitals

Chapter Contents

Section 24.1

Birth Defects of the Genitals and Urinary Tract

There are many birth defects that involve the genitals and urinary tract. These defects can affect the kidneys (organs that filter wastes from the blood and form urine), ureters (tubes leading from the kidneys to the bladder), bladder (sac that holds urine), urethra (the tube that drains urine out of the body from the bladder), and the male and female genitals. For boys, the genitals include the penis, prostate gland, and testes. For girls, the genitals include the vagina, uterus, fallopian tubes, and ovaries.

Abnormalities of the genitals and urinary tract are among the most common birth defects, affecting as many as one in ten babies. Some of these abnormalities are minor problems that may cause no symptoms (such as having two ureters leading from one kidney to the bladder), and go undiagnosed unless the child has an x-ray, ultrasound examination or surgery for a related or unrelated problem. Other abnormalities can cause problems such as urinary tract infections, blockages, pain, and kidney damage or failure.

What is the cause of genital and urinary tract defects?

A few genital and urinary tract defects or disorders are inherited from parents who have the disorder or carry the gene for it. Specific causes of most of these conditions are unknown, however. Genetics and environmental factors presumably play various roles during development of these organs. A family with an affected child should consult a genetic counselor, geneticist or a physician who is familiar with genetic disorders. These experts can discuss what is known about the cause of the specific defect and what the risks may be that the defect or disorder will occur again in subsequent offspring.

How are urinary tract defects diagnosed?

Many urinary tract defects can be diagnosed before or after birth with an ultrasound examination, which uses sound waves to examine internal organs of the fetus. After birth, ultrasound and/or a number of other tests may be recommended to provide more information on how well the kidneys and other urinary tract structures are functioning.

What are the most common urinary tract defects?

Some of the most common urinary tract defects include: renal agenesis, hydronephrosis, polycystic kidney disease, multicystic kidneys, low urinary tract obstruction, bladder exstrophy and epispadias, hypospadias, and ambiguous genitals.

What is renal agenesis?

Renal agenesis is the absence of one or both kidneys. About 1 in 4,000 babies is born with neither kidney (bilateral renal agenesis). Tragically, about one-third of these babies are stillborn and the rest die in the first days of life. There is no treatment that can save them.

Babies with bilateral renal agenesis often have birth defects affecting other organs, such as the heart and lungs. A fetus that has no kidneys cannot produce urine, a major part of the amniotic fluid that is crucial for normal fetal lung expansion and development. Therefore, most of these deaths result from underdeveloped lungs. Lack of amniotic fluid also contributes to the abnormal facial features and limb defects seen in these babies.

Up to 20 times as many babies (about one in 550) are born with a single kidney (unilateral renal agenesis). These babies often can live normal lives, although they may be at increased risk for kidney infections, kidney stones, high blood pressure, and kidney failure. Some affected babies, however, have other birth defects involving the urinary tract, genitals or other organs. These children may face a variety of health problems, depending upon the specific birth defects involved.

What is hydronephrosis?

Hydronephrosis involves swelling of one or both kidneys, with accumulation of urine that cannot flow out of the kidney(s) because of a blockage somewhere in the urinary tract. Significant hydronephrosis is diagnosed in about 1 in 500 pregnancies during a prenatal ultrasound examination.

The blockage that causes hydronephrosis often is caused by a flap of tissue near where urine empties from the bladder (posterior urethral valves). In severe cases, the fetus's bladder becomes swollen with urine, and the urine backs up and may damage or destroy the kidneys. When hydronephrosis is diagnosed before birth, the doctor will monitor the fetus with repeated ultrasound examinations to see if the condition is worsening. Some babies with severe hydronephrosis are sick at birth, with breathing problems, urinary tract infections, and kidney failure. Once these problems have been treated, the urinary blockage can be surgically corrected (although some kidney damage may remain). Many mild cases of hydronephrosis resolve without surgery.

Occasionally, hydronephrosis can become life-threatening before birth. In such cases, a small tube called a shunt may be inserted into the fetus's bladder to drain urine into the amniotic fluid until birth, when the blockage can be repaired. Prenatal treatment of these obstructions has been the most successful form of fetal surgery to date.

Urinary blockages also commonly occur where the ureter connects to the kidney (ureteropelvic junction obstruction). This condition varies in severity, with some cases causing kidney failure in newborns and infants, and others improving without treatment. Surgery often is recommended in the first year or two of life to relieve the obstruction and prevent further kidney damage, urinary tract infections, and pain.

What is polycystic kidney disease?

Polycystic kidney disease (PKD) is an inherited disorder that results in the growth of numerous cysts in the kidneys, reduced kidney function and, often, kidney failure. There are two main forms of the disorder: autosomal dominant and autosomal recessive PKD. Besides kidney failure, both forms can cause frequent urinary tract infections, pain, high blood pressure, and other problems.

Autosomal dominant PKD is one of the most common genetic disorders, affecting between 1 in 200 and 1 in 1,000 individuals of all ages. It most often is inherited from a parent who has the disease, although up to one-quarter of cases occur in individuals without a family history of the disease. Symptoms usually begin between the ages of 30 and 40, although children can sometimes be affected.

Autosomal recessive PKD is a rare form of the disease that affects children, with cysts sometimes developing before birth. About 1 in 10,000 to 1 in 40,000 babies are born with the disorder. Severely affected babies die in the first days of life, while others with a milder version may live into their teens or twenties. This form of PKD is inherited when both parents (who are unaffected) pass along the gene for the disorder to their child.

Drug treatment can control PKD-related problems such as high blood pressure and urinary tract infections. If kidney failure develops, the patient is treated regularly with a procedure called dialysis that does the kidney's job to cleanse the blood, and sometimes treated with a kidney transplant.

Kidney cysts are a feature of certain other disorders. These include multicystic kidneys, which affect about 1 in 4,000 babies. This disorder, which varies greatly in severity, can cause death in the newborn period when both kidneys are affected. It is believed that multicystic kidneys result from an obstruction in the urinary tract during the early stages of development. Babies with only one affected kidney may have few consequences, such as urinary tract infections. While the affected kidney often does not function (and, in some cases, may need to be removed), an affected child can live a normal life with one healthy kidney.

Kidney cysts also can be a feature of a number of genetic syndromes. In many cases, such cysts cause few or no problems.

What are bladder exstrophy and epispadias?

Bladder exstrophy is a malformation of the bladder in which the bladder is turned inside out and located on the outside of the abdomen. In addition, the skin on the lower abdomen does not form properly, the pelvic bones are widely spaced, and there may be genital abnormalities. Bladder exstrophy, which occurs in about 1 in 30,000 births, affects boys about five times more often than girls.

Epispadias is a related defect involving the urethra and genitals. It often accompanies bladder exstrophy, but may occur by itself. In boys, the urethra often is short and split, with an opening on the upper surface of the penis. The penis itself appears short and flat. In girls, the clitoris may be split, and the urinary opening also is abnormally placed. Up to half of children with epispadias have bladder control problems.

Bladder exstrophy and epispadias can be repaired surgically. Many affected children require a number of surgeries over the first several years of life to achieve bladder control and normal-appearing genitals. In children with bladder exstrophy, the first surgery usually is performed within 48 hours of birth to close the bladder and replace it in the pelvis, close the abdominal wall and bring the pelvic bones into their correct position. Genital repair often is done during this procedure in girls, but repair of the penis usually is done at between the ages of one and two years. Additional surgery to control urine leakage may be done around three years of age. Studies show that about 85 percent of affected children can control their bladders following these surgeries.

What is hypospadias?

Hypospadias is a common birth defect of the penis that affects nearly one percent of baby boys. The urethra does not extend to the tip of the penis; instead, the opening of the urethra is located somewhere along the underside of the penis.

Hypospadias generally is diagnosed during the newborn examination in the hospital nursery. Affected boys should not be circumcised because the foreskin (which is removed by circumcision) may be needed to help surgically repair the defect. Surgery, which extends the urethra to the tip of the penis, usually is performed between the ages of 9 and 15 months. Without surgery, most affected boys would have to urinate sitting down and, as adults, would suffer pain during intercourse.

What are ambiguous genitals?

Babies who are born with ambiguous genitals have external genital organs that do not appear clearly male or female, or have features of both. For example, a girl may be born with a large clitoris that resembles a penis, or a boy may have testicles with female-like external genitals. An estimated 1 in 1,000 to 1 in 2,000 babies are affected.

There are many causes of ambiguous genitals, including chromosomal and genetic disorders, hormonal disturbances, enzyme deficiencies, and unexplained abnormalities of the fetal tissues that are destined to become the genitals. The most common cause of ambiguous genitals is an inherited disorder called congenital adrenal hyperplasia (CAH) which, in severe forms, also can disturb kidney function and may cause death. CAH involves an enzyme deficiency that causes the adrenal glands to produce excess amounts of male hormones (androgens). The excess androgens cause the clitoris of a girl with CAH to grow too large, resembling a penis. The disorder, which can be diagnosed with blood tests, requires lifelong treatment with the missing hormones. Affected girls may require surgery to correct the appearance of their genitals. (CAH can be diagnosed before birth with a prenatal test called chorionic villus sampling, allowing for prenatal drug treatment that sometimes can prevent genital defects.)

Another common cause of ambiguous genitals is androgen insensitivity syndrome. Affected babies have male chromosomes (XY) but, due to genetic defects, their cells do not respond or respond incompletely to androgens (male hormones). Babies with complete androgen insensitivity have testes (which usually remain inside the abdomen) and female external genitals, although they do not have a uterus or ovaries. These children are almost always raised as girls and have a completely normal female appearance, although they need treatment with hormones to undergo pubertal changes. Babies with partial androgen sensitivity have cells that partially respond to androgens, and often have ambiguous external genitals.

A number of chromosomal abnormalities also can result in ambiguous genitals. These include gonadal dysgenesis, in which the baby has normal male chromosomes (XY), with either female internal and external genital organs, or ambiguous external genitals and some combination of male and female internal organs.

When a child is born with ambiguous genitals, various diagnostic studies need to be done in an attempt to define the baby's gender. These will include physical examination, blood tests (including chromosomal analysis and measurement of the levels of various hormones), urine tests and, sometimes, ultrasound examination or surgery to look at the internal organs. A team of medical specialists will use these tests to help determine whether the baby is developing more like a male or female, and may recommend assigning a gender for the baby. They may then recommend hormone therapy or reconstructive surgery on the genitals. Doctors often recommended that a boy with a very underdeveloped penis and other genital ambiguities undergo reconstructive surgery and be raised as a girl. More recently, in such cases, doctors are somewhat more likely to suggest that the parents raise the child as a girl, but to hold off on surgery to see how the child is developing—and, very importantly, whether the child feels more like a boy or girl. These situations can be extremely difficult for the child and family, so ongoing psychological counseling is strongly recommended.

References

Bernstein, J. The kidneys and the urinary tract, in: Rudolph, A.M. et al (eds.), *Rudolph's Pediatrics*, 20th edition. Stamford, CT, Appleton & Lange, 1996, pages 1347-1405.

Fausto-Sterling, A. The five sexes revisited. *The Sciences*, July/August 2000, pages 19-23.

Hendricks, M. Into the hands of babes. *Johns Hopkins Magazine*, September 2000, pages 12-17.

National Institute of Diabetes and Digestive and Kidney Diseases. *Polycystic Kidney Disease.* NIH Publication No. 96-4008, 1998.

Thomas, D.F.M. *Urological Disease in the Fetus and Infant: Diagnosis and Management.* Oxford, England, Butterworth Heinemann, 1997.

Section 24.2

Ureterocele

Most of us are born with two ureters, one to drain the urine from each kidney into the bladder. Yet what if the portion of the ureter closest to the bladder becomes enlarged because the ureter opening is very tiny and obstructs urine outflow? That is the case for people with a ureterocele. Luckily, medicine has given urologists a range of diagnostic tests and surgical techniques to deal with this abnormality. So read below to see how your urologist might correct this condition.

What happens under normal conditions?

Within the urinary tract, the kidneys filter and remove waste and water from the blood to produce urine. The urine travels from the kidneys down two narrow tubes called the ureters, where it is then stored in the bladder. Normally, the attachment between the ureters and the bladder is a one-way flap valve that allows unimpeded urinary flow into the bladder but prevents urine from flowing backward (vesicoureteral reflux) into the kidneys. Approximately one out of 125 people may have two ureters draining a single kidney. One ureter drains the upper part of the kidney and the second ureter drains the lower portion. This "duplicated collecting system" is not a problem as long as each ureter enters the bladder normally. When the bladder empties, urine flows out of the body through the urethra, a tube at the bottom of the bladder. The opening of the urethra is at the end of the penis in boys and in front of the vagina in girls.

What is a ureterocele?

A ureterocele is a birth defect that affects the kidney, ureter, and bladder. When a person has a ureterocele, the portion of the ureter closest to the bladder swells up like a balloon because the ureter opening is very tiny and obstructs urine outflow. As the urine flow is obstructed, urine backs up in the ureter. Approximately one in 2,000 persons are affected by this condition. In 90 percent of girls the ureterocele occurs in the upper half of a duplicated urinary tract. Approximately half of boys have a duplicated urinary tract and half have a single system. Ureteroceles may be "ectopic" when a portion protrudes through the bladder outlet into the urethra, or "orthotopic" when they remain entirely within the bladder. In five to ten percent of cases there is a ureterocele on both sides (bilateral). The majority of ureteroceles are diagnosed in children less than two years of age, although occasionally older children or adults are found to have a ureterocele.

What are some complications of a ureterocele?

This condition often predisposes an individual to a kidney infection. Vesicoureteral reflux is also common, particularly in individuals with a duplication of the urinary tract, because the ureterocele distorts the normal one-way valve attachment between the ureter and bladder. In addition, reflux on the opposite side is common for similar reasons. In rare cases, a ureterocele may prevent the passage of kidney stones. Also, the ureterocele may be so large that it completely obstructs the flow of urine from the bladder into the urethra. Occasionally, in girls, the ureterocele may sink and protrude out from the opening of the urethra.

What are some symptoms of a ureterocele?

Symptoms can include flank or back pain, urinary tract infection, fever, painful urination, foul-smelling urine, abdominal pain, blood in the urine (hematuria), and/or excessive urination.

How is a ureterocele diagnosed?

Although doctors can and often do detect ureteroceles during prenatal ultrasounds, they may not be diagnosed until a patient is being evaluated for another medical condition like a urinary tract infection.

Ultrasonography is the first imaging test used in evaluation. Additional imaging studies may also be necessary to help delineate the anatomy. One such test is a voiding cystourethrogram (VCUG), which is an x-ray examination of the bladder and lower urinary tract. A catheter is inserted through the urethra, the bladder is filled with a water-soluble dye, and then the catheter is withdrawn. Several x-ray images of the bladder and urethra are captured as the patient empties the bladder. These images allow radiologists to diagnose any abnormalities in the flow of urine through the body.

In individuals with a ureterocele, it is also important to evaluate the function of the kidneys, specifically to determine whether the affected portion of the kidney has any function. In most cases, this evaluation is performed with a renal scan.

Abdominal CT scans, MRI tests and excretory urograms are additional studies that may also be performed in the evaluation of a patient with a ureterocele. These tests are usually performed in situations where the urinary tract anatomy is extremely ambiguous and will allow the surgeon to better identify anatomical variations.

What are some treatment options?

Timing of therapy and form of treatment are based on the age of the patient, whether the affected portion of the kidney is functioning and whether vesicoureteral reflux is present. In some cases, more than one procedure is necessary. In rare cases, observation (no treatment) may be recommended.

Because a ureterocele predisposes an individual to a kidney infection, usually an antibiotic is prescribed until the ureterocele and its complicating features have been treated. The following are available treatment options:

Transurethral puncture: A form of minimally invasive therapy is to puncture and decompress the ureterocele using a cystoscope that is inserted through the urethra. The procedure usually takes 15 to 30 minutes, and often can be done on an outpatient basis. In some cases, this treatment is unsuccessful if the ureterocele wall is thick and difficult to recognize. The advantage of this treatment is that there is no surgical incision. Risks include failure to adequately decompress the ureterocele, possibly causing urine to flow into the ureterocele, which could necessitate an open operation. In addition, there is a slight risk of causing an obstructive flap valve with the ureterocele, which can make it difficult to urinate.

Upper pole nephrectomy: Often, if the upper half of the kidney does not function because of the ureterocele and there is no vesicoureteral reflux, removal of the affected portion of the kidney is recommended. In many cases, this operation is performed through a small incision under the rib cage. In some cases it may be performed laparoscopically.

Nephrectomy: If the entire kidney does not function because of the ureterocele, removal of the kidney is recommended. Usually this can be done laparoscopically, although at some centers it is performed through a very small incision under the rib cage.

Removal of the ureterocele and ureteral reimplantation: If it is deemed necessary to remove the ureterocele, then an operation is performed in which the bladder is opened, the ureterocele is removed, the floor of the bladder and bladder neck are reconstructed, and the ureters are reimplanted in such a way to create a non-refluxing connection between the ureters and the bladder. The operation is performed through a small lower abdominal incision. The success rate with this procedure is 90 to 95 percent and the complications include persistent ureteral obstruction.

Ureteropyelostomy or upper-to-lower ureteroureterostomy: If the upper portion of the ureter shows significant function, one option is to connect the obstructed upper portion to the non-obstructed lower portion of the ureter or pelvis of the kidney. The operation is done through a small lower abdominal incision. The success rate with this procedure is 95 percent.

Frequently Asked Questions

Is there any way to prevent this condition?

There is no known prevention for this condition; it is present at birth but may not be discovered until later in life.

My baby was diagnosed with a ureterocele on a prenatal ultrasound. She seems very healthy. Is it absolutely necessary for her to undergo treatment?

In the past, most children with a ureterocele had their condition detected following a serious kidney infection, which often required hospitalization for intravenous antibiotics. Consequently, it would be unusual for her not to develop a urinary tract infection unless her ureterocele was treated.

My doctor has recommended that my daughter take antibiotic prophylaxis because she has a ureterocele and urinary reflux. Is it safe to take antibiotics every day?

Many children and adults take a low dose of an antibiotic every day to prevent urinary tract infections. This form of therapy has been used for over 35 years and has proven to be relatively safe, as long as the dose is maintained at one-fourth to one-half the full dose. One needs to weigh the risk of taking the antibiotic against the risk of a serious kidney infection if the antibiotic were not taken.

My child was diagnosed with a ureterocele and it was punctured through a small scope. Now there is reflux into the ureterocele and the lower part of the kidney also. Will more surgery be necessary?

In most cases, if there is reflux up the ureter into the lower part of the kidney and/or the ureterocele, the reflux is unlikely to disappear with time and removal of the ureterocele and ureteral reimplantation is often necessary.

Section 24.3

Urachal Anomalies

Before birth, there is a connection between the belly button and the bladder. This connection, called the urachus, normally disappears before birth. But what happens if part of the urachus remains after birth? Read on to learn more about what problems can arise.

What happens under normal conditions?

The bladder, located in the lower abdomen, is formed from structures located in the lower half of the developing fetus that are directly connected to the umbilical cord. After the first few weeks of gestation, this thick pathway to and from the placenta contains blood vessels, a merged channel to the future intestine, and a tubular structure called the allantois. The internal part of the allantois is connected to the top of the developing bladder, and in ordinary circumstances, collapses and becomes a cord-like structure called the urachus. The formation and regression of this connection from the top of the bladder to the belly button are completed by the middle of the second trimester of pregnancy (approximately 20 weeks).

Although the urachus is easily seen by a surgeon whenever an operation inside the abdomen or around the bladder is performed, it is a remnant of development that serves no further purpose but can be a source of specific health problems. Such problems are rare and usually seen in childhood, but occasionally can be seen for the first time in adults.

What are the symptoms of urachal abnormalities?

Because this remnant of early development is found between the belly button and the top of the bladder, diseases of the urachus can appear anywhere in that space. In newborns and infants, persistent

271

drainage or "wetness" of the belly button can be a sign of a urachal problem. However, the most common detectable problem at the belly button is a granuloma, a reddened area that is present because the base of the umbilical cord stump did not heal properly.

Urachal abnormalities can also be seen without persistent umbilical drainage—35 percent of urachal problems are manifestations of an enclosed urachal cyst or infected urachal cyst (abscess). This type of problem is seen more often in older children and adults. Instead of visible belly button drainage, the symptoms of such a cyst consist of lower abdominal pain, fever, a lump that can be felt, pain with urination, urinary tract infection or hematuria.

How are urachal abnormalities treated?

A umbilical granuloma is usually treated by chemical cauterization in the office of the primary care provider. The condition is a superficial abdominal wall problem that heals after treatment and has no long-term implications; it is not caused by a urachal problem.

In contrast to the simple granuloma, persistent umbilical wetness needs to be further evaluated. Approximately 65 percent of all urachal problems appear as a sinus or drainage opening at the belly button. Most of those are not connected all the way to the bladder, but a small percentage represent an open pathway from the bladder to belly button, called a patent urachus. The drainage can be analyzed for urea and creatinine levels, which would be high if the fluid was primarily made of urine from a bladder connection instead of inflammatory tissue fluid. There can be associated redness from the drainage itself. Skin infection—indicated by tenderness, fever or spreading redness of the surrounding skin—can occur and requires prompt antibiotic treatment and possible hospitalization. This is called omphalitis and can be caused by bacteria that have become involved with a urachal sinus or the other embryologic structure in the belly button that was once connected to the intestinal system and might also be persistent. Once inflammation is controlled, the nature and extent of an opening at the belly button can be determined by a sinogram. This involves placing a small tube into the sinus opening and allowing contrast material to flow in while taking x-rays to determine the direction and extent of the channel. If the channel follows the expected pathway toward the top of the bladder, the diagnosis is urachal sinus. Treatment should be directed toward complete surgical removal of the urachus and all of its connections, including a small amount of the top of the bladder. Leaving any portion of the structure allows for the possible development of a future malignancy. Less than one percent of all bladder malignancies occur in the urachus, but once the urachus has become a potential problem, it should be removed.

When there is no draining sinus to investigate, an ultrasound of the lower abdomen will show the typical findings of a fluid-filled, enclosed lump in the location of the urachus. In an adult, where the rare possibility of malignancy could be present, an abdominal and pelvic CT scan might be helpful. Again, complete removal of the urachus is important. Simple needle or other drainage of the cyst will result in recurrence in at least one-third of patients, since the linings and structures are still present. About 80 percent of infected cysts are populated by *Staphylococcus aureus*, and one-third contain multiple types of bacteria. Almost all the time, such an infected cyst stays confined to its predetermined anatomical location; rarely, an infected cyst can drain into the peritoneal cavity and present with additional signs of peritonitis and febrile illness.

Therefore, most urachal problems can be characterized by the physical examination and a sinogram or ultrasound. Sometimes a combination of these is needed, and occasionally it is useful to obtain a voiding cystourethrogram. This is done when the draining urachus is associated with outlet obstruction of the bladder, which would also need to be treated. This possibility is usually determined by the age, gender and physical examination of the patient. There are also situations where a direct look inside the bladder (cystoscopy) can add a bit more information to the diagnostic picture, but most urologists recommend that the basic course of action be determined by the previously described approach.

What can be expected after treatment for urachal abnormalities?

After complete surgical removal of a troublesome urachus with no immediate postoperative problems, there should be no further issues and no need for follow-up or evaluation on a regular basis.

Frequently Asked Questions

Besides the problems that have already been outlined, are there other diseases that appear at the belly button?

As you might expect, there have been rare reports of other inflammatory problems involving the structures that are contained in the umbilical cord. These include infections of the remnant blood vessels. In addition, the vitelline duct, which is supposed to regress in its course between the belly button and the small intestine, sometimes has its own remnant problems. The sinogram that is useful for identifying urachal problems will also serve to identify a likely vitelline duct problem.

Occasionally, an intra-abdominal process such as appendicitis or ovarian cyst can mimic some of the symptoms of a urachal problem.

Are urachal abnormalities hereditary?

No. There is no evidence that they are inherited.

After my baby's umbilical cord stump came off, his belly button was extremely red. Is this normal or does he need immediate evaluation?

Some redness is expected after the stump falls away. Dabbing a small amount of alcohol on the site with a Q-tip twice a day will usually allow complete healing in two to three days. If the redness fails to improve or worsens, contact your primary care provider.

Section 24.4

Ureteropelvic Junction Obstruction

Alternative names: UP junction obstruction; obstruction of the ureteropelvic junction

Definition: Ureteropelvic junction (UPJ) obstruction involves a blockage in the area where a ureter, one of the tubes that carries urine from the kidney to the bladder, attaches to the part of the kidney known as the renal pelvis.

Causes, Incidence, and Risk Factors

UPJ obstruction is generally a congenital (present from before birth) condition caused by narrowing of the connection between the ureter and the renal pelvis, which is part of the kidney. This blockage causes urine to build up in the renal pelvis, damaging the kidney.

UPJ obstruction is the most frequently diagnosed cause of urinary obstruction in children. It is now commonly diagnosed during prenatal ultrasound studies that show a dilated renal pelvis or a condition called hydronephrosis.

When recognized before the baby is born, UPJ obstruction may require surgical correction in the first few days after birth. Less severe cases may not require surgery until later in life, and some cases do not require surgery at all.

UPJ obstruction may be recognized after birth when an abdominal mass is found on examination, or if the infant develops a urinary tract infection associated with fever. Back pain and blood in the urine may also be signs of UPJ obstruction.

Symptoms

- Back or flank pain
- Urinary tract infection with fever
- Bloody urine (hematuria)
- Lump in the abdomen (abdominal mass)

Signs and Tests

Maternal pregnancy ultrasound may show hydronephrosis in the fetus.

Tests after birth may include the following:

- Creatinine clearance
- BUN [blood urea nitrogen]
- Electrolytes
- IVP [intravenous pyelogram]
- Nuclear scan of kidneys
- Voiding cystourethrogram

Treatment

Surgical correction of the obstruction allows urine to flow normally. Open surgery is usually performed in infants, although adults may be treated with less-invasive procedures:

- **Percutaneous technique:** the obstruction is corrected via a small incision in the side.

- **Endoscopic technique:** the obstruction is cleared via a small instrument inserted through the urethra.

These procedures involve much smaller incisions than traditional open surgery.

A tube called a stent may be placed to drain urine from the kidney until the patient heals. A nephrostomy tube, which is placed in the patient's side to drain urine, may also be required for a short time after the surgery.

Expectations (Prognosis)

Rapid decompression of the kidney immediately following birth may substantially improve kidney function in an infant with UPJ obstruction diagnosed before the child is born. Early recognition and repair may also preserve future kidney function.

Most patients do well with no long-term consequences, although a small number of patients will require dialysis at some point in their lives as a result of this problem.

Complications

Permanent loss of kidney function (kidney failure) is a possible complication of UPJ obstruction.

Calling Your Healthcare Provider

Call your healthcare provider if your infant has bloody urine, fever, a lump in the abdomen or if the baby seems to have back pain or pain in the flanks (the area towards the sides of the body between the ribs and the pelvis).

Section 24.5

Vesicoureteral Reflux

National Kidney and Urologic Diseases Information Clearinghouse
(NKUDIC), a service of the National Institute of Diabetes and Digestive
and Kidney Diseases (NIDDK), National Institutes of Health (NIH), Pub.
No. 03-4555, April 2003.

Urine normally flows in one direction—down from the kidneys,
through tubes called ureters, to the bladder. Vesicoureteral reflux
(VUR) is the abnormal flow of urine from the bladder back into the
ureters.

VUR is most commonly diagnosed in infancy and childhood after
the patient has a urinary tract infection (UTI). About one-third of
children with UTI are found to have VUR. VUR can lead to infection
because urine that remains in the child's urinary tract provides a place
for bacteria to grow. But sometimes the infection itself is the cause of
VUR.

There are two types of VUR. Primary VUR occurs when a child is
born with an impaired valve where the ureter joins the bladder. This
happens if the ureter did not grow long enough during the child's development in the womb. The valve does not close properly, so urine
backs up (refluxes) from the bladder to the ureters, and eventually
to the kidneys. This type of VUR can get better or disappear as the
child gets older. The ureter gets longer as the child grows, and the
function of the valve improves.

Secondary VUR occurs when there is a blockage anywhere in the
urinary system. The blockage may be caused by an infection in the
bladder that leads to swelling of the ureter. This also causes a reflux
of urine to the kidneys.

Infection is the most common symptom of VUR. As the child gets
older, other symptoms, such as bedwetting, high blood pressure, protein in the urine, and kidney failure, may appear.

Common tests to show the presence of urinary tract infection include urine tests and cultures. Because no single test can tell everything about the urinary tract that might be important to know, more
than one of the following imaging tests may be needed:

- **Kidney and bladder ultrasound:** A test that uses sound waves to examine the kidney and bladder. This test shows shadows of the kidney and bladder that may point out certain abnormalities. The test cannot reveal all important urinary abnormalities or measure how well a kidney works.

- **Voiding cystourethrogram (VCUG):** A test that examines the urethra and bladder while the bladder fills and empties. A liquid that can be seen on x-rays is placed in the bladder through a catheter. Pictures are taken when the bladder is filled and when the child urinates. This test can reveal abnormalities of the inside of the urethra and bladder. The test can also determine whether the flow of urine is normal when the bladder empties.

- **Intravenous pyelogram:** A test that examines the whole urinary tract. A liquid that can be seen on x-rays is injected into a vein. The substance travels into the kidneys and bladder, revealing possible obstructions.

- **Nuclear scans:** A number of tests using radioactive materials that are usually injected into a vein to show how well the kidneys work, their shape, and whether urine empties from the kidneys normally. Each kind of nuclear scan gives different information about the kidneys and bladder. Nuclear scans expose a child to about the same amount of radiation as a conventional x-ray. At times, it can be even less.

The goal for treatment of VUR is to prevent any kidney damage from occurring. Infections should be treated at once with antibiotics to prevent the infection from moving into the kidneys. Antibiotic therapy usually corrects reflux caused by infection. Sometimes surgery is needed to correct primary VUR.

Chapter 25

Urethral Stricture

The urethra is an important part of the urinary tract. While its primary job in both genders is to pass urine outside the body, this channel also has an important role in ejaculating semen from the reproductive tract of men. Most of us will undergo few, if any, problems with our urethra, but a few of us may experience the discomfort and dysfunction associated with urethral stricture disease. What is this and how can it be treated? The information below should help you talk with your urologist.

What happens under normal conditions?

During urination, the bladder empties through the urethra and out of the body. Urine passes through an opening called the bladder neck into a portion of the urethra surrounded by the prostate, called the prostatic urethra. The next segment of the urethra is called the membranous urethra and it contains a muscle called the external urinary sphincter. This sphincter allows a patient to voluntarily hold urine and to stop during urination. Together, the prostatic urethra and the membranous urethra make up the posterior urethra, and are approximately one to two inches long. The urine then enters the bulbar urethra, followed by the penile urethra. The penile urethra is the segment that runs along the bottom surface of the penis. The exit at the tip of the penis is called the meatus. The bulbar urethra, penile urethra, and meatus make up the anterior urethra, which is nine to ten inches long.

What is a urethral stricture?

A urethral stricture is a scar in or around the urethra, which can block the flow of urine, and is a result of inflammation, injury or infection.

Who is at risk for urethral strictures?

Urethral strictures are more common in men because their urethras are longer than those in women. Thus men's urethras are more susceptible to disease or injury. A person is rarely born with urethral strictures.

What are some causes of urethral stricture?

Stricture disease may occur anywhere from the bladder to the tip of the penis. The common causes of stricture are trauma to the urethra and gonorrheal infection. However, in many cases, no cause can be identified. Stricture of the posterior urethra is often caused by a urethral injury associated with a pelvic bone fracture (e.g., motor vehicle or industrial accident). Patients who sustain posterior urethral injuries from pelvic fracture generally suffer a disruption of the urethra, where the urethra is cut and separated. These patients are completely unable to urinate and must have a catheter to realign the urethra. The catheter is placed through the penis up into the bladder to allow urine to drain until a repair can be performed. Trauma such as straddle injuries, direct trauma to the penis, and catheterization can result in strictures of the anterior urethra. In adults, urethral strictures may occur after prostate surgery, removal of kidney stones, urinary catheterization or other instrumentation. In children, urethral strictures most often follow reconstructive surgery for congenital abnormalities of the penis and urethra, cystoscopy, and urethral catheter drainage.

What are the symptoms of urethral strictures?

Some symptoms that may be an indication of urethral strictures can include the following:

- painful urination

- slow urine stream

- decreased urine output

- spraying of the urine stream

- blood in the urine

- abdominal pain

- urethral discharge

How are urethral strictures diagnosed?

Simply put, the urethra is like a garden hose. When there is a kink or narrowing along the hose, no matter how short or long, flow can be significantly reduced. When a stricture becomes narrow enough to decrease urine flow, the patient will develop symptoms. Frequent urination, urinary tract infections, and inflammation or infections of the prostate and scrotal contents (epididymis) may occur. With long-term severe obstruction, damage to the kidneys can occur.

Evaluation of patients with urethral stricture disease includes a physical examination, urethral imaging (x-rays or ultrasound), and sometimes urethroscopy. The retrograde urethrogram is an invaluable test to evaluate and document the stricture. Combined with antegrade urethrogram, length of the stricture can be determined. The retrograde urethrogram is performed as an outpatient x-ray procedure and can indicate the number, position, length, and severity of the stricture(s). This study involves insertion of contrast dye (fluid that can be seen on an x-ray) into the urethra at the tip of the penis. No needles or catheters are used. The retrograde urethrogram study allows doctors to see the entire urethra and outlines the area of narrowing at the stricture. Ultrasound is performed by placing a small, pencil-like ultrasound wand on the skin over the stricture to view it and surrounding tissue. Urethroscopy is a procedure where the doctor gently places a small, flexible, lubricated telescope into the urethra and advances it to the stricture. This study permits the doctor to see the urethra between the tip of the penis and the stricture. All of these tests can be performed in an office setting and will allow the urologist to provide treatment recommendations.

In the case of urethral trauma, once emergency treatment has been provided, the evaluation of patients with posterior urethral disruptions involves a retrograde urethrogram, and if a suprapubic catheter is present, injection of contrast dye through this tube at the same time. Contrast injected from below fills the urethra up to the injured area, and contrast injected from above fills the bladder and the urethra down to the stricture. These two films together allow the surgeon to determine the gap between the two ends in order to plan the surgical repair.

How can urethral strictures be prevented?

The most important preventive measure is to avoid injury to the urethra and pelvis. Also, if a patient is performing self-catheterization they should exercise care, to liberally instill lubricating jelly into the urethra, and to use the smallest possible catheter necessary for the shortest period of time.

Acquired strictures may be a result of inflammation caused by sexually transmitted diseases (STDs). Although gonorrhea was once the most common cause of inflammatory strictures, antibiotic therapy has proven effective in reducing the number of resulting strictures. *Chlamydia* is now the more common cause, but strictures caused by this infection may be prevented by avoiding contact with infected individuals or by using condoms.

What are some treatment options?

Treatment options for urethral stricture disease are varied and selection depends upon the length, location, and degree of scar tissue associated with the stricture. Options include enlarging the stricture by gradual stretching (dilation), cutting the stricture with a laser or knife through a telescope (urethrotomy), and surgical removal (excision) of the stricture with reconnection and reconstruction with grafts.

Dilation: This is usually performed in the urologist's office under local anesthetic and involves stretching the stricture using progressively larger dilators called "sounds." Alternatively, the stricture can be dilated with a special balloon on a catheter. Dilation is rarely a cure and needs to be periodically repeated. If the stricture recurs too rapidly the patient may be taught how to insert a catheter into the urethra periodically to prevent early closure.

Pain, bleeding, and infection are the main problems associated with dilation procedures. Occasionally, a "false passage" or second urethral channel may be formed from traumatic passage of the "sound."

Urethrotomy: This procedure involves use of a specially designed cystoscope that is advanced along the urethra until the stricture is encountered. A knife blade or laser operating from the end of the cystoscope is then used to cut the stricture, creating a gap in the narrowing.

A catheter may be placed into the urethra to hold the cleft open for a period of time after the procedure to allow healing in the open position. The suggested length of time for leaving a catheter tube draining after stricture treatment can vary.

Urethral stent: This procedure involves placement of a metallic stent that has the appearance of a circular chain link fence. The stent is placed into the urethra through the penis using a specially designed cystoscopic insertion tool after the urethra is widened. The stent expands within the widened stricture and prevents the urethra from closing. The lining of the urethra eventually covers the stent, which remains in place permanently. This treatment has the advantage of being "minimally invasive." However, it is only suited to very select strictures and frequently causes significant swelling around the device. Removal of these devices is very difficult and may result in a more significant stricture.

Open surgical urethral reconstruction: Many different reconstructive procedures have been used to treat strictures, some of which require one or two operations. In all cases, the choice of repair is influenced by the characteristics of the stricture, and no single repair is appropriate for all situations. Open reconstruction of a short urethral stricture may involve surgery to remove the stricture and reconnect the two ends (anastomotic urethroplasty). When the stricture is too long and this repair is not possible, tissue can be transferred to enlarge the segment to normal (substitution procedures). Substitution repairs may need to be performed in stages in difficult circumstances.

Anastomotic Procedures

These are usually reserved for urethral strictures of two centimeters or less where the urethra can be reconnected after removing the stricture. This procedure involves a cut between the scrotum and rectum. This is usually performed as an outpatient procedure or with a brief hospitalization. A small, soft catheter will be left in the penis for 10 to 21 days and removed after an x-ray is performed to ensure healing of the repair.

Substitution Procedures

A.   *Free graft procedures:* Strictures significantly longer than two centimeters may be repaired with a free graft procedure to enlarge the urethra. The graft may be skin (usually removed from the shaft of the penis) or buccal mucosa removed from inside the cheek. Brief hospitalization and catheterization for two or three weeks are usually required after this procedure.

B. *Skin flap procedures:* When a long stricture is associated with severe scarring and a free graft would not survive, flaps of skin can be rotated from the penis to ensure survival of the newly created urethra. These procedures are complex and require a surgeon experienced in plastic surgery techniques. Brief hospitalization and catheterization for two or three weeks are usually required after this procedure.

C. *Staged procedure:* When sufficient local tissue is not available for a skin flap procedure and local tissue factors are not suitable for a free graft, a staged procedure may be required. The first stage in a staged procedure focuses on opening the underside of the urethra to expose the complete length of the stricture. A graft is secured to the edges of the opened urethra and allowed to heal and mature over a period of three months to a year. During that time, patients urinate through a new opening behind the stricture, which in some cases will require the patient to sit down to urinate. The second stage is performed several months after the graft around the urethra has healed and is soft and flexible. At this stage the graft is formed into a tube and the urethra is returned to normal. A small, soft catheter will be left in the penis for 10 to 21 days.

What are the possibilities of recurrence?

Because urethral strictures can recur at any time after surgery, patients should be monitored by a urologist. After removal of the catheter, follow up of the repair should be performed intermittently with physical examination and x-ray studies being performed as necessary. Sometimes, the doctor will perform urethroscopy to evaluate the repaired area. Some patients will have recurrence of stricture at the site of the prior repair. These are sometimes mild and require no intervention, but if they cause obstruction they can be treated with urethrotomy or dilation. A repeat open surgical repair may be needed for significant recurrent strictures.

Frequently Asked Questions

Can urethral strictures be treated with medicine?

No.

What can occur if no treatment is taken?

The patient would have to continue to tolerate problems with urination. Urinary and/or testicular infections and stones can develop. Also, there is a risk that urinary retention may occur which can cause the bladder to enlarge and also lead to kidney problems.

Is there a risk of infecting others with urethral strictures?

Urethral strictures are not contagious but the underlying cause, like an STD, may be contagious.

Chapter 26

Benign Urethral Lesions

The urethra is an important part of the urinary tract. While its primary job in both genders is to pass urine outside the body, this channel also has an important role in ejaculating semen from the reproductive tract of men. Most of us will undergo few, if any, problems with our urethra. But a few of us may experience the discomfort and dysfunction associated with benign urethral lesions. What are they and can they be treated? The information below should help you talk with your urologist.

What happens under normal conditions?

The urethra is a tube-like organ whose function is to transport urine from the bladder out of the body. In males, the urethra begins at the bladder and extends through the prostate gland, perineum and the entire length of the penis. In females, the urethra is much shorter and extends from the bladder to just in front of the vagina and opens outside the body. Normally, urine flow is painless and can be controlled, the stream is strong, the urine is clear, and there is never any visible blood in the urine.

What are some causes of benign urethral lesions?

Causes can include abscesses, pelvic fractures, straddle injuries, infections or injury caused by surgical instruments (e.g., catheters, cystoscopes, resectoscopes, etc.).

What are some types of benign urethral lesions?

Benign neoplasms: Linked to the presence of genital warts on the penile shaft, these lesions are often the product of human papillomavirus (HPV). Urethral wart-like growths are suspected when there is bleeding from the urethra, a visible lesion on the opening of the urethra or changes in the urinary stream, accompanied by a history of genital warts.

Balanitis xerotica obliterans (BXO): BXO is a chronic condition with unknown causes that affects the end of the penis and is marked by pale, shiny, whitish skin around the opening of the urethra. The scarring and thinning of the membrane begin (in most cases) in young adulthood and can progress, leading to a narrowing of the urethra and difficulty passing urine. Other symptoms include soreness and itching in the area and sometimes ulceration.

Urethral stricture disease: Results in scar tissue or inflammation at one or more points in the urethra and of variable severity. Complications of urethral stricture disease include but are not limited to a decrease in urine flow rate, frequent urination, urinary tract infections, bleeding, and inflammation/infection of the prostate. Diagnosis is usually made by urinalysis, retrograde urethrogram, and cystoscopy.

Urethral polyps: A urethral polyp is an irregularity that is usually present at birth. It is usually composed of fibrous tissue but may include some smooth muscle, small cysts or nerve tissue all covered by a thin protective layer of tissue. Symptoms include a lump in the vulva, blood in the urine or a blockage. Urethral polyps are diagnosed with cystoscopy, a fiber-optic technique that allows a urologist to readily view the polyp, and a voiding cystourethrogram (VCUG). By combining an x-ray of the urethra with dye in the area, the doctor can easily view the structures.

Paraurethral cyst: Also known as Skene glands, paraurethral glands are located in the urethrovaginal wall at the opening into the urethra in females. A paraurethral cyst will be evident to a doctor by its appearance—a glistening, tense and bulging yellowish-white mass reducing the size of the urethral opening. Other symptoms include a misdirected urinary stream and possibly painful urination.

Urethral caruncle: Urethral caruncles are polypoid (or stalk-like) masses, hanging from one area of the external urethral opening. The primary sign of this problem is a thin, reddish membrane protruding from one portion of the urethral opening. Other symptoms include bleeding and urination problems such as frequency, urgency, and pain. A urethral caruncle is usually spotted during an examination for another condition. They are relatively common in the urethral epithelium of women who do not use hormone replacement therapy (HRT) after menopause. Marked by a purplish mucosal mass, this condition can cause a variety of symptoms, including difficult or painful urination, blood in the urine, and tenderness around the opening of the urethra.

Urethral prolapse: A rare and more bothersome abnormality of the female urethra than other benign lesions is called urethral prolapse, which occurs most commonly in young girls though it also may surface at any age. It is marked by the urethra's membrane and underlying spongy tissue protruding out the opening of the urethra. This leads to pain, vaginal bleeding, and occasionally urine retention. A diagnosis is usually made by simple physical examination.

How are benign lesions treated?

The nature and location of any benign lesion will influence how it is treated. Abscesses, urethral injuries, and infections require immediate attention. A urologist has a variety of medications and procedures to deal with these lesions.

Abscesses linked to gonococcal urethritis can be treated successfully today with antibiotics. Additionally, your urologist may drain the abscess and divert the urine flow until your condition improves and you can urinate normally.

Treating urethral stricture disease is based on the accurate delineation of individual scars. The cornerstone of this process is urethrography, an imaging technique that utilizes retrograde instillation of a contrast dye into the urethra to determine the length and location of the strictures. If these strictures are very dense or if they completely destroy the channel, a more detailed urination study through an incision above the pubic bone may be necessary.

Urethral strictures are often treated by increasing the diameter of the channel either through dilation or endoscopic incision. Techniques such as direct vision internal urethrotomy (DVIU), are very successful for short strictures (less than two centimeters), particularly in the bulbar and membranous regions of the urethra.

Dilation performed under local anesthetic jelly utilizes a series of increasingly large tubes or dilators that are passed from the urethral opening into the bladder. The insertion of the dilators may be conducted under the guide of a urethroscope. Dilation produces some discomfort, usually made worse by tighter, dense strictures. The urologist may place a urethral catheter into the urethra 24 hours or longer after to drain the bladder.

DVIU is also carried out under general anesthesia, although some urologists elect to perform it with a local anesthetic in the office. In either case, with the aid of a cystoscope, the surgeon makes a deep incision through the stricture with a small endoscopic knife. By making a single cut through the scarred stricture, the doctor exposes healthy epithelial tissue beneath, which should allow the urethra to re-cover itself. Long strictures, as well as any scars in the pendulous urethra, respond less well to DVIU or dilation. Instead, those scars, along with completely destroyed urethras, can be dealt with by surgical reconstruction, which has varying results.

A surgical procedure called urethroplasty is performed by making an incision in the penis and then removing the stricture. Your doctor will then probably follow up by rejoining the tissue at the ends of the urethra or inserting a skin graft to partially or completely restore the urethra at the stricture. While this procedure requires no overnight hospital stay, a catheter will remain in place for approximately three weeks.

Permanent, implantable metal stents have been employed for bulbar urethral strictures. But while initial clinical trials have yielded promising results in men exhibiting shorter scars (two centimeters or less) with some co-factors, the stent's application is limited. Because the brace is permanent once inserted, it has been most successful in patients with bulbar urethral scars, strictures that are otherwise difficult to manage due to the poor quality of the corpus spongiosum. Skin grafts and repeated urethrotomy, urethral incision repairs, often tried in those circumstances have resulted in recurrent stricture disease.

Treating benign neoplasms is difficult. Lasers can be used to destroy visible lesions connected to this condition. Some physicians advocate topical cream treatments. But as of now, no technique reliably eliminates the condition or prevents the virus from recurring in the future.

Local antibacterial and anti-inflammatory agents are used to treat BXO.

Treatment for urethral polyps consists of removing the polyp using cystourethroscopy, a minimally-invasive technique using a fiberoptic instrument that allows the urologist to peer into the space and, with additional miniaturized instruments, remove the growth.

In the case of paraurethral cysts, no treatment is necessary if there are no symptoms since they usually spontaneously rupture and decompress. If, however, a blockage develops, the urologist may pierce the cyst with a scalpel blade to relieve the milky drainage.

For patients with a urethral caruncle but no symptoms, the primary treatment option is reassurance but may also include topical estrogen cream or hormone replacement therapy (HRT). If the caruncle is large or small and causing problems, the urologist will probably choose to remove the growth and cauterize the base.

Treatment for a urethral prolapse consists of surgically removing the prolapsed tissue and repositioning the membrane using stitches to prevent further protrusions.

What can be expected after treatment for benign urethral lesions?

Benign lesions associated with human papillomavirus (HPV) and gonorrhea are notoriously difficult to address, even though antibiotics are effective in controlling the problem. So it is not uncommon to repeat treatment because such urethral lesions resurface.

After either dilation or direct vision internal urethrotomy (DVIU), you can expect some blood alongside the Foley catheter and occasionally in the urine draining from it. If you have heavy bleeding, your urologist may elect a large-bore catheter, which will probably be left in for a longer period.

The main complications associated with both dilation and internal urethrotomy are high rates of stricture. Recurrence depends on the length of the stricture, with shorter ones usually doing better with these therapies than longer ones. For instance, scars less than two centimeters in length have a 50 percent long-term cure rate with DVIU. Several studies have suggested that daily, intermittent catheterization up to three months after the procedure may reduce recurrence.

Strictures more than a centimeter, on the other hand, exhibit success rates significantly lower than 50 percent. In addition, the chance for long-term cure with either DVIU or dilation is very low. Nevertheless, in some men DVIU or dilation may be appropriate, even though

291

the urologist knows that intermittent catheterization or a repeat procedure will be necessary.

Complications associated with urethroplasty can include recurrent stricture disease, bleeding, infection, and lower extremity complications due to patient positioning. Three weeks after surgery, your doctor will probably order a voiding cystourethrogram, a contrast imaging study of your urethra, to determine if the area is healing properly.

Doctors usually follow any stricture procedure with uroflow studies to monitor the force of the urine stream from the urethra as well as other factors. In addition, repeat radiographic studies are commonly performed at three- and 12-month intervals after a urethroplasty to monitor any recurrence. While most strictures develop within a year of surgery, they have been known to show up ten years later.

Chapter 27

Benign Disorders of the Prostate

Chapter Contents

Section 27.1

What You Need to Know about Prostate Problems

Excerpted from "What I Need to Know about Prostate Problems," National Kidney and Urologic Diseases Information Clearinghouse (NKUDIC), a service of the National Institute of Diabetes and Digestive and Kidney Diseases (NIDDK), National Institutes of Health (NIH), Pub. No. 05-4806, November 2004.

What is the prostate?

The prostate is part of a man's sex organs. It's about the size of a walnut and surrounds the tube called the urethra, located just below the bladder.

The urethra has two jobs: to carry urine from the bladder when you urinate and to carry semen during a sexual climax, or ejaculation. Semen is a combination of sperm plus fluid that the prostate adds.

What are prostate problems?

For men under 50, the most common prostate problem is prostatitis.

For men over 50, the most common prostate problem is prostate enlargement. This condition is also called benign prostatic hyperplasia or BPH. Older men are at risk for prostate cancer as well, but this disease is much less common than BPH. More information about prostate cancer is available from the National Cancer Institute.

What is prostatitis?

"Prostatitis" means that the prostate is inflamed; it could be swollen, red, and warm. If you have prostatitis, you may have a burning feeling when you urinate, or you may have to urinate more often. Or you may have a fever or just feel tired.

Inflammation in any part of the body is usually a sign that the body is fighting germs or repairing an injury. Some kinds of prostatitis are caused by germs, or bacteria. If you have bacterial prostatitis, your doctor can look through a microscope and find bacteria in a sample of your urine. Your doctor can then give you an antibiotic medicine to fight the bacteria.

If you keep getting infections, you may have a defect in your prostate that allows bacteria to grow. This defect can usually be corrected by surgery.

Most of the time, doctors don't find any bacteria in men with prostatitis. If you have urinary problems, the doctor will look for other possible causes, such as a kidney stone or cancer.

If no other causes are found, the doctor may decide that you have a condition called nonbacterial prostatitis.

Antibiotics will not help nonbacterial prostatitis. You may have to work with your doctor to find a treatment that's good for you. Changing your diet or taking warm baths may help. Your doctor may give you a medicine called an alpha blocker to relax the muscle tissue in the prostate. No single solution works for everyone with this condition.

What is prostate enlargement, or BPH?

If you're a man over 50 and have started having problems urinating, the reason could be an enlarged prostate, or BPH. As men get older, their prostate keeps growing. As it grows, it squeezes the urethra. Since urine travels from the bladder through the urethra, the pressure from the enlarged prostate may affect bladder control.

If you have BPH, you may have one or more of these problems:

- A frequent and urgent need to urinate (You may get up several times a night to go to the bathroom.)

- Trouble starting a urine stream (Even though you feel you have to rush to get to the bathroom, you find it hard to start urinating.)

- A weak stream of urine

- A small amount of urine each time you go

- The feeling that you still have to go, even when you have just finished urinating

- Leaking or dribbling

- Small amounts of blood in your urine

You may barely notice that you have one or two of these symptoms, or you may feel as though urination problems have taken over your life.

Is BPH a sign of cancer?

No. It's true that some men with prostate cancer also have BPH, but that doesn't mean that the two conditions are always linked. Most men with BPH don't develop prostate cancer. However, because the early symptoms are the same for both conditions, you should see a doctor to evaluate these symptoms.

Is BPH a serious disease?

By itself, BPH is not a serious condition, unless the symptoms are so bothersome that you can't enjoy life. But BPH can lead to serious problems. One problem is urinary tract infections.

If you can't urinate at all, you should get medical help right away. Sometimes this happens suddenly to men after they take an over-the-counter cold or allergy medicine.

In rare cases, BPH and its constant urination problems can lead to kidney damage.

Section 27.2

Types of Prostatitis

"Prostatitis: Disorders of the Prostate," National Kidney and Urologic Diseases Information Clearinghouse (NKUDIC), a service of the National Institute of Diabetes and Digestive and Kidney Diseases (NIDDK), National Institutes of Health (NIH), Pub. No. 04-4553, December 2003.

Prostatitis may account for up to 25 percent of all office visits by young and middle-aged men for complaints involving the genital and urinary systems. The term prostatitis actually encompasses four disorders:

- **Acute bacterial prostatitis** is the least common of the four types but also the easiest to diagnose and treat effectively. Men with this disease often have chills, fever, pain in the lower back and genital area, urinary frequency and urgency often at night, burning or painful urination, body aches, and a demonstrable infection of the urinary tract as evidenced by white blood cells and bacteria in the urine. The treatment is an appropriate antibiotic.

- **Chronic bacterial prostatitis**, also relatively uncommon, is acute prostatitis associated with an underlying defect in the prostate, which becomes a focal point for bacterial persistence in the urinary tract. Effective treatment usually requires identifying and removing the defect and then treating the infection with antibiotics. However, antibiotics often do not cure this condition.

- **Chronic prostatitis**, chronic pelvic pain syndrome, is the most common but least understood form of prostatitis. It is found in men of any age, its symptoms go away and then return without warning, and it may be inflammatory or noninflammatory. In the inflammatory form, urine, semen, and other fluids from the prostate show no evidence of a known infecting organism but do contain the kinds of cells the body usually produces to fight infection. In the noninflammatory form, no evidence of inflammation, including infection-fighting cells, is present.

  Antibiotics will not help nonbacterial prostatitis. You may have to work with your doctor to find a treatment that's good for you. Changing your diet or taking warm baths may help. Your doctor may give you a medicine called an alpha blocker to relax the muscle tissue in the prostate. No single solution works for everyone with this condition.

- **Asymptomatic inflammatory prostatitis** is the diagnosis when the patient does not complain of pain or discomfort but has infection-fighting cells in his semen. Doctors usually find this form of prostatitis when looking for causes of infertility or testing for prostate cancer.

Section 27.3

Prostate Enlargement: Benign Prostatic Hyperplasia

National Kidney and Urologic Diseases Information Clearinghouse (NKUDIC), a service of the National Institute of Diabetes and Digestive and Kidney Diseases (NIDDK), National Institutes of Health (NIH), Pub. No. 04-3012, February 2004.

Benign Prostatic Hyperplasia (BPH): A Common Part of Aging

It is common for the prostate gland to become enlarged as a man ages. Doctors call the condition benign prostatic hyperplasia (BPH), or benign prostatic hypertrophy.

As a man matures, the prostate goes through two main periods of growth. The first occurs early in puberty, when the prostate doubles in size. At around age 25, the gland begins to grow again. This second growth phase often results, years later, in BPH.

Though the prostate continues to grow during most of a man's life, the enlargement doesn't usually cause problems until late in life. BPH rarely causes symptoms before age 40, but more than half of men in their sixties and as many as 90 percent in their seventies and eighties have some symptoms of BPH.

As the prostate enlarges, the layer of tissue surrounding it stops it from expanding, causing the gland to press against the urethra like a clamp on a garden hose. The bladder wall becomes thicker and irritable. The bladder begins to contract even when it contains small amounts of urine, causing more frequent urination. Eventually, the bladder weakens and loses the ability to empty itself. Urine remains in the bladder. The narrowing of the urethra and partial emptying of the bladder cause many of the problems associated with BPH.

Many people feel uncomfortable talking about the prostate, since the gland plays a role in both sex and urination. Still, prostate enlargement is as common a part of aging as gray hair. As life expectancy rises, so does the occurrence of BPH. In the United States in 2000, there were 4.5 million visits to a physician for BPH.

Why BPH Occurs

The cause of BPH is not well understood. No definite information on risk factors exists. For centuries, it has been known that BPH occurs mainly in older men and that it doesn't develop in men whose testes were removed before puberty. For this reason, some researchers believe that factors related to aging and the testes may spur the development of BPH.

Throughout their lives, men produce both testosterone, an important male hormone, and small amounts of estrogen, a female hormone. As men age, the amount of active testosterone in the blood decreases, leaving a higher proportion of estrogen. Studies done with animals have suggested that BPH may occur because the higher amount of estrogen within the gland increases the activity of substances that promote cell growth.

Another theory focuses on dihydrotestosterone (DHT), a substance derived from testosterone in the prostate, which may help control its growth. Most animals lose their ability to produce DHT as they age. However, some research has indicated that even with a drop in the blood's testosterone level, older men continue to produce and accumulate high levels of DHT in the prostate. This accumulation of DHT may encourage the growth of cells. Scientists have also noted that men who do not produce DHT do not develop BPH.

Some researchers suggest that BPH may develop as a result of "instructions" given to cells early in life. According to this theory, BPH occurs because cells in one section of the gland follow these instructions and "reawaken" later in life. These "reawakened" cells then deliver signals to other cells in the gland, instructing them to grow or making them more sensitive to hormones that influence growth.

Symptoms

Many symptoms of BPH stem from obstruction of the urethra and gradual loss of bladder function, which results in incomplete emptying of the bladder. The symptoms of BPH vary, but the most common ones involve changes or problems with urination, such as the following:

- a hesitant, interrupted, weak stream

- urgency and leaking or dribbling

- more frequent urination, especially at night

The size of the prostate does not always determine how severe the obstruction or the symptoms will be. Some men with greatly enlarged glands have little obstruction and few symptoms while others, whose glands are less enlarged, have more blockage and greater problems.

Sometimes a man may not know he has any obstruction until he suddenly finds himself unable to urinate at all. This condition, called acute urinary retention, may be triggered by taking over-the-counter cold or allergy medicines. Such medicines contain a decongestant drug, known as a sympathomimetic. A potential side effect of this drug may be to prevent the bladder opening from relaxing and allowing urine to empty. When partial obstruction is present, urinary retention also can be brought on by alcohol, cold temperatures, or a long period of immobility.

It is important to tell your doctor about urinary problems such as those described above. In eight out of ten cases, these symptoms suggest BPH, but they also can signal other, more serious conditions that require prompt treatment. These conditions, including prostate cancer, can be ruled out only by a doctor's exam.

Severe BPH can cause serious problems over time. Urine retention and strain on the bladder can lead to urinary tract infections, bladder or kidney damage, bladder stones, and incontinence. If the bladder is permanently damaged, treatment for BPH may be ineffective. When BPH is found in its earlier stages, there is a lower risk of developing such complications.

Diagnosis

You may first notice symptoms of BPH yourself, or your doctor may find that your prostate is enlarged during a routine checkup. When BPH is suspected, you may be referred to a urologist, a doctor who specializes in problems of the urinary tract and the male reproductive system. Several tests help the doctor identify the problem and decide whether surgery is needed. The tests vary from patient to patient, but the following are the most common.

Digital Rectal Exam (DRE)

This exam is usually the first test done. The doctor inserts a gloved finger into the rectum and feels the part of the prostate next to the rectum. This exam gives the doctor a general idea of the size and condition of the gland.

Prostate Specific Antigen (PSA) Blood Test

To rule out cancer as a cause of urinary symptoms, your doctor may recommend a PSA blood test. PSA, a protein produced by prostate cells, is frequently present at elevated levels in the blood of men who have prostate cancer. The U.S. Food and Drug Administration has approved a PSA test for use in conjunction with a digital rectal exam to help detect prostate cancer in men age 50 or older and for monitoring prostate cancer patients after treatment. However, much remains unknown about the interpretation of PSA levels, the test's ability to discriminate cancer from benign prostate conditions, and the best course of action following a finding of elevated PSA.

A fact sheet titled "Questions and Answers about the Prostate-Specific Antigen (PSA) Test" can be found on the National Cancer Institute website at http://cis.nci.nih.gov/fact/5_29.htm.

Rectal Ultrasound

If there is a suspicion of prostate cancer, your doctor may recommend a test with rectal ultrasound. In this procedure, a probe inserted in the rectum directs sound waves at the prostate. The echo patterns of the sound waves form an image of the prostate gland on a display screen.

Urine Flow Study

Sometimes the doctor will ask a patient to urinate into a special device that measures how quickly the urine is flowing. A reduced flow often suggests BPH.

Cystoscopy

In this exam, the doctor inserts a small tube through the opening of the urethra in the penis. This procedure is done after a solution numbs the inside of the penis so all sensation is lost. The tube, called a cystoscope, contains a lens and a light system, which help the doctor see the inside of the urethra and the bladder. This test allows the doctor to determine the size of the gland and identify the location and degree of the obstruction.

Treatment

Men who have BPH with symptoms usually need some kind of treatment at some time. However, a number of recent studies have questioned the need for early treatment when the gland is just mildly enlarged. These studies report that early treatment may not be needed because the symptoms of BPH clear up without treatment in as many as one-third of all mild cases. Instead of immediate treatment, they suggest regular check-ups to watch for early problems. If the condition begins to pose a danger to the patient's health or causes a major inconvenience to him, treatment is usually recommended.

Since BPH may cause urinary tract infections, a doctor will usually clear up any infection with antibiotics before treating the BPH itself. Although the need for treatment is not usually urgent, doctors generally advise going ahead with treatment once the problems become bothersome or present a health risk.

The following section describes the types of treatment that are most commonly used for BPH.

Drug Treatment

Over the years, researchers have tried to find a way to shrink or at least stop the growth of the prostate without using surgery. The Food and Drug Administration (FDA) has approved four drugs to relieve common symptoms associated with an enlarged prostate.

Finasteride, FDA-approved in 1992 (marketed under the name Proscar), and dutasteride, FDA-approved in 2001 (marketed as Avodart), inhibit production of the hormone DHT, which is involved with prostate enlargement. The use of either of these drugs can either prevent progression of growth of the prostate or actually shrink the prostate in some men.

FDA also approved the drugs terazosin (marketed as Hytrin) in 1993, doxazosin (marketed as Cardura) in 1995, tamsulosin (marketed as Flomax) in 1997, and alfuzosin (marketed as Uroxatral) in 2003 for the treatment of BPH. All four drugs act by relaxing the smooth muscle of the prostate and bladder neck to improve urine flow and to reduce bladder outlet obstruction. The four drugs belong to the class known as alpha blockers. Terazosin and doxazosin were developed first to treat high blood pressure. Tamsulosin and alfuzosin were developed specifically to treat BPH.

NIDDK's Medical Therapy of Prostatic Symptoms (MTOPS) Trial recently found that using finasteride and doxazosin together is more effective than either drug alone to relieve symptoms and prevent BPH progression. The two-drug regimen reduced the risk of BPH progression by 67 percent, compared to 39 percent for doxazosin alone and 34 percent for finasteride alone.

Minimally Invasive Therapy

Because drug treatment is not effective in all cases, researchers in recent years have developed a number of procedures that relieve BPH symptoms but are less invasive than conventional surgery.

Transurethral microwave procedures: In May 1996, FDA approved the Prostatron, a device that uses microwaves to heat and destroy excess prostate tissue. In the procedure called transurethral microwave thermotherapy (TUMT), the Prostatron sends computer-regulated microwaves through a catheter to heat selected portions of the prostate to at least 111 degrees Fahrenheit. A cooling system protects the urinary tract during the procedure.

A similar microwave device, the Targis System, received FDA approval in September 1997. Like the Prostatron, the Targis System delivers microwaves to destroy selected portions of the prostate and uses a cooling system to protect the urethra. A heat-sensing device inserted in the rectum helps monitor the therapy.

Both procedures take about one hour and can be performed on an outpatient basis without general anesthesia. Neither procedure has been reported to lead to impotence or incontinence.

Although microwave therapy does not cure BPH, it reduces urinary frequency, urgency, straining, and intermittent flow. It does not correct the problem of incomplete emptying of the bladder. Ongoing

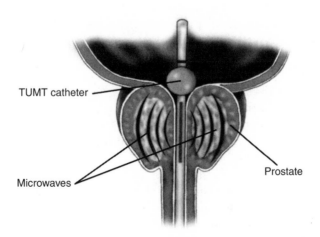

Figure 27.1. In TUMT, microwaves heat part of the prostate.

research will determine any long-term effects of microwave therapy and who might benefit most from this therapy.

Transurethral needle ablation: In October 1996, FDA approved VidaMed's minimally invasive Transurethral Needle Ablation (TUNA) System for the treatment of BPH.

The TUNA System delivers low-level radiofrequency energy through twin needles to burn away a well-defined region of the enlarged prostate. Shields protect the urethra from heat damage. The TUNA System improves urine flow and relieves symptoms with fewer side effects when compared with transurethral resection of the prostate (TURP). No incontinence or impotence has been observed.

Surgical Treatment

Most doctors recommend removal of the enlarged part of the prostate as the best long-term solution for patients with BPH. With surgery for BPH, only the enlarged tissue that is pressing against the urethra is removed; the rest of the inside tissue and the outside capsule are left intact. Surgery usually relieves the obstruction and incomplete emptying caused by BPH. The following section describes the types of surgery that are used.

Transurethral surgery: In this type of surgery, no external incision is needed. After giving anesthesia, the surgeon reaches the prostate by inserting an instrument through the urethra.

A procedure called TURP (transurethral resection of the prostate) is used for 90 percent of all prostate surgeries done for BPH. With TURP, an instrument called a resectoscope is inserted through the penis. The resectoscope, which is about 12 inches long and ½ inch in diameter, contains a light, valves for controlling irrigating fluid, and an electrical loop that cuts tissue and seals blood vessels.

During the 90-minute operation, the surgeon uses the resectoscope's wire loop to remove the obstructing tissue one piece at a time. The pieces of tissue are carried by the fluid into the bladder and then flushed out at the end of the operation.

Most doctors suggest using TURP whenever possible. Transurethral procedures are less traumatic than open forms of surgery and require a shorter recovery period.

Another surgical procedure is called transurethral incision of the prostate (TUIP). Instead of removing tissue, as with TURP, this procedure widens the urethra by making a few small cuts in the bladder neck, where the urethra joins the bladder, and in the prostate gland itself. Although some people believe that TUIP gives the same relief as TURP with less risk of side effects such as retrograde ejaculation, its advantages and long-term side effects have not been clearly established.

Open surgery: In the few cases when a transurethral procedure cannot be used, open surgery, which requires an external incision, may be used. Open surgery is often done when the gland is greatly enlarged, when there are complicating factors, or when the bladder has been damaged and needs to be repaired. The location of the enlargement within the gland and the patient's general health help the surgeon decide which of the three open procedures to use.

With all the open procedures, anesthesia is given and an incision is made. Once the surgeon reaches the prostate capsule, he scoops out the enlarged tissue from inside the gland.

Laser surgery: In March 1996, FDA approved a surgical procedure that employs side-firing laser fibers and Nd: YAG lasers to vaporize

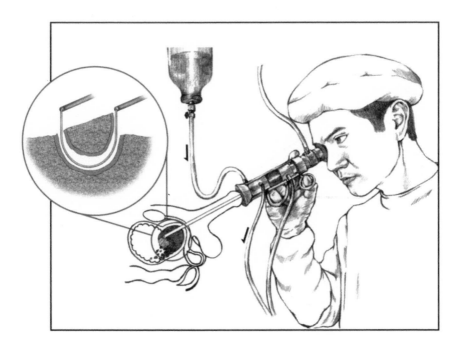

Figure 27.2. In TURP, a wire loop cuts away pieces of the prostate.

obstructing prostate tissue. The doctor passes the laser fiber through the urethra into the prostate using a cystoscope and then delivers several bursts of energy lasting 30 to 60 seconds. The laser energy destroys prostate tissue and causes shrinkage. Like TURP, laser surgery requires anesthesia and a hospital stay. One advantage of laser surgery over TURP is that laser surgery causes little blood loss. Laser surgery also allows for a quicker recovery time. But laser surgery may not be effective on larger prostates. The long-term effectiveness of laser surgery is not known.

Your Recovery after Surgery in the Hospital

If you have surgery, you'll probably stay in the hospital depending on the type of surgery you had and how quickly you recover.

At the end of surgery, a special catheter is inserted through the opening of the penis to drain urine from the bladder into a collection bag. Called a Foley catheter, this device has a water-filled balloon on the end that is placed in the bladder, which keeps it in place.

This catheter is usually left in place for several days. Sometimes, the catheter causes recurring painful bladder spasms the day after surgery. These may be difficult to control, but they will eventually disappear.

You may also be given antibiotics while you are in the hospital. Many doctors start giving this medicine before or soon after surgery

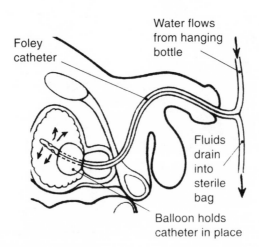

Figure 27.3. *Foley catheter.*

to prevent infection. However, some recent studies suggest that antibiotics may not be needed in every case, and your doctor may prefer to wait until an infection is present to give them.

After surgery, you will probably notice some blood or clots in your urine as the wound starts to heal. If your bladder is being irrigated (flushed with water), you may notice that your urine becomes red once the irrigation is stopped. Some bleeding is normal, and it should clear up by the time you leave the hospital. During your recovery, it is important to drink a lot of water (up to eight cups a day) to help flush out the bladder and speed healing.

Do's and Don'ts

Take it easy the first few weeks after you get home. You may not have any pain, but you still have an incision that is healing—even with transurethral surgery, where the incision can't be seen. Since many people try to do too much at the beginning and then have a setback, it is a good idea to talk to your doctor before resuming your normal routine. During this initial period of recovery at home, avoid any straining or sudden movements that could tear the incision. Here are some guidelines:

- Continue drinking a lot of water to flush the bladder.
- Avoid straining when moving your bowel.
- Eat a balanced diet to prevent constipation. If constipation occurs, ask your doctor if you can take a laxative.
- Don't do any heavy lifting.
- Don't drive or operate machinery.

Getting Back to Normal

Even though you should feel much better by the time you leave the hospital, it will probably take a couple of months for you to heal completely. During the recovery period, the following are some common problems that can occur.

Problems Urinating

You may notice that your urinary stream is stronger right after surgery, but it may take awhile before you can urinate completely normally again. After the catheter is removed, urine will pass over the surgical wound on the prostate, and you may initially have some discomfort or feel a sense of urgency when you urinate. This problem will gradually lessen, though, and after a couple of months you should be able to urinate less frequently and more easily.

Inability to Control Urination (Incontinence)

As the bladder returns to normal, you may have some temporary problems controlling urination, but long-term incontinence rarely occurs. Doctors find that the longer problems existed before surgery, the longer it will take for the bladder to regain its full function after the operation.

Bleeding

In the first few weeks after transurethral surgery, the scab inside the bladder may loosen, and blood may suddenly appear in the urine. Although this can be alarming, the bleeding usually stops with a short period of resting in bed and drinking fluids. However, if your urine is so red that it is difficult to see through or if it contains clots or if you feel any discomfort, be sure to contact your doctor.

Sexual Function after Surgery

Many men worry about whether surgery for BPH will affect their ability to enjoy sex. Some sources state that sexual function is rarely affected, while others claim that it can cause problems in up to 30 percent of all cases. However, most doctors say that even though it takes awhile for sexual function to return fully, with time, most men are able to enjoy sex again.

Complete recovery of sexual function may take up to one year, lagging behind a person's general recovery. The exact length of time depends on how long after symptoms appeared that BPH surgery was done and on the type of surgery. Following is a summary of how surgery is likely to affect the following aspects of sexual function.

Erections

Most doctors agree that if you were able to maintain an erection shortly before surgery, you will probably be able to have erections afterward. Surgery rarely causes a loss of erectile function. However, surgery cannot usually restore function that was lost before the operation.

Ejaculation

Although most men are able to continue having erections after surgery, a prostatectomy frequently makes them sterile (unable to father children) by causing a condition called "retrograde ejaculation" or "dry climax."

During sexual activity, sperm from the testes enters the urethra near the opening of the bladder. Normally, a muscle blocks off the entrance to the bladder, and the semen is expelled through the penis. However, the coring action of prostate surgery cuts this muscle as it widens the neck of the bladder. Following surgery, the semen takes the path of least resistance and enters the wider opening to the bladder rather than being expelled through the penis. Later it is harmlessly flushed out with urine. In some cases, this condition can be treated with a drug called pseudoephedrine, found in many cold medicines, or imipramine. These drugs improve muscle tone at the bladder neck and keep semen from entering the bladder.

Orgasm

Most men find little or no difference in the sensation of orgasm, or sexual climax, before and after surgery. Although it may take some time to get used to retrograde ejaculation, you should eventually find sex as pleasurable after surgery as before.

Many people have found that concerns about sexual function can interfere with sex as much as the operation itself. Understanding the surgical procedure and talking over any worries with the doctor before surgery often help men regain sexual function earlier. Many men also find it helpful to talk to a counselor during the adjustment period after surgery.

Further Treatment

In the years after your surgery, it is important to continue having a rectal exam once a year and to have any symptoms checked by your doctor.

Since surgery for BPH leaves behind a good part of the gland, it is still possible for prostate problems, including BPH, to develop again. However, surgery usually offers relief from BPH for at least 15 years. Only ten percent of the men who have surgery for BPH eventually need a second operation for enlargement. Usually these are men who had the first surgery at an early age.

Sometimes, scar tissue resulting from surgery requires treatment in the year after surgery. Rarely, the opening of the bladder becomes scarred and shrinks, causing obstruction. This problem may require a surgical procedure similar to transurethral incision (see section on Surgical Treatment). More often, scar tissue may form in the urethra and cause narrowing. This problem can usually be solved during an office visit when the doctor stretches the urethra.

Prostatic Stents

Stents are small devices inserted through the urethra to the narrowed area and allowed to expand, like a spring. The stent pushes back the prostatic tissue, widening the urethra. FDA approved the UroLume Endoprosthesis in 1996 to relieve urinary obstruction in men and improve the ability to urinate. The device is approved for use in men for whom other standard surgical procedures to correct urinary obstruction have failed.

BPH and Prostate Cancer: No Apparent Relation

Although some of the signs of BPH and prostate cancer are the same, having BPH does not seem to increase the chances of getting prostate cancer. Nevertheless, a man who has BPH may have undetected prostate cancer at the same time or may develop prostate cancer in the future. For this reason, the National Cancer Institute and the American Cancer Society recommend that all men over 40 have a rectal exam once a year to screen for prostate cancer.

After BPH surgery, the tissue removed is routinely checked for hidden cancer cells. In about one out of ten cases, some cancer tissue is found, but often it is limited to a few cells of a nonaggressive type of cancer, and no treatment is needed.

Section 27.4

Studying Therapies for Benign Prostatic Hyperplasia

This section contains information from "Minimally Invasive Surgical Therapies (MIST) Treatment Consortium for Benign Prostatic Hyperplasia (BPH)," March 15, 2004, and "NIH Launches New Study to Compare Prostate Surgery and Drugs," August 19, 2004, National Institute of Diabetes and Digestive and Kidney Diseases (NIDDK) of the National Institutes of Health (NIH).

Minimally Invasive Surgical Therapies (MIST) Treatment Consortium for Benign Prostatic Hyperplasia (BPH)

Background

The Division of Kidney and Urologic and Hematologic Diseases of the National Institute of Diabetes and Digestive and Kidney Diseases (NIDDK) has had a substantial and longstanding interest in evaluating the effectiveness of treatment strategies for the symptoms of benign prostatic hyperplasia (BPH). For many years, transurethral resection of the prostate (TURP) has been the standard surgical therapy for this condition. However, during the past decade, a number of technical innovations have allowed the development of new surgical treatments that aim to achieve the same long-term outcomes of TURP but with less morbidity, lower costs, office-based treatment or shorter length of hospital stay, and more rapid recovery. These new, "minimally-invasive" surgical approaches include laser therapy, hyperthermia and thermotherapy, transurethral electrovaporization, microwave therapy, and transurethral needle ablation. Newer techniques are appearing regularly. Published reports on the outcomes of these minimally-invasive therapies are highly variable in their quality, and rigorously conducted randomized clinical trials have only rarely been conducted.

To assess the long-term safety and effectiveness of these new therapies, the NIDDK has formed a consortium of seven Prostate Evaluation Treatment Centers and a Biostatistical Coordinating Center to develop and conduct randomized, controlled, clinical trials that will give a clearer picture of the benefits and risks of these methods. The seven clinical centers are Baylor College of Medicine, Columbia University, Mayo Clinic, Milwaukee College of Medicine, Northwestern University, University of Colorado Health Science Center, and Texas Southwestern Medical Center. The Data Coordinating Center is at George Washington University.

Clinical Trial

The first trial to be conducted by the MIST consortium will evaluate the safety and effectiveness of transurethral needle ablation (TUNA), transurethral microwave therapy (TUMT), and combined medical therapy with alfuzosin, an alpha blocker, and finasteride, an alpha-reductase inhibitor. The primary outcome is treatment failure, determined by an objective set of criteria, within 36 months. The recruitment goal is 714 patients (238 per treatment group). Recruitment began in [April] 2004 (http://www.clinicaltrials.gov). The trial will end in July 2008 with the last yearly follow-up exam. The results of the first trial will provide both physicians and patients with the knowledge needed to make the most appropriate choices for long-term management of BPH.

NIH Launches New Study to Compare Prostate Surgery and Drugs

The Minimally Invasive Surgical Therapies (MIST) Consortium for Benign Prostatic Hyperplasia (BPH) has launched a new study to compare long-term benefits and risks of transurethral needle ablation (TUNA) and transurethral microwave thermotherapy (TUMT) to a regimen of the alpha-1 inhibitor alfuzosin and the 5-alpha reductase inhibitor finasteride. The National Institute of Diabetes and Digestive and Kidney Diseases (NIDDK) at NIH, part of the Department of Health and Human Services, is investing more than $15 million in the study.

TUNA and TUMT use heat to destroy part of the enlarged prostate to improve urine flow and symptoms. Early studies suggest that these procedures reduce the occurrence of erection or bladder control side effects, which occur more often with the traditional surgery for BPH, known as transurethral resection of the prostate (TURP). TUNA and TUMT are said to be minimally invasive in part because they typically are done with local anesthesia and men go home the same day, whereas TURP requires general anesthesia and an overnight hospital stay. As for drug therapy, a recently published large randomized study showed that a regimen of finasteride (Proscar) and the alpha-1 inhibitor doxazosin (Cardura) prevents progression of BPH in a significant percentage of symptomatic men and it helps men at high risk avoid surgery.

"It's easy to see why drug therapy, TUNA and TUMT have been embraced by many urologists and patients," said Leroy M. Nyberg Jr., Ph.D., M.D., director of NIDDK's urology trials. "Yet, we don't know which treatment is more effective in the long run and, for the most part, who would be better served by the drug combination versus one of the minimally invasive therapies."

By July 2006, researchers plan to have recruited and randomly assigned more than 700 men with moderate to severe symptoms and no prior prostate surgery to one of the three MIST therapies. The men, age 50 and over, will be followed closely for three to five years, until about July 2009, to see who develops urinary retention, urinary tract infection or unacceptable incontinence after treatment; who needs more treatment; and whose symptoms don't improve by at least 30 percent after treatment.

Consortium members recruiting patients are Baylor College of Medicine in Houston; Columbia University in New York City; Mayo Clinic in Rochester, MN; Medical College of Wisconsin in Milwaukee; Northwestern University in Chicago; University of Colorado Health Sciences Center in Denver; and the University of Texas Southwestern Medical Center in Dallas. George Washington University Biostatistics Center in Rockville, MD, provides overall coordination for the study and data collection and analysis. For contact information visit http://www.mistbph.org.

BPH is increasingly common after age 50. Mild symptoms may wax and wane on their own, but Nyberg predicts that as more baby boomers cross into their 50s, physicians are likely to start seeing more men who are up frequently at night using the bathroom, a typical symptom of BPH along with embarrassing episodes of needing to go right away (urgency), daytime frequency, and occasional episodes of unavoidable wetting. Over time, the progressive symptoms associated with BPH can have a significant impact on quality of life for the individual as well as his close family members.

In 2000, BPH accounted for about 8 million office visits, 117,000 trips to emergency rooms, 105,000 hospital stays and 87,400 TURPs. BPH also cost patients and insurers about $1.1 billion, without considering nutritional supplements and 2.2 million prescriptions, according to NIDDK's Urologic Diseases in America interim compendium, released spring [2004].

MIST will also compare TUNA to TUMT and seeks to identify men best suited for each of the three therapies. Changes in sexual function, ejaculation, bladder changes, PSA, prostate size and shape, and ratio of various prostate tissues; and pain before, during and after surgery, among other parameters, will be tracked in search of characteristics predicting likely outcome and effectiveness of therapies.

"Having a protocol to fit the man to the therapy without having to try each treatment along the way should translate into lower costs and more-satisfied patients," said John W. Kusek, Ph.D., a clinical trials expert at NIDDK.

MIST therapies are approved by FDA, but relative benefits, risks and cost have never been compared. Further, there have been few rigorously conducted randomized trials of the minimally invasive surgical approaches.

"Previous studies of TUMT and TUNA haven't looked at side-effects and symptom relief long-term but, after we've finished MIST, men and their doctors should be a lot smarter about the options," said Kusek.

Other support for MIST comes from Diagnostic Ultrasound, Bothell, Washington; Urologix Inc. and Medtronic, both in Minneapolis; Merck & Co., Whitehouse Station, New Jersey; and Sanofi-Synthelabo Inc., New York.

Part Five

Disorders of the Kidneys

Chapter 28

Genetic and Congenital Disorders that Affect the Kidneys

Chapter Contents

Section 28.1

Polycystic Kidney Disease

National Kidney and Urologic Diseases Information Clearinghouse (NKUDIC), a service of the National Institute of Diabetes and Digestive and Kidney Diseases (NIDDK), National Institutes of Health (NIH), Pub. No. 05-4008, December 2004.

Polycystic kidney disease (PKD) is a genetic disorder characterized by the growth of numerous cysts in the kidneys. The cysts are filled with fluid. PKD cysts can slowly replace much of the mass of the kidneys, reducing kidney function and leading to kidney failure.

The kidneys are two organs, each about the size of a fist, located in the upper part of a person's abdomen, toward the back. The kidneys filter wastes from the blood to form urine. They also regulate amounts of certain vital substances in the body.

When PKD causes kidneys to fail—which usually happens after many years—the patient requires dialysis or kidney transplantation. About one-half of people with the major type of PKD progress to kidney failure, also called end-stage renal disease (ESRD).

PKD can cause cysts in the liver and problems in other organs, such as the heart and blood vessels in the brain. These complications help doctors distinguish PKD from the usually harmless "simple" cysts that often form in the kidneys in later years of life.

In the United States, about 500,000 people have PKD, and it is the fourth leading cause of kidney failure. Medical professionals describe two major inherited forms of PKD and a noninherited form:

- **Autosomal dominant PKD** is the most common inherited form. Symptoms usually develop between the ages of 30 and 40, but they can begin earlier, even in childhood. About 90 percent of all PKD cases are autosomal dominant PKD.

- **Autosomal recessive PKD** is a rare inherited form. Symptoms of autosomal recessive PKD begin in the earliest months of life, even in the womb.

- **Acquired cystic kidney disease (ACKD)** develops in association with long-term kidney problems, especially in patients who

318

have kidney failure and who have been on dialysis for a long time. Therefore it tends to occur in later years of life. It is not an inherited form of PKD.

What is autosomal dominant PKD?

Autosomal dominant PKD is one of the most common inherited disorders. The phrase "autosomal dominant" means that if one parent has the disease, there is a 50 percent chance that the disease will pass to a child. At least one parent must have the disease for a child to inherit it. Either the mother or father can pass it along, but new mutations may account for one-fourth of new cases. In some rare cases, the cause of autosomal dominant PKD occurs spontaneously in the child soon after conception—in these cases the parents are not the source of this disease.

Many people with autosomal dominant PKD live for decades without developing symptoms. For this reason, autosomal dominant PKD is often called "adult polycystic kidney disease." Yet, in some cases, cysts may form earlier, even in the first years of life.

The disease is thought to occur equally in men and women and equally in people of all races. However, some studies suggest that it occurs more often in whites than in blacks and more often in females than in males.

The cysts grow out of nephrons, the tiny filtering units inside the kidneys. The cysts eventually separate from the nephrons and continue to enlarge. The kidneys enlarge along with the cysts (which can number in the thousands), while retaining roughly their kidney shape. In fully developed PKD, a cyst-filled kidney can weigh as much as 22 pounds. High blood pressure occurs early in the disease, often before cysts appear.

What are the symptoms of autosomal dominant PKD?

The most common symptoms are pain in the back and the sides (between the ribs and hips), and headaches. The dull pain can be temporary or persistent, mild or severe.

People with autosomal dominant PKD also can experience the following:

- urinary tract infections
- hematuria (blood in the urine)
- liver and pancreatic cysts
- abnormal heart valves
- high blood pressure
- kidney stones

- aneurysms (bulges in the walls of blood vessels) in the brain
- diverticulosis (small sacs on the colon)

How is autosomal dominant PKD diagnosed?

To diagnose autosomal dominant PKD, a doctor typically observes three or more kidney cysts using ultrasound imaging. The diagnosis is strengthened by a family history of autosomal dominant PKD and the presence of cysts in other organs.

In most cases of autosomal dominant PKD, the person's physical condition appears normal for many years, even decades, so the disease can go unnoticed. Physical checkups and blood and urine tests may not lead to diagnosis. The slow, undetected progression is why some people live for many years without knowing they have autosomal dominant PKD.

Once cysts have formed, however, diagnosis is possible with imaging technology. Ultrasound, which passes sound waves through the body to create a picture of the kidneys, is used most often. Ultrasound imaging employs no injected dyes or radiation and is safe for all patients, including pregnant women. It can also detect cysts in the kidneys of a fetus.

More powerful and expensive imaging procedures such as computed tomography (CT scan) and magnetic resonance imaging (MRI) also can detect cysts, but they usually are not required for diagnosis because ultrasound provides adequate information. CT scans require x-rays and sometimes injected dyes.

A genetic test can detect mutations in the *PKD1* and *PKD2* genes. Although this test can detect the presence of the autosomal dominant PKD mutations before cysts develop, its usefulness is limited by two factors: it cannot predict the onset or ultimate severity of the disease, and no absolute cure is available to prevent the onset of the disease. On the other hand, a young person who knows of a PKD gene mutation may be able to forestall the disease through diet and blood pressure control. The test may also be used to determine whether a young member of a PKD family can safely donate a kidney to a parent. Anyone considering genetic testing should receive counseling to understand all the implications of the test.

How is autosomal dominant PKD treated?

Although a cure for autosomal dominant PKD is not available, treatment can ease the symptoms and prolong life.

Pain: A doctor will first suggest over-the-counter pain medications, such as aspirin or Tylenol. For most but not all cases of severe pain, surgery to shrink cysts can relieve pain in the back and flanks. However, surgery provides only temporary relief and usually does not slow the disease's progression toward kidney failure.

Headaches that are severe or that seem to feel different from other headaches might be caused by aneurysms, or swollen blood vessels, in the brain. Headaches also can be caused by high blood pressure. People with autosomal dominant PKD should see a doctor if they have severe or recurring headaches—even before considering over-the-counter pain medications.

Urinary tract infections: Patients with autosomal dominant PKD tend to have frequent urinary tract infections, which can be treated with antibiotics. People with the disease should seek treatment for urinary tract infections immediately, because infection can spread from the urinary tract to the cysts in the kidneys. Cyst infections are difficult to treat because many antibiotics do not penetrate into the cysts. However, some antibiotics are effective.

High blood pressure: Keeping blood pressure under control can slow the effects of autosomal dominant PKD. Lifestyle changes and various medications can lower high blood pressure. Patients should ask their doctors about such treatments. Sometimes proper diet and exercise are enough to keep blood pressure low.

End-stage renal disease: Because kidneys are essential for life, people with ESRD must seek one of two options for replacing kidney functions: dialysis or transplantation. In hemodialysis, blood is circulated into an external machine, where it is cleaned before re-entering the body; in peritoneal dialysis, a fluid is introduced into the abdomen, where it absorbs wastes, and it is then removed. Transplantation of healthy kidneys into ESRD patients has become a common and successful procedure. Healthy (non-PKD) kidneys transplanted into PKD patients do not develop cysts.

What is autosomal recessive PKD?

Autosomal recessive PKD is caused by a particular genetic flaw that is different from the genetic flaw that causes autosomal dominant PKD. Parents who do not have PKD can have a child with the disease if both parents carry the abnormal gene and both pass the gene to their baby. The chance of this happening (when both parents carry the abnormal gene) is one in four. If only one parent carries the abnormal gene, the baby cannot get the disease.

The symptoms of autosomal recessive PKD can begin before birth, so it is often called "infantile PKD." Children born with autosomal recessive PKD usually develop kidney failure within a few years. Severity of the disease varies. Babies with the worst cases die hours or days after birth. Children with an infantile version may have sufficient renal function for normal activities for a few years. People with the juvenile version may live into their teens and twenties and usually will have liver problems as well.

What are the symptoms of autosomal recessive PKD?

Children with autosomal recessive PKD experience high blood pressure, urinary tract infections, and frequent urination. The disease usually affects the liver, spleen, and pancreas, resulting in low blood-cell counts, varicose veins, and hemorrhoids. Because kidney function is crucial for early physical development, children with autosomal recessive PKD are usually smaller than average size.

How is autosomal recessive PKD diagnosed?

Ultrasound imaging of the fetus or newborn baby reveals cysts in the kidneys, but does not distinguish between the cysts of autosomal recessive and autosomal dominant PKD. Ultrasound examination of kidneys of relatives can be helpful; for example, a parent or grandparent with autosomal dominant PKD cysts could help confirm diagnosis of autosomal dominant PKD in a fetus or child. (It is extremely rare, although not impossible, for a person with autosomal recessive PKD to become a parent.) Because autosomal recessive PKD tends to scar the liver, ultrasound imaging of the liver also aids in diagnosis.

How is autosomal recessive PKD treated?

Medicines can control high blood pressure in autosomal recessive PKD, and antibiotics can control urinary tract infections. Eating increased amounts of nutritious food improves growth in children with autosomal recessive PKD. In some cases, growth hormones are used. In response to kidney failure, autosomal recessive PKD patients must receive dialysis or transplantation.

What are genetic diseases?

Genes are segments of DNA, the long molecules that reside in the nuclei of your body's cells. The genes, through complex processes, cause chemical activities that lead to growth and maintenance of the body.

At conception, DNA (and therefore genes) from both parents are passed to the child.

A genetic disease occurs when one or both parents pass abnormal genes to a child at conception. If receiving an abnormal gene from just one parent is enough to produce a disease in the child, the disease is said to have dominant inheritance. If receiving abnormal genes from both parents is needed to produce disease in the child, the disease is said to be recessive.

The chance of acquiring a dominant disease (one gene copy is enough) is higher than the chance of acquiring a recessive disease (two gene copies are needed). A child who receives only one gene copy for a recessive disease at conception will not develop the genetic disease (such as autosomal recessive PKD), but could pass the gene to the following generation.

What is acquired cystic kidney disease (ACKD)?

ACKD develops in kidneys with long-term damage and bad scarring, so it often is associated with dialysis and end-stage renal disease. About 90 percent of people on dialysis for five years develop ACKD. People with ACKD can have any underlying kidney disease, such as glomerulonephritis or kidney disease of diabetes.

The cysts of ACKD may bleed. Kidney tumors, including kidney (renal) cancer, can develop in people with ACKD. Renal cancer is rare yet occurs at least twice as often in ACKD patients as in the general population.

How is ACKD diagnosed?

Patients with ACKD usually seek help because they notice blood in their urine (hematuria). The cysts bleed into the urinary system, which discolors urine. Diagnosis is confirmed using ultrasound, CT scan, or MRI of the kidneys.

How is ACKD treated?

Most ACKD patients are already receiving treatment for kidney problems. In rare cases, surgery is used to stop bleeding of cysts and to remove tumors or suspected tumors.

Hope through Research

Scientists have begun to identify the processes that trigger formation of PKD cysts. Advances in the field of genetics have increased our understanding of the abnormal genes responsible for autosomal dominant and autosomal recessive PKD. Scientists have located two genes associated with autosomal dominant PKD. The first was located in 1985 on chromosome 16 and labeled *PKD1*. *PKD2* was localized to chromosome 4 in 1993. Within three years, the scientists had isolated the proteins these two genes produce—polycystin-1 and polycystin-2.

When both of these genes are normal, the proteins they produce work together to foster normal kidney development and inhibit cyst formation. A mutation in either *PKD1* or *PKD2* can lead to cyst formation, but evidence suggests that the disease development also requires other factors, in addition to the mutation in one of the PKD genes.

Genetic analyses of most families with PKD confirm mutations in either the *PKD1* or *PKD2* gene. In rare cases, however, families with PKD have been found to have normal *PKD1* and *PKD2* genes. As a result, researchers theorize that a *PKD3* gene exists, but that gene has not been mapped or identified.

Researchers recently identified the autosomal recessive PKD gene (called *PKHD1*) on chromosome 6. No genetic test kit is yet available to detect mutations in *PKHD1*.

Researchers have bred mice with a genetic disease that parallels both inherited forms of human PKD. Studying these mice will lead to greater understanding of the genetic and nongenetic mechanisms involved in cyst formation. In 2000, scientists reported that a cancer drug was successful in inhibiting cyst formation in mice with the PKD gene. In 2003, scientists also demonstrated that another compound, one that blocks function of a kidney receptor, inhibits cyst formation in mice with the *ADPKD* or *ARPKD* gene. The scientists hope that further testing will lead to safe and effective treatments for humans.

Section 28.2

Primary Hyperoxaluria

Hyperoxaluria and Oxalosis

Hyperoxaluria is a condition where too much oxalate is present in the urine. Oxalate is the salt form of oxalic acid, and is a natural end product of metabolism. Oxalate does not appear to be needed for any human body process and normally, more than 90 percent is excreted by the healthy kidney, with a small amount of excretion into the lower gut. Since oxalate and calcium are continuously excreted by the kidney into the urine, it can combine with calcium causing formations of calcium-oxalate crystals and grow into a kidney stone.

Kidney stones are more common in adults, occurring in ten percent of men and three percent of women during their lifetimes. Kidney stones are rare in children and uncommon in teenagers, though can occur at any age. Calcium oxalate stones are the most common type of stone formed by individuals who have kidney stone disease. Increased oxalate in the urine can come from eating too much oxalate in foods, over-absorption of oxalate from the intestinal tract associated with intestinal diseases (enteric hyperoxaluria), and abnormalities of oxalate production (primary hyperoxaluria).

Hyperoxaluria is uncommon. In some people the cause of the excess urine oxalate is not known, but may result from changes in the way kidneys handle normal amounts of body oxalate. In its many forms it can be found among all ages, from infants to people in their 70s. The highest amounts of oxalate in the urine however are seen in diseases in which the liver produces too much oxalate—this occurs in primary hyperoxaluria.

Because of the low solubility of oxalate, increased concentrations of oxalate in body fluids, including the urine, can lead to the deposition of calcium oxalate (oxalosis) in the kidney tissue (nephrocalcinosis) or urinary tract (urolithiasis, nephrolithiasis, kidney stones). Oxalosis occurs after the kidneys fail and the excess oxalate builds up in the blood and then deposits oxalate salts in the eyes, blood vessels, bones, muscles, heart, and other major organs.

Primary Hyperoxaluria Type I and Type II

Primary hyperoxaluria (PH) is a rare genetic (inherited) disorder that is present at birth. Primary hyperoxaluria comes in many forms, of which only two, type I and type II are well characterized. Type I and type II are both autosomal recessive diseases. Although type I is more common than type II, it is still a rare disease with an estimated frequency of somewhere between 1 in 100,000 and 1 in 1,000,000.

In type I and type II PH, the enzyme in the liver is defective but the organ that suffers is the kidney. In a person with type I, the liver creates too little of the enzyme alanine-glyoxylate aminotransferase or AGT. In patients with type I, the deficiency of AGT causes increased amounts of oxalate and glycolate to be formed in the body. Unfortunately, oxalate cannot be further metabolized, and it can only be eliminated from the body by the kidney by urinary excretion. This leads to an increase in urinary excretion, producing both hyperoxaluria and hyperglycolic aciduria.

In type II, the liver is missing a different enzyme called glyoxylate reductase or GR also called, hydroxypyruvate reductase or HPR. Like AGT, GR is also found mainly in liver cells. Very large amounts of oxalate are produced when there is too little of the enzyme in the liver which leads to increased urinary excretion. Type II patients frequently have high concentrations of glyceric acid in the urine in addition to hyperoxaluria. Over time, large amounts of oxalate in the urine can cause kidney stones.

Patients with primary hyperoxaluria typically present kidney stones, anywhere from birth to the mid-20s. But hyperoxaluria may go unrecognized until age 30 to 40. When very large amounts of oxalate are present in the urine, such as in primary hyperoxaluria, the kidneys can be damaged to the point that they stop working (renal failure). In some patients the first symptom may be kidney failure. Oxalosis occurs after the kidneys fail and the excess oxalate builds up in the blood, and then spreads to the eyes, bones, muscles, blood vessels, heart, and other major organs.

Milder forms of hyperoxaluria can cause kidney stones without other associated problems. Severe hyperoxaluria not only causes kidney stones but if left untreated, can lead to serious illness and even death. Among patients with primary hyperoxaluria, about 50 percent will have kidney failure by age 15, and about 80 percent will have kidney failure by age 30. For that reason, it is critical that primary hyperoxaluria be diagnosed and treated as early as possible.

Other Forms of Primary Hyperoxaluria

Other forms of PH certainly exist and a number of individuals have been described with very high urine oxalate who have normal AGT and GR activities. However, reasons for the marked increase in oxalate in these patients (whether it is due to a different liver enzyme defect or to problems in the kidney) has not yet been identified.

Chronic Kidney Disease, Kidney Failure, and Oxalosis

The kidneys, when working normally, are very efficient at eliminating excess oxalate that is produced by the liver or absorbed from the intestinal tract. In patients with good kidney function, blood concentrations of oxalate are kept normal or near the normal range, and it is only in the urine and the kidney tissue that high concentrations of oxalate occur. It is the high concentration of oxalate in the urine (hyperoxaluria) that causes stones to form, and over time causes damage to kidney tissue.

As time passes, kidney function may be reduced by 50 percent or more. When that occurs, and the kidney can no longer eliminate excess oxalate efficiently, blood levels of oxalate begin to rise. When blood oxalate concentrations reach a critical level, the amount of oxalate in the blood is high enough to form complexes with calcium leading to calcium oxalate deposits in multiple body tissues (called oxalosis).

Oxalosis can involve many different organs. Most common in patients with primary hyperoxaluria with associated kidney failure are deposits in small blood vessels which can cause painful skin ulcers that do not heal, deposits in bone marrow causing anemia, deposits in bone tissue causing failure to grow in children and fractures in adults and children, and calcium oxalate deposits in the heart causing abnormalities of heart rhythm or poor heart function.

Oxalosis will become progressively more severe as long as the blood oxalate concentration remains high, and can lead to death. For this reason, prompt recognition of the problem and prompt treatment are essential. Kidney dialysis can remove oxalate from the blood, but in most patients with primary hyperoxaluria dialysis cannot keep pace with the very large amount of oxalate produced. Definitive treatment of kidney failure and oxalosis in patients with primary hyperoxaluria is transplantation.

Section 28.3

Alport Syndrome

© 2005 A.D.A.M., Inc. Reprinted with permission. Updated January 19, 2004, by Irfan A. Agha, M.D.

Alternative names: hereditary nephritis, hematuria—nephropathy—deafness, hemorrhagic familial nephritis, hereditary deafness and nephropathy

Definition: Alport syndrome is an inherited disorder (usually X-linked) involving damage to the kidney, blood in the urine, and in some families, loss of hearing. The disorder may also include eye defects.

Causes, Incidence, and Risk Factors

Alport syndrome is very similar to hereditary nephritis. There may be nerve deafness and congenital eye abnormalities associated with Alport syndrome. The cause is a mutation in a gene for collagen. The disorder is uncommon, and most often affects males since the genetic defect is typically found on the X chromosome.

In women, the disorder is usually mild, with minimal or no symptoms. Women can transmit the gene for the disorder to their children, even if the woman has no symptoms of the disorder. In men, the symptoms are more severe and progress faster.

The disorder causes chronic glomerulonephritis with destruction of the glomeruli in the kidneys. Initially, there are no symptoms. Progressive destruction of the glomeruli causes blood in the urine and decreases the effectiveness of the kidney's filtering system.

There is progressive loss of kidney function and accumulation of fluids and wastes in the body, with eventual progression to end-stage renal disease (ESRD) at an early age. ESRD, caused by Alport syndrome, often develops between adolescence and age 40.

Risk factors include having a family history of Alport syndrome, nephritis, end-stage renal disease in male relatives, hearing loss before age 30, bloody urine, glomerulonephritis, and similar disorders.

Symptoms

- Abnormal urine color
- Blood in the urine
- Loss of hearing, more common in males
- Decrease or loss of vision, more common in males
- Cough
- Ankle, feet, and leg swelling
- Swelling, overall
- Swelling around the eyes

Note: There may be no symptoms in some cases. Symptoms of chronic renal failure or heart failure may be present or may develop.

Signs and Tests

Examination is nonspecific, except for blood in the urine. Minute amounts of blood (microscopic hematuria) is present from birth in nearly all affected males. The blood pressure may be elevated. Examination of the eyes may show fundus (posterior inner part of eye) or lens changes, cataracts, or lens protrusion (lenticonus). Examination of the ears shows no structural changes.

- Urinalysis shows blood, protein, and other abnormalities.
- BUN [blood urea nitrogen], creatinine are elevated.
- Red blood cell count, hematocrit may decrease.
- Hematuria test is positive.
- Audiometry may show nerve deafness.
- Renal biopsy shows chronic glomerulonephritis with the classical changes of Alport syndrome.

Treatment

Treatment goals include monitoring and controlling progression of the disease and treatment of symptoms. The most important task is strict control of high blood pressure.

Treatment of chronic renal failure will become necessary. This may include dietary modifications, fluid restriction, and other treatments. Ultimately, chronic renal failure progresses to end-stage renal disease, requiring dialysis or transplantation.

Surgical repair of cataracts (cataract extraction), or repair of the anterior lenticonus is possible.

Loss of hearing is likely to be permanent. Counseling and education to increase coping skills can be helpful. Learning new skills such as lip reading or sign language may be of some benefit. Hearing aids are helpful. Young men with Alport syndrome should use hearing protection in noisy environments.

Genetic counseling may be recommended because of the inherited pattern of the disorder.

Expectations (Prognosis)

In women, there is usually a normal life span with no manifestation except for blood in the urine. Rarely, women exhibit hypertension, edema, and nerve deafness as a complication of pregnancy.

In men, deafness, visual difficulties, and renal failure are likely by age 50.

Complications

- Chronic renal failure
- End-stage renal disease
- Permanent deafness
- Decrease or loss of vision

Calling Your Healthcare Provider

Call for an appointment with your healthcare provider if symptoms indicating Alport syndrome may be present, or if there is a history of Alport syndrome and children are planned.

Call your healthcare provider if urine output decreases or stops. This may be a symptom of chronic renal failure.

Prevention

This uncommon disorder is inherited. Awareness of risk factors, such as a family history of the disorder, may allow the condition to be detected early.

Section 28.4

Bartter Syndrome

"Bartter's Syndrome," © 2005 A.D.A.M., Inc. Reprinted with permission. Updated November 10, 2004, by John Goldenring, M.D.

Alternative names: Potassium wasting

Definition: Bartter syndrome involves a group of symptoms and signs:

* Enlargement of certain kidney cells

* Alkalosis associated with reduced potassium (hypokalemic alkalosis)

* Increased production of the hormone aldosterone

There is no elevation of blood pressure with Bartter syndrome, which usually occurs with kidney disease.

Causes, Incidence, and Risk Factors

The exact cause of Bartter syndrome is not known. In some cases, it may be genetic and the condition is present from before birth (congenital).

The condition is thought to be caused by a defect in the kidney's ability to reabsorb potassium. As a result, an excessive amount of potassium is excreted from the body. This is also known as potassium wasting.

Symptoms

This disease usually occurs in childhood. Symptoms include muscle cramping and weakness, constipation, increased frequency of urination, and growth failure.

Signs and Tests

The diagnosis of Bartter syndrome is usually made by finding low levels of potassium in the blood. The potassium level is usually less than 2.5 mEq/L. Other signs of this syndrome include the following:

- Normal blood pressure
- Low blood chloride
- Metabolic alkalosis (blood is more alkaline than normal)
- High blood levels of the hormones renin and aldosterone (both are involved in the regulation of potassium by the kidney)
- High levels of potassium and chloride in the urine

These same signs and symptoms can also occur in people who have taken excessive amounts of diuretics or laxatives. Urine tests can be done to exclude these causes.

In Bartter syndrome, a biopsy of the kidney typically shows overgrowth of cells called the juxtaglomerular apparatus. However, this is not found in all patients, especially in young children.

Treatment

Bartter syndrome is treated by keeping the blood potassium level above 3.5 mEq/L. This is achieved through a diet rich in potassium. Some patients also require salt and magnesium supplements.

Expectations (Prognosis)

The long-term prognosis for patients with Bartter syndrome is not certain. Infants who experience severe growth failure typically grow normally with treatment. Studies are being done to see if these children have decreased mental functioning, which can occur if potassium levels are abnormal for too long. While most patients remain well with ongoing treatment, some develop kidney failure.

Complications

Kidney failure is a possible complication.

Calling Your Healthcare Provider

Call your healthcare provider if your child is not growing well, is urinating frequently, and is having muscle cramps.

Chapter 29

Kidney Diseases in Children

Chapter Contents

Section 29.1

Childhood Kidney Diseases

This information, from "Kidney Diseases in Childhood," was provided by KidsHealth, one of the largest resources online for medically reviewed health information written for parents, kids, and teens. For more articles like this one, visit www.KidsHealth.org, or www.TeensHealth.org. © 2001 The Nemours Center for Children's Health Media, a division of The Nemours Foundation. Reviewed by Laszlo Hopp, M.D., May 2001.

The kidneys play a critical role in overall health. Acting like a water filter that separates out harmful minerals and chemicals, the kidneys process about 200 quarts of blood in an adult every day to produce about 1 to 2 quarts of urine, which is made up of waste products and extra water. Urine leaves the kidneys (almost all people are born with two) through tubes called ureters, which empty into the bladder. Without the kidneys, waste products would build up in the blood and damage the body.

The filtration process occurs in microscopic units inside the kidneys called nephrons; each kidney has about a million nephrons. As they remove waste products and extra water, the nephrons return chemicals the body needs (such as sodium, phosphorus, and potassium) to the blood. Each chemical is vital to overall health and must be in proper balance. Too much or too little can be harmful.

The kidneys also produce three important hormones: erythropoietin (uh-rith-ro-poy-uh-tin), which stimulates the bone marrow to make red blood cells; renin, which helps regulate blood pressure; and the active form of vitamin D, which helps control the calcium balance in the body and maintain healthy bones.

When something goes wrong with the hormones or filtering process, it could indicate a kidney disease. What are kidney diseases, and how can they be treated?

What are kidney diseases?

Kidney diseases can include congenital malformations (birth defects), obstructions of the urinary tract, and disease of the kidney tissue itself. The most common kidney diseases in children are congenital abnormalities, such as:

- **Posterior urethral valve obstruction,** a narrowing or obstruction of the urethra (the tube that carries urine out of the body from the bladder).

- **Fetal hydronephrosis,** a dilatation or enlargement of one or both of a fetus' kidneys due to an abnormality in the developing urinary tract. Hydronephrosis can also occur in infancy or childhood due to a blockage in the urinary tract or vesicoureteral reflux (VUR), which occurs when the mechanism that prevents urine from backing up from the bladder to the kidneys does not develop or function properly.

Cystic kidney diseases usually are congenital (the child is born with it). One form of cystic kidney disease is polycystic kidney disease (PKD), which is the presence of numerous fluid-filled cysts in the kidneys. The cysts can replace much of the mass of the kidneys and can lead to kidney failure. Some forms of PKD are inherited.

Another form of cystic kidney disease is multicystic kidney disease, in which a developmentally abnormal kidney (dysplastic kidney) grows large cysts and eventually stops functioning. Although PKD always affects both kidneys, multicystic kidney disease frequently affects only one.

Some other diseases affecting the kidneys are:

- **Renal tubular acidosis,** a condition in which the kidneys do not properly regulate the amount of acid in the body.

- **Wilms tumor,** a type of childhood cancer that involves the kidney.

- **Nephritis,** an inflammation or infection of the filtering unit of the kidney.

- **Nephrosis,** a change in nephrons that is not inflammatory; nephrotic syndrome occurs when large amounts of protein are lost from the body through the urine, usually as a result of nephrosis.

What causes kidney diseases?

Just about every parent feels guilty when there's a diagnosis of a kidney disease in his or her child. Doctors emphasize that, in children, these diseases typically are not the result of anything a parent did or didn't do. In some cases, nephritis is inherited or may be the result of an infection, but more often, the cause is unknown.

"Despite women taking every possible precaution during their pregnancies, [congenital abnormalities] can occur," says Barry L. Warshaw, MD, associate professor of pediatrics at Emory School of Medicine in Atlanta, Georgia. "Some disorders are genetic, but it can be recessive and you have no way of knowing that."

Repeated kidney and urinary tract infections, sickle cell anemia, lupus, high blood pressure, and diabetes can also cause kidney damage; so can a serious injury like a car accident or a major fall.

When to call the doctor?

The signs and symptoms of urinary tract or kidney disease can be diverse and include:

- fever.

- swelling around the eyes, feet, and ankles.

- burning or pain during urination.

- significant increase in the frequency of urination.

- difficulty in controlling urination in children who are mature enough to use the toilet.

- recurrence of nighttime bedwetting (in children who have been dry for several months).

- blood in the urine.

- high blood pressure.

"I ask families, 'How do you do in the car on the road? Can you make it from place to place or do you have to stop to go to the bathroom?'" Dr. Warshaw says. "If you do and that's new, it's something that needs to be evaluated."

One sign of urethral valve obstruction in newborn boys is poor urinary stream. "Most boys can give you a nice hose effect," Dr. Warshaw explains. With obstructed valves, the urine may only dribble out.

Another sign of possible kidney disease that should be brought to your child's doctor's attention is the presence of edema (swelling, especially around the eyes, face, feet, and ankles), which may be present in nephrotic syndrome.

How are kidney diseases diagnosed?

If your child's doctor suspects a kidney disease in your child, he or she may order urine tests, blood tests, imaging studies, or a biopsy to help make a diagnosis. Your child's doctor may also consult with or refer your child to a nephrologist, a doctor who specializes in the diagnosis and treatment of kidney diseases.

With urinalysis (a type of urine test), your child's doctor can quickly detect abnormalities (such as too many red blood cells) that may signal inflammation or irritation in the urinary tract. Urinalysis can also detect excess white blood cells, which are most commonly associated with bladder and kidney infections. Urinalysis also can reveal the presence of casts, cylindrical structures made up of cells and/or protein that form in the kidney's nephrons when some kidney diseases are present. The absence of casts doesn't eliminate the possibility of a kidney disease, but their presence suggests it.

Some tests, such as creatinine clearance, involve collecting urine over a 24-hour period, but the difficulty in collecting such a sample in young children (especially those still in diapers) limits their use.

Certain blood tests tell doctors how well the kidneys are filtering waste products and balancing the bloodstream's chemical makeup. Creatinine and blood urea nitrogen (BUN) are two common blood level tests that doctors use to monitor kidney function.

Two other important diagnostic tools a doctor may use during an initial physical exam are blood pressure and growth measurements. Along with the heart, the kidneys are the most important organ in the body in determining blood pressure. High blood pressure in a child is an important sign that the kidneys need to be evaluated. Accurate growth measurements can provide a clue in diagnosing some kidney diseases because children with chronic kidney disease often grow poorly.

Your child's doctor may use a kidney biopsy to evaluate your child's kidney function. A biopsy is a procedure in which a small piece of the kidney tissue is removed with a needle. Performed while a child is under anesthesia, it's a simple procedure that can help make an accurate diagnosis of the kidney problem in about nine out of 10 cases. It's especially helpful in the diagnosis of nephritis and nephrosis.

In addition to doing a physical examination, the doctor will ask you about any concerns and symptoms you have, your past health, your family's health, any medications you're taking, any allergies you may have, and other issues. This is called the medical history.

In addition to standard x-rays, other imaging studies a doctor may use to help diagnose kidney diseases include:

Ultrasound: Of all the studies, ultrasound is the most commonly used. Painless and requiring no x-ray exposure or special preparation, a renal ultrasound shows details of the anatomy of the kidneys and bladder. It can rule out or diagnose obstructions, developmental abnormalities, tumors, and stones in the kidneys and urinary tract.

Computerized tomography (CT): A CT scan is often helpful in revealing the anatomy of the kidneys or bladder and, in some cases, is better than ultrasound for finding kidney stones. It can show if the kidneys have developed properly or if the flow of urine is blocked by a stone or a developmental abnormality.

Renal nuclear scan: A renal nuclear scan involves having special radioactive material injected into a vein. The radiation dose is similar to that of a simple x-ray. The scan shows how the kidneys compare to each other in size, shape, and function. It also can detect scarring or other evidence of recurrent or chronic kidney infection.

Cystoscopy: Cystoscopy is not commonly performed but can detect bladder abnormalities by inserting a small fiberoptic videoscope into the bladder.

Voiding cystourethrogram (VCUG): VCUG is commonly used to evaluate the bladder and the ureters. This procedure involves putting a dye into the bladder to see whether there's an obstruction or abnormal backflow of urine when a child urinates (called vesicoureteral reflux, or VUR).

Section 29.2

Hemolytic Uremic Syndrome

National Kidney and Urologic Diseases Information Clearinghouse (NKUDIC), a service of the National Institute of Diabetes and Digestive and Kidney Diseases (NIDDK), National Institutes of Health (NIH), Pub. No. 04-4570, December 2003.

Hemolytic (HEE-mo-LIT-ik) uremic (yoo-REE-mik) syndrome, or HUS, is one of the most common causes of sudden, short-term kidney failure in children. In severe cases, this acute kidney failure may require several sessions of dialysis to take over the kidneys' job of filtering wastes from the blood, but most children recover without permanent damage to their health.

Most cases of HUS occur after an infection of the digestive system by *Escherichia coli* bacterium, which is found in contaminated foods like meat, dairy products, and juice. Some people have contracted HUS after swimming in pools or lakes contaminated with feces. Washing and cooking foods adequately, avoiding undercooked meats, and avoiding unclean swimming areas are the best ways to protect your children from this disease.

The infection of the digestive tract is called gastroenteritis and may cause the child to vomit and have stomach cramps and bloody diarrhea. Most children who experience gastroenteritis recover fully in two or three days and do not develop HUS. In a few children, however, HUS develops when the bacteria lodged in the digestive system make toxins that enter the bloodstream and start to destroy red blood cells.

Symptoms of HUS may not become apparent until a week after the digestive problems. The child remains pale, tired, and irritable. Other symptoms include small, unexplained bruises or bleeding from the nose or mouth that may occur because the toxins also destroy the platelets, cells that normally help clotting.

You may notice that your child's urine output decreases. Urine formation slows because the damaged red blood cells clog the tiny blood vessels in the kidneys, making them work harder to remove wastes and extra fluid from the blood. The body's inability to rid itself of excess fluid and wastes may in turn cause high blood pressure or swelling of the face, hands, feet, or the entire body. This progression to acute kidney failure occurs in about half the cases of HUS.

Call your child's doctor immediately if you notice unexplained bruises, unusual bleeding, swollen limbs or generalized swelling, extreme fatigue, or decreased urine output in your child. You should call your doctor or visit an emergency room if your child goes 12 hours without urinating.

Treatments, which consist of maintaining normal salt and water levels in the body, are aimed at easing the immediate symptoms and preventing further complications. Blood transfusions (packed red blood cells) are sometimes necessary, and high blood pressure may need treatment. Only the most severe cases require dialysis. Some children may sustain significant kidney damage that slowly develops into permanent kidney failure and will then require long-term peritoneal dialysis or hemodialysis or a kidney transplant. Most children recover completely with no long-term consequences.

Some parents feel a sense of responsibility for their child's illness after a case of HUS. While the disease may ultimately have been preventable, caregivers should not feel guilty because the insidious course of the disease cannot be predicted from the initial bacterial infection, which many children experience without developing HUS. Caregivers who see that their children receive the appropriate medical care should rest assured that they have done all that any caring parent could do.

Chapter 30

Diabetes Insipidus

Diabetes insipidus (DI) is characterized by excretion of large amounts of dilute urine, which disrupts your body's water regulation. To make up for lost water, you may feel the need to drink large amounts of water. You are likely to urinate frequently, even at night, which can disrupt sleep or, on occasion, cause bedwetting. Because of the excretion of abnormally large volumes of dilute urine, you may quickly become dehydrated if you do not drink enough water. Children with DI may be irritable or listless and, in some cases, may have fever, vomiting, or diarrhea. In its clinically significant forms, it is a rare disease.

Diabetes Insipidus versus Diabetes Mellitus

DI should not be confused with diabetes mellitus, which results from insulin deficiency or resistance leading to high blood glucose. Diabetes insipidus and diabetes mellitus are unrelated, although they can have similar signs and symptoms, like excessive thirst and excessive urination.

Diabetes mellitus (DM) is far more common than DI and receives more news coverage. DM has two forms, referred to as type 1 diabetes (formerly called juvenile diabetes, or insulin-dependent diabetes

National Kidney and Urologic Diseases Information Clearinghouse (NKUDIC), a service of the National Institute of Diabetes and Digestive and Kidney Diseases (NIDDK), National Institutes of Health (NIH), Pub. No. 03-4620, June 2003.

mellitus, or IDDM) and type 2 diabetes (formerly called adult-onset diabetes, or noninsulin-dependent diabetes mellitus, or NIDDM). DI is a different form of illness altogether.

Normal Fluid Regulation in the Body

Your body has a complex system for balancing the volume and composition of body fluids. Your kidneys remove extra body fluids from your bloodstream. This fluid waste is stored in the bladder as urine. If your fluid regulation system is working properly, your kidneys make less urine to conserve fluid when the body is losing water. Your kidneys also make less urine at night when the body's metabolic processes are slower.

In order to keep the volume and composition of body fluids balanced, the rate of fluid intake is governed by thirst, and the rate of excretion is governed by the production of antidiuretic hormone (ADH), also called vasopressin. This hormone is made in the hypothalamus, a small gland located in the base of the brain. ADH is stored in the nearby pituitary gland and released from it into the bloodstream when necessary. When ADH reaches the kidneys, it directs the kidneys to concentrate the urine by returning excess water to the bloodstream and therefore make less urine.

DI occurs when this precise system for regulating the kidneys' handling of fluids is disrupted. The most common form of clinically serious DI, central DI, results from damage to the pituitary gland, which disrupts the normal storage and release of ADH. Another form, nephrogenic DI, results when the kidneys are unable to respond to ADH. Rarer forms occur because of a defect in the thirst mechanism (dipsogenic DI) or during pregnancy (gestational DI).

A specialist should determine which form of DI is present before starting any treatment.

Central DI

Damage to the pituitary gland can be caused by different diseases as well as by head injuries, neurosurgery, or genetic disorders. To treat the resulting ADH deficiency, a synthetic hormone called desmopressin can be taken by an injection, a nasal spray, or a pill. While taking desmopressin, you should drink fluids or water only when you are thirsty and not at other times. This is because the drug prevents water excretion and water can build up now that your kidneys are making less urine and are less responsive to changes in body fluids.

Nephrogenic DI

The kidneys' ability to respond to ADH can be impaired by drugs (like lithium, for example) and by chronic disorders including polycystic kidney disease, sickle cell disease, kidney failure, partial blockage of the ureters, and inherited genetic disorders. Sometimes the cause of nephrogenic DI is never discovered.

Desmopressin will not work for this form of DI. Instead, you may be given a drug called hydrochlorothiazide (also called HCTZ) or indomethacin. HCTZ is sometimes combined with amiloride. Again, you should drink fluids only when you are thirsty and not at other times.

Dipsogenic DI

A third type of DI is caused by a defect in or damage to the thirst mechanism, which is located in the hypothalamus. This defect results in an abnormal increase in thirst and fluid intake that suppresses ADH secretion and increases urine output. Desmopressin or other drugs should not be used to treat dipsogenic DI because they may decrease urine output but not thirst and fluid intake. This fluid "overload" can lead to water intoxication, a condition that lowers the concentration of sodium in the blood and can seriously damage the brain.

Gestational DI

A fourth type of DI occurs only during pregnancy. Gestational DI occurs when an enzyme made by the placenta destroys ADH in the mother. The placenta is the system of blood vessels and other tissue that develops with the fetus. The placenta allows exchange of nutrients and waste products between mother and fetus.

Most cases of gestational DI can be treated with desmopressin. In rare cases, however, an abnormality in the thirst mechanism causes gestational DI, and desmopressin should not be used.

Diagnosis

Because DM is more common and because DM and DI have similar symptoms, a healthcare provider may suspect that a patient with DI has DM. But testing should make the diagnosis clear.

Your physician must determine which type of DI is involved before proper treatment can begin. Diagnosis is based on a series of tests, including urinalysis and a fluid deprivation test.

Table 30.1. Comparison of Diabetes Insipidus and Diabetes Mellitus

	Central diabetes insipidus	Nephrogenic diabetes insipidus	Diabetes mellitus
How common is the disease?	Uncommon	Uncommon	Common
What causes the disease?	The mechanism for secreting vasopressin malfunctions.	The kidneys are unable to respond to the diuretic hormone vasopressin. It is acquired or may be inherited by male children.	Enough of the hormone insulin is not secreted, or the body's cells do not respond to it. Heredity, stress, obesity, pregnancy, and drugs can also lead to diabetes mellitus.
What do these hormones do and why are they important?	Vasopressin is a diuretic hormone that controls water metabolism. It is made in the hypothalamus (a part of the brain) and is stored and secreted by the posterior pituitary gland (also in the brain).	It causes tubules within the kidney to reabsorb water. Water that is not absorbed is released as urine.	Insulin is made in the pancreas, where it controls carbohydrate metabolism. It controls sugar (glucose) levels in the body.
What are the signs and symptoms of the disease?	Sudden or gradual urination of large amounts of clear, colorless fluid, followed by excessive thirst (polydipsia). Dehydration can occur if fluid balance is not maintained.	Same as central diabetes insipidus: polyuria followed by polydipsia.	Excessive urination (polyuria), excessive thirst (polydipsia), excessive appetite (polyphagia). May be sudden or gradual with no symptoms. Tiredness, weight gain or loss, skin infections that do not heal.
What diagnostic tests can be used to detect the disease?	Water deprivation test/vasopressin test. Hypertonic saline infusion test.	Water deprivation test/vasopressin test. Hypertonic saline infusion test.	Fast blood sugar—24 hr. post-prandial test. Glucose tolerance test.
What treatments are used to combat the disease?	Balance fluid intake and urine output. Replace antidiuretic hormone, vasopressin, find, if possible, underlying brain disease.	Balance urine output with fluid intake. Diuretics.	Correct sugar/insulin intake. Prevent progression of disease. Diet. Oral medication.

Source: "Diabetes Insipidus: What Kind of Diabetes Is That?" Patient Information Publications, Warren Grant Magnuson Clinical Center, National Institutes of Health, 1998.

Urinalysis is the physical and chemical examination of urine. The urine of a person with DI will be less concentrated. Therefore, the salt and waste concentrations are low, and the amount of water excreted is high. A physician evaluates the concentration of urine by testing its specific gravity or osmolality.

A fluid deprivation test helps determine whether DI is caused by (1) excessive intake of fluid, (2) a defect in ADH production, or (3) a defect in the kidneys' response to ADH. This test measures changes in body weight, urine output, and urine composition when fluids are withheld. Sometimes measuring blood levels of ADH during this test is also necessary.

In some patients, an MRI (magnetic resonance imaging) of the brain may be necessary as well.

Chapter 31

Kidney Stones

Chapter Contents

Section 31.1

What You Should Know about Kidney Stones

"Kidney Stones in Adults," National Kidney and Urologic Diseases Information Clearinghouse (NKUDIC), a service of the National Institute of Diabetes and Digestive and Kidney Diseases (NIDDK), National Institutes of Health (NIH), Pub. No. 05-2495, December 2004.

Kidney stones, one of the most painful of the urologic disorders, are not a product of modern life. Scientists have found evidence of kidney stones in a 7,000-year-old Egyptian mummy. Unfortunately, kidney stones are one of the most common disorders of the urinary tract. In 2000, patients made 2.7 million visits to healthcare providers and more than 600,000 patients went to emergency rooms for kidney stone problems. Men tend to be affected more frequently than women.

Most kidney stones pass out of the body without any intervention by a physician. Stones that cause lasting symptoms or other complications may be treated by various techniques, most of which do not involve major surgery. Also, research advances have led to a better understanding of the many factors that promote stone formation.

What is the urinary tract?

The urinary tract, or system, consists of the kidneys, ureters, bladder, and urethra. The kidneys are two bean-shaped organs located below the ribs toward the middle of the back. The kidneys remove extra water and wastes from the blood, converting it to urine. They also keep a stable balance of salts and other substances in the blood. The kidneys produce hormones that help build strong bones and help form red blood cells.

Narrow tubes called ureters carry urine from the kidneys to the bladder, an oval-shaped chamber in the lower abdomen. Like a balloon, the bladder's elastic walls stretch and expand to store urine. They flatten together when urine is emptied through the urethra to outside the body.

What is a kidney stone?

A kidney stone is a hard mass developed from crystals that separate from the urine and build up on the inner surfaces of the kidney. Normally, urine contains chemicals that prevent or inhibit the crystals from forming. These inhibitors do not seem to work for everyone, however, so some people form stones. If the crystals remain tiny enough, they will travel through the urinary tract and pass out of the body in the urine without being noticed.

Kidney stones may contain various combinations of chemicals. The most common type of stone contains calcium in combination with either oxalate or phosphate. These chemicals are part of a person's normal diet and make up important parts of the body, such as bones and muscles.

A less common type of stone is caused by infection in the urinary tract. This type of stone is called a struvite or infection stone. A bit less common is the uric acid stone. Cystine stones are rare.

Urolithiasis is the medical term used to describe stones occurring in the urinary tract. Other frequently used terms are urinary tract

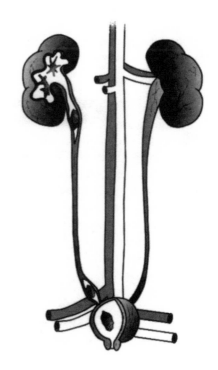

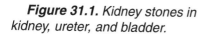

Figure 31.1. Kidney stones in kidney, ureter, and bladder.

stone disease and nephrolithiasis. Doctors also use terms that describe the location of the stone in the urinary tract. For example, a ureteral stone (or ureterolithiasis) is a kidney stone found in the ureter. To keep things simple, however, the term "kidney stones" is used throughout this text.

Gallstones and kidney stones are not related. They form in different areas of the body. If you have a gallstone, you are not necessarily more likely to develop kidney stones.

Who gets kidney stones?

For unknown reasons, the number of people in the United States with kidney stones has been increasing over the past 30 years. The prevalence of stone-forming disease rose from 3.8 percent in the late 1970s to 5.2 percent in the late 1980s and early 1990s. White Americans are more prone to develop kidney stones than African Americans. Stones occur more frequently in men. The prevalence of kidney stones rises dramatically as men enter their 40s and continues to rise into their 70s. For women, the prevalence of kidney stones peaks in their 50s. Once a person gets more than one stone, others are likely to develop.

What causes kidney stones?

Doctors do not always know what causes a stone to form. While certain foods may promote stone formation in people who are susceptible, scientists do not believe that eating any specific food causes stones to form in people who are not susceptible.

A person with a family history of kidney stones may be more likely to develop stones. Urinary tract infections, kidney disorders such as cystic kidney diseases, and certain metabolic disorders such as hyperparathyroidism are also linked to stone formation. In addition, more than 70 percent of people with a rare hereditary disease called renal tubular acidosis develop kidney stones.

Cystinuria and hyperoxaluria are two other rare, inherited metabolic disorders that often cause kidney stones. In cystinuria, too much of the amino acid cystine, which does not dissolve in urine, is voided. This can lead to the formation of stones made of cystine. In patients with hyperoxaluria, the body produces too much of the salt oxalate. When there is more oxalate than can be dissolved in the urine, the crystals settle out and form stones.

Hypercalciuria is inherited. It is the cause of stones in more than half of patients. Calcium is absorbed from food in excess and is lost into the urine. This high level of calcium in the urine causes crystals of calcium oxalate or calcium phosphate to form in the kidneys or urinary tract.

Other causes of kidney stones are hyperuricosuria which is a disorder of uric acid metabolism, gout, excess intake of vitamin D, urinary tract infections, and blockage of the urinary tract. Certain diuretics which are commonly called water pills or calcium-based antacids may increase the risk of forming kidney stones by increasing the amount of calcium in the urine.

Calcium oxalate stones may also form in people who have a chronic inflammation of the bowel or who have had an intestinal bypass operation, or ostomy surgery. As mentioned above, struvite stones can form in people who have had a urinary tract infection. People who take the protease inhibitor indinavir, a drug used to treat HIV infection, are at risk of developing kidney stones.

What are the symptoms?

Kidney stones often do not cause any symptoms. Usually, the first symptom of a kidney stone is extreme pain, which occurs when a stone

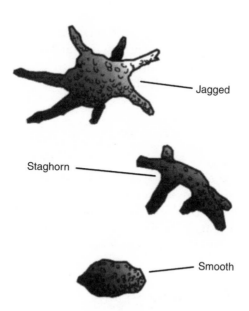

Figure 31.2. *Shapes of various stones. Sizes are usually smaller than shown here.*

acutely blocks the flow of urine. The pain often begins suddenly when a stone moves in the urinary tract, causing irritation or blockage. Typically, a person feels a sharp, cramping pain in the back and side in the area of the kidney or in the lower abdomen. Sometimes nausea and vomiting occur. Later, pain may spread to the groin.

If the stone is too large to pass easily, pain continues as the muscles in the wall of the tiny ureter try to squeeze the stone along into the bladder. As a stone grows or moves, blood may appear in the urine. As the stone moves down the ureter closer to the bladder, you may feel the need to urinate more often or feel a burning sensation during urination.

If fever and chills accompany any of these symptoms, an infection may be present. In this case, you should contact a doctor immediately.

How are kidney stones diagnosed?

Sometimes "silent" stones—those that do not cause symptoms—are found on x-rays taken during a general health exam. If they are small, these stones would likely pass out of the body unnoticed. More often, kidney stones are found on an x-ray or sonogram taken on someone who complains of blood in the urine or sudden pain. These diagnostic images give the doctor valuable information about the stone's size and location. Blood and urine tests help detect any abnormal substance that might promote stone formation.

The doctor may decide to scan the urinary system using a special test called a CT (computed tomography) scan or an IVP (intravenous pyelogram). The results of all these tests help determine the proper treatment.

How are kidney stones treated?

Fortunately, surgery is not usually necessary. Most kidney stones can pass through the urinary system with plenty of water (two to three quarts a day) to help move the stone along. Often, you can stay home during this process, drinking fluids and taking pain medication as needed. The doctor usually asks you to save the passed stone(s) for testing. (You can catch it in a cup or tea strainer used only for this purpose.)

How can I prevent kidney stones?

If you've had more than one kidney stone, you are likely to form another; so prevention is very important. To prevent stones from forming, your doctor must determine their cause. He or she will order laboratory tests, including urine and blood tests. Your doctor will also ask about your medical history, occupation, and eating habits. If a stone has been removed, or if you've passed a stone and saved it, the laboratory should analyze it because its composition helps in planning treatment.

You may be asked to collect your urine for 24 hours after a stone has passed or been removed. The sample is used to measure urine volume and levels of acidity, calcium, sodium, uric acid, oxalate, citrate, and creatinine (a product of muscle metabolism). Your doctor will use this information to determine the cause of the stone. A second 24-hour urine collection may be needed to determine whether the prescribed treatment is working.

Lifestyle changes: A simple and most important lifestyle change to prevent stones is to drink more liquids—water is best. If you tend to form stones, you should try to drink enough liquids throughout the day to produce at least two quarts of urine in every 24-hour period.

People who form calcium stones used to be told to avoid dairy products and other foods with high calcium content. But recent studies have shown that foods high in calcium, including dairy products, may help prevent calcium stones. Taking calcium in pill form, however, may increase the risk of developing stones.

You may be told to avoid food with added vitamin D and certain types of antacids that have a calcium base. If you have very acidic urine, you may need to eat less meat, fish, and poultry. These foods increase the amount of acid in the urine.

To prevent cystine stones, you should drink enough water each day to dilute the concentration of cystine that escapes into the urine, which may be difficult. More than a gallon of water may be needed every 24 hours, and a third of that must be drunk during the night.

Foods and drinks containing oxalate: People prone to forming calcium oxalate stones may be asked by their doctor to cut back on certain foods if their urine contains an excess of oxalate.

• beets	• rhubarb
• chocolate	• spinach
• coffee	• strawberries
• cola	• tea
• nuts	• wheat bran

353

People should not give up or avoid eating these foods without talking to their doctor first. In most cases, these foods can be eaten in limited amounts.

Medical therapy: The doctor may prescribe certain medications to prevent calcium and uric acid stones. These drugs control the amount of acid or alkali in the urine, key factors in crystal formation. The drug allopurinol may also be useful in some cases of hyperuricosuria.

Doctors usually try to control hypercalciuria, and thus prevent calcium stones, by prescribing certain diuretics, such as hydrochlorothiazide. These drugs decrease the amount of calcium released by the kidneys into the urine by favoring calcium retention in bone. They work best when sodium intake is low. Very rarely, patients with hypercalciuria may be given the drug sodium cellulose phosphate, which binds calcium in the intestines and prevents it from leaking into the urine.

If cystine stones cannot be controlled by drinking more fluids, your doctor may prescribe drugs such as Thiola and Cuprimine, which help reduce the amount of cystine in the urine.

For struvite stones that have been totally removed, the first line of prevention is to keep the urine free of bacteria that can cause infection. Your urine will be tested regularly to be sure that no bacteria are present. If struvite stones cannot be removed, your doctor may prescribe a drug called acetohydroxamic acid (AHA). AHA is used with long-term antibiotic drugs to prevent the infection that leads to stone growth.

People with hyperparathyroidism sometimes develop calcium stones. Treatment in these cases is usually surgery to remove the parathyroid glands (located in the neck). In most cases, only one of the glands is enlarged. Removing the glands cures the patient's problem with hyperparathyroidism and with kidney stones as well.

Will I need surgical treatment?

Surgery should be reserved as an option for cases where other approaches have failed. Surgery may be needed to remove a kidney stone if any of the following occurs:

- It does not pass after a reasonable period of time and causes constant pain.
- It is too large to pass on its own or is caught in a difficult place.
- It blocks the flow of urine.
- It causes ongoing urinary tract infection.

- It damages kidney tissue or causes constant bleeding.
- It has grown larger (as seen on follow-up x-ray studies).

Until 20 years ago, surgery was necessary to remove a stone. It was very painful and required a recovery time of four to six weeks. Today, treatment for these stones is greatly improved, and many options do not require major surgery.

Section 31.2

Treating Kidney Stones

Excerpted from "Surgical Management of Stones," © 2005 American Urological Association Education and Research, Inc. All rights reserved. For current information on urological health topics, visit www.UrologyHealth .org. Reprinted with permission. Reviewed August 2003.

Deciding on Appropriate Treatment

How are kidney stones treated?

Stone size, the number of stones, and their location are perhaps the most important factors in deciding the appropriate treatment for a patient with kidney stones. The composition of a stone, if known, can also affect the choice of treatments. Options for surgical treatment of stones include the following:

Shock wave lithotripsy (SWL): This is a completely non-invasive form of treatment in which an energy source generates a shock wave that is directed at a urinary stone within the kidney or ureter. Shock waves are transmitted to the patient either through a water bath, which the patient is placed in, or using a water-filled cushion that is placed against the skin. Ultrasound or fluoroscopy is used to locate the stone and focus the shock waves. The repeated force caused by the shock waves fragments the stone into small pieces.

SWL is most often performed under heavy sedation, although general anesthesia is sometimes used. Once the treatment is completed, the small stone particles then pass down the ureter and are eventually urinated away. In certain cases, a stent may need to be placed up the ureter just prior to SWL to assist in stone fragment passage.

Certain types of stone (cystine, calcium oxalate monohydrate) are resistant to SWL and usually require another treatment. In addition, larger stones (generally greater than 2.5 centimeters) may break into large pieces that can still block the kidney. Stones located in the lower portion of the kidney also have a decreased chance of passage.

Ureteroscopy (URS): This treatment involves the use of a very small, fiberoptic instrument called a ureteroscope, which allows access to stones in the ureter or kidney. The ureteroscope allows your

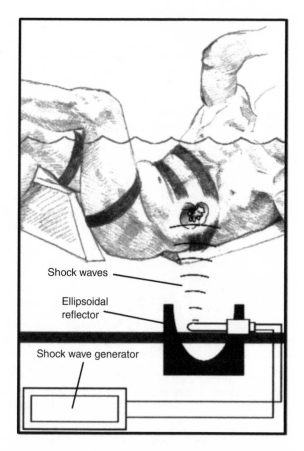

Figure 31.3. *Extracorporeal shockwave lithotripsy (Source: NIDDK).*

urologist to directly visualize the stone by progressing up the ureter via the bladder. No incisions are necessary but general anesthesia is used.

Once the stone is seen through the ureteroscope, a small, basket-like device can be used to grasp smaller stones and remove them. If a stone is too large to remove, a laser, spark-generating probe or air-driven (pneumatic) probe can be passed through a channel built into the ureteroscope and the stone can be fragmented. A straightforward case is complete once the stone has been shattered appropriately. However, if extensive manipulation was required to reach and/or treat the stone, your urologist may choose to place a stent within the ureter to allow the post-operative swelling to subside.

Percutaneous nephrolithotomy (PNL): PNL is the treatment of choice for large stones located within the kidney that will not be effectively treated with either SWL or URS. General anesthesia is required to perform a PNL. The main advantage of this approach compared to traditional open surgery is that only a small incision (about one centimeter) is required in the flank. The urologist then places a guide wire through the incision. The wire is inserted into the kidney under fluoroscopic guidance and directed down the ureter. A passage is then created around the wire using dilators to provide access into the kidney.

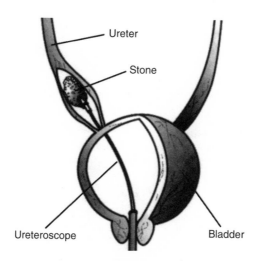

Figure 31.4. *Ureteroscopic stone removal (Source: NIDDK).*

An instrument called a nephroscope is then passed into the kidney to visualize the stone. Fragmentation can then be done using an ultrasonic probe or a laser. Because the tract allows passage of larger instruments, your urologist can suction out or grasp the stone fragments as they are produced. This results in a higher clearance of stone fragments than with SWL or URS. Once the procedure is complete, a tube is left in the flank to drain the kidney for several days.

Open surgery: A large incision is required in order to expose the kidney or portion of ureter that is involved with the stone. The portion of kidney overlying the stone or the ureteral wall is then surgically cut and the stone removed. At present, open surgery is used only for very complicated cases of stone disease.

What can be expected after treatment for kidney stones?

Recovery times vary depending upon treatment, with the less invasive procedures allowing shorter recovery periods and quicker return to activity.

Shock Wave Lithotripsy (SWL): Patients generally go home the same day as the procedure and are able to resume a normal activity level in two to three days. Fluid intake is encouraged, as larger quantities of urine can help stone fragments to pass. Because the fragments need to pass spontaneously down the ureter, some flank pain can be anticipated. It is possible that the stone may not have shattered well

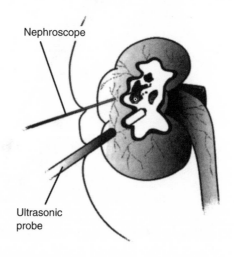

Figure 31.5. Percutaneous nephrolithotomy (Source: NIDDK).

Nephroscope

Ultrasonic probe

enough to pass all of the fragments. If so, a repeat SWL treatment or other option may be required. If a stent was placed prior to SWL, this will need to be removed in your urologist's office within a few weeks. Stents are usually well tolerated by patients but can occasionally cause some bladder irritation and frequent urination.

Ureteroscopy (URS): Patients normally go home the same day and can resume normal activity in two to three days. As with SWL, if your urologist places a stent, it will need to be removed in approximately one week.

Percutaneous nephrolithotomy (PNL): After PNL, patients usually spend two to three days in the hospital. Your urologist may choose to have additional x-rays done while you are still in the hospital to determine if any stone fragments are still present. If some remain, your urologist may want to look back into the kidney with a nephroscope to remove them. This secondary procedure usually can be done with sedation and through the existing tract into the kidney. Once the stones have been removed, the stent coming out of the flank is removed and the patient can be discharged. Normal activity can be resumed after approximately one to two weeks.

Open surgery: Because these procedures are the most invasive and painful, patients often spend up to five to seven days in the hospital. Full recovery may take up to six weeks.

Postoperatively, your urologist will encourage a high fluid intake, to keep the daily volume of urine produced greater than two liters a day. In addition, you may need to undergo additional blood and urine tests to determine specific risk factors for stone formation and help minimize the chance for future stones. Although stone recurrence rates differ with each individual, a good estimate to keep in mind is a 50 percent chance of redeveloping a stone within a five-year period.

Frequently Asked Questions

What are the risks or potential complications of the various treatments?

Each treatment has its own inherent risks. Some risks that can be associated with all surgical procedures are the possibility of bleeding and infection. It is extremely rare for patients undergoing shock wave lithotripsy (SWL) or ureteroscopy (URS) to have any problems with blood loss or infection. The probability is higher with more invasive treatments such as percutaneous nephrolithotomy (PNL) or open surgery. In most cases, patients do not require transfusion unless the procedure is unusually difficult.

With SWL, except in emergencies, patients must avoid aspirin, nonsteroidal anti-inflammatory drugs such as ibuprofen or other blood thinners, as these can cause significant bleeding around the kidney. It is important that these medications be stopped at least one week prior to treatment if possible. SWL is generally a very safe treatment. Long-term follow up of patients has shown a slight increase in blood pressure, but no lasting adverse effect on kidney function has been noted.

In URS, there is a small possibility that the ureteral wall could be damaged or torn during the procedure. If this occurs, placement of a stent for two to three weeks is usually sufficient to allow the damaged area to heal. A complete tear of the ureter is very rare and requires open surgery to repair.

When PNL is performed, there is a small chance of air or fluids forming around a lung if the access channel is made toward the upper portion of the kidney. These entities are treated with a chest tube, which allows drainage of the fluid from around the lung. Other rare complications include injury to the bowel and injury to blood vessels within the kidney.

Will I have significant pain after the procedure?

Some discomfort is inevitable after surgical intervention for stones. The degree of discomfort is directly related to the invasiveness of the procedure. If needed, your urologist will prescribe medication to help control the pain during the recovery period.

What are signs of a problem postoperatively?

It is not uncommon for a patient to have a low-grade fever for the first 48 hours after surgery. However, if the fever continues or rises above 101.5° F (38.5° C) it could be a sign of active infection and should be reported to your urologist. Flank discomfort is also common after surgical interventions. However, if the pain becomes increasingly worse or unbearable, despite medication, your urologist should be notified.

How many times will I need to be treated?

The answer to this question depends on the size of stone and the treatment used. The chances for re-treatment are highest after SWL if the stone is large, extremely hard or in the lower portion of the kidney. PNL and open surgery tend to produce the highest stone-free rates.

Where can I get more information?

American Urological Association (AUA) Guidelines Patient Guides: *The Management of Ureteral Stones*, and *The Management of Staghorn Kidney Stones*. [See Chapter 53, "Directory of Urinary and Kidney Disorders Organizations," for contact information for the American Urological Association.]

Section 31.3

Shattering Myths about Kidney Stones

"Shattering Myths about Kidney Stones," a report from The NIH *Word on Health*, Consumer Health Information Based on Research from the National Institutes of Health (NIH), November 2002.

Kidney stones. Just mention them and people cringe—and for good reason. They are one of the most painful conditions a person can have. Chances are you know someone who's had them. More people are developing kidney stones, and researchers are trying to find out why and what can be done to prevent them.

But what exactly is a kidney stone? Kidney stones are hard masses developed from crystals that build up in the kidney, the organ that makes urine. These crystals can contain various combinations of chemicals, but are most often made of calcium in combination with either oxalate or phosphate. These chemicals are part of a normal diet and make up important parts of the body, such as bones and muscles. The crystals normally remain tiny enough to travel through the urinary tract and pass out of the body in the urine without being noticed. But in some people, the crystals stick together and continue to build up to form kidney stones.

Many people have misconceptions about kidney stones. Some think that stones occur only rarely and mainly in people who are already ill. But now we know that's changing. Get the facts about how research is offering new hope to those who suffer from this increasingly common condition.

Myth: Kidney stones are rare.

Fact: Kidney stones are one of the most common disorders of the urinary tract.

The National Institute of Health (NIH)'s National Institute of Diabetes and Digestive and Kidney Diseases (NIDDK) estimates that up to ten percent of Americans will have a kidney stone at some point in their lives, and most will be between the ages of 20 and 40.

Over the past 20 years, the number of people with kidney stones has been increasing. Scientists don't have an explanation for this, but they think it may be related to diet and lifestyle. "Kidney stones are becoming a common occurrence in adults, and it looks like a combination of environmental and genetic factors may be responsible," says Dr. Thomas Hostetter, director of NIDDK's National Kidney Disease Education Program.

Myth: Only men get kidney stones.

Fact: Women get kidney stones too. Even children can get them. Although men tend to develop kidney stones more frequently than women, the number of women with kidney stones has been increasing. Even children can have kidney stones, although less often than adults.

"Most children with kidney stones usually have a genetic or metabolic disease that makes them more likely to form stones," explains Dr. Hostetter. If you have a family history of kidney stones, you are also more likely to develop them. Some people with a family history are believed to have a defective gene that results in excess calcium in their urine. NIDDK researchers are attempting to find out more about the genes responsible for this disorder, and to see if there are any other unusual factors that make these families more susceptible to kidney stones.

Myth: Eating certain foods will cause kidney stones to develop.

Fact: Not usually. In general, scientists don't think that eating any specific foods causes stones to form in people who are not already susceptible. Dr. Hostetter says that, in some people, a diet high in protein may lead to kidney stones because extra protein causes calcium to be excreted from the body, raising calcium levels in the urine. For a person without any history of kidney stones, a diet with moderate amounts of protein should be followed, he advises.

People with urinary tract infections, kidney disorders such as cystic kidney diseases, and certain rare, inherited metabolic disorders are also more likely to develop kidney stones. In some of these susceptible people, the foods they eat can have an influence on the development of their kidney stones. For example, if you are at higher risk for kidney stones, your doctor may tell you to limit or avoid foods containing higher levels of oxalate, which include chocolate, coffee, beer, dairy products, and some fruits and vegetables.

Myth: Most kidney stones are formed from calcium, so calcium in the diet should be reduced.

Fact: That used to be what doctors thought, but no longer. For years, doctors thought a low-calcium diet was the best way to prevent kidney stones, especially in those who already had stones. But recent research has reversed that thinking. Dr. Hostetter explains that several studies have shown that low-calcium diets are not effective, and may actually be harmful, since they tend to increase the likelihood of low-bone density and osteoporosis.

Researchers now believe that more rather than less calcium is better. Recent studies have shown that a diet with normal amounts of calcium is probably best. Over a period of five years, scientists studied a group of men with recurrent kidney stones and found that those who had normal calcium levels in their diet were less likely to form new stones than men who were on a low-calcium diet.

Dr. Hostetter explains that calcium is important because it binds to oxalate and removes it from the body. He adds, "The men also restricted their intake of animal protein and salt, which may explain why they had fewer stones."

Researchers are continuing to study the benefits of this diet. But for now, drinking that glass of milk and cutting back on the hamburgers and chips may help reduce your risk of kidney stones.

Myth: Most people with kidney stones have to undergo surgery.

Fact: Thankfully, this isn't true any longer. The good news is that most kidney stones pass out of the body without any help. For those that require treatment, there are now a number of options that can be tried before surgery is considered. Major surgery is now usually the last resort for treating kidney stones.

For some people, drinking plenty of water may be all that's needed to help kidney stones pass easily from the urinary tract. Sometimes pain killers and diuretics, medicines that increase the flow of urine, are given as well. Depending on the type of stone you have, your doctor may recommend a special diet to help reduce or eliminate substances in the urine that can lead to kidney stones. Your doctor may also prescribe medications that can control the amount of calcium and other chemicals in your urine that can form kidney stones. NIH researchers are currently working to develop new drugs with fewer side effects.

If your kidney stones do not pass, you may need extracorporeal shock wave lithotripsy, commonly known as lithotripsy, a technique that uses shock waves produced outside the body to hit and break up the stones so they can pass out of the body. In some cases where stones are quite large or their location will not allow for lithotripsy, you may need surgery or urethroscopy, where a small fiberoptic instrument is placed into the ureter to remove the stones. Today, even with surgery, treatment is so improved that most stones can be removed without a long recovery time.

Myth: Once a person has kidney stones, there's nothing that can be done to prevent future stones.

Fact: Most people can take action to reduce their risk of getting more stones.

It's true that once you have a kidney stone, you are more likely to have others down the road, but there are some things that you can do to help prevent this from happening.

As with other chronic conditions, the best treatment for kidney stones is prevention. Drinking plenty of water throughout the day is one of the best ways to prevent future stones from forming. Your doctor may also want to run some laboratory tests and take a medical history to determine the factors that need to be changed to reduce the risk of future stones. A special diet and/or medicines may also be prescribed for you. The most important thing you can do is to ask your doctor what you can do to prevent kidney stones from recurring.

Myth: If a person has kidney stones, he or she is more likely to have gallstones.

Fact: Not even close. Gallstones and kidney stones are not related at all. They form in different areas of the body. Typically, those at risk for developing gallstones are a different group from those who have kidney stones. Women, Native and Mexican Americans, people over 60, and those on frequent diets are more likely to have gallstones.

Health experts say that by taking an active role in your health you may be able to reduce your risk of getting kidney stones. Dr. Hostetter concludes, "Maintaining a healthy diet with normal amounts of calcium, drinking adequate amounts of fluids, and seeing your doctor for regular check-ups are a good prescription for all of us."

—by Mary Sullivan

Chapter 32

Solitary Kidney

Most people have two kidneys, one on each side of the spinal column in the back just below the rib cage. Each kidney is about the size of a fist and contains about one million nephrons. The nephrons are microscopic filtering "baskets" that transfer wastes from the blood to the collecting tubules of the urinary system.

A person may have only one kidney for one of three main reasons.

- A person may be born with only one kidney, a condition known as renal agenesis. Many people with this condition lead normal, healthy lives and only discover that they have one kidney when they have an x-ray or sonogram or surgery for some unrelated condition.

- Some people must have one kidney removed to treat cancer or other diseases or injuries. The operation to remove a kidney is called a nephrectomy.

- A growing number of people are donating a kidney to be transplanted into a family member or friend whose kidneys have failed.

Most people can live a normal, healthy life with one kidney. Taking precautions is wise to protect the kidney function you do have.

National Kidney and Urologic Diseases Information Clearinghouse (NKUDIC), a service of the National Institute of Diabetes and Digestive and Kidney Diseases (NIDDK), National Institutes of Health (NIH), Pub. No. 04-5390, May 2004.

Possible Effects of Solitary Kidney

If having a single kidney does affect your health, the changes are likely to be so small and happen so slowly that you won't notice them. Over long periods of time, however, these gradual changes may require specific measures or treatments. Changes that may result from a single kidney include the following:

- **High blood pressure:** Kidneys help maintain a healthy blood pressure by regulating how much fluid flows through the bloodstream and by making a hormone called renin that works with other hormones to expand or contract blood vessels. Many people who lose or donate a kidney are found to have slightly higher blood pressure after several years.

- **Proteinuria:** Excessive protein in the urine, a condition known as proteinuria, can be a sign of kidney damage. People are often found to have higher-than-normal levels of protein in their urine after they have lived with one kidney for several years.

- **Reduced GFR:** The glomerular filtration rate (GFR) shows how efficiently your kidneys are removing wastes from your bloodstream. People have a reduced GFR if they have only one kidney.

You can have high blood pressure, proteinuria, and reduced GFR and still feel fine. As long as these conditions are under control, they will probably not affect your health or longevity. Schedule regular checkups with your doctor to monitor these conditions.

How You Can Protect Your Kidneys

Monitoring

Your doctor should monitor your kidney function by checking your blood pressure and testing your urine and blood once a year.

- Normal blood pressure is considered to be 120/80 or lower. You have high blood pressure if it is over 140/90. People with kidney disease or one kidney should keep their blood pressure below 130/80. Controlling blood pressure is especially important because high blood pressure can damage kidneys.

- Your doctor may use a strip of special paper dipped into a little cup of your urine to test for protein. The color of the "dipstick" indicates the presence or absence of protein. A more sensitive test for proteinuria involves laboratory measurement and calculation of the protein-to-creatinine ratio. A high protein-to-creatinine ratio in urine (greater than 30 milligrams of albumin per 1 gram of creatinine) shows that kidneys are leaking protein that should be kept in the blood.

* Measuring GFR used to require an injection of a contrast medium like iothalamate into the bloodstream followed by a 24-hour urine collection to see how much of the medium was filtered through the kidneys in that time. In recent years, however, scientists have discovered that they can estimate a person's GFR based on the amount of creatinine in a small blood sample. The new GFR calculation uses the patient's creatinine measurement along with weight, age, and values assigned for sex and race. Some medical laboratories may calculate GFR at the same time they measure and report creatinine values. If your GFR stays consistently below 60, you are considered to have chronic kidney disease.

Controlling Blood Pressure

If your blood pressure is above normal, you should work with your doctor to keep it below 130/80. Great care should be taken in selecting blood pressure medicines for people with a solitary kidney. Angiotensin-converting enzyme (ACE) inhibitors and angiotensin receptor blockers (ARBs) are two classes of blood pressure medicine that protect kidney function and reduce proteinuria. But these medicines may be harmful to someone with renal artery stenosis (RAS), which is the hardening of the arteries that enter the kidneys. Diuretics can help control blood pressure by removing excess fluid in the body. Controlling your blood pressure may require a combination of two or more medicines, plus changes in diet and activity level.

Eating Sensibly

Having a single kidney does not mean that you have to follow a special diet. You simply need to make healthy choices, including fruits, vegetables, grains, and low-fat dairy foods. Limit your daily salt (sodium) intake to 2,000 milligrams or less if you already have high blood pressure. Reading nutrition labels on packaged foods to learn how much sodium is in one serving and keeping a sodium diary can help. Limit alcohol and caffeine intake as well.

Avoid high-protein diets. Protein breaks down into the waste materials that the kidneys must remove, so excessive protein puts an extra burden on the kidneys. Eating moderate amounts of protein is still important for proper nutrition. A dietitian can help you find the right amount of protein in your diet.

Avoiding Injury

Some doctors may advise patients with a solitary kidney to avoid contact sports like boxing, football, and hockey. One study indicated that motor vehicle collisions and bike riding accidents were more likely than sports injuries to seriously damage the kidneys. In recent years, athletes with a single working kidney have participated in sports competition at the highest levels. Having a solitary kidney should not automatically disqualify you from sports participation. Children should be encouraged to engage in some form of physical activity, even if contact sports are ruled out. Protective gear such as padded vests worn under a uniform can make limited contact sports like basketball or soccer safe. Doctors, parents, and patients should consider the risks of any activity and decide whether the benefits outweigh those risks.

Hope through Research

In recent years, researchers have learned much about kidney disease. The National Institute of Diabetes and Digestive and Kidney Diseases (NIDDK) sponsors several programs aimed at understanding kidney failure and finding treatments to stop its progression. NIDDK's Division of Kidney, Urologic, and Hematologic Diseases supports basic research into normal kidney development in the embryo and the genetic causes of birth defects that may result in a solitary kidney. New imaging techniques can help to diagnose solitary kidney before birth.

Chapter 33

Glomerular Diseases

Many diseases affect kidney function by attacking the glomeruli, the tiny units within the kidney where blood is cleaned. Glomerular diseases include many conditions with a variety of genetic and environmental causes, but they fall into two major categories:

- **Glomerulonephritis** (gloh-MAIR-yoo-loh-neh-FRY-tis) describes the inflammation of the membrane tissue in the kidney that serves as a filter, separating wastes and extra fluid from the blood.

- **Glomerulosclerosis** (gloh-MAIR-yoo-loh-skleh-ROH-sis) describes the scarring or hardening of the tiny blood vessels within the kidney.

Although glomerulonephritis and glomerulosclerosis have different causes, they can both lead to end-stage renal disease (ESRD).

The Glomeruli

Blood enters the kidneys through arteries that branch inside the kidneys into tiny clusters of looping blood vessels. Each cluster is called a glomerulus, which comes from the Greek word meaning filter.

National Kidney and Urologic Diseases Information Clearinghouse (NKUDIC), a service of the National Institute of Diabetes and Digestive and Kidney Diseases (NIDDK), National Institutes of Health (NIH), Pub. No. 04-4358, December 2003.

The plural form of the word is glomeruli. There are approximately one million glomeruli, or filters, in each kidney. The glomerulus is attached to the opening of a small fluid-collecting tube called a tubule. Blood is filtered in the glomerulus, and extra water and wastes pass into the tubule and become urine. Eventually, the urine drains from the kidneys into the bladder through larger tubes called ureters.

Each glomerulus-and-tubule unit is called a nephron. Each kidney is composed of about one million nephrons. In healthy nephrons, the glomerular membrane that separates the blood vessel from the tubule allows waste products and extra water to pass into the tubule while keeping blood cells and protein in the bloodstream.

How Glomerular Diseases Interfere with Kidney Function

Glomerular diseases damage the glomeruli, letting protein and sometimes red blood cells leak into the urine. Sometimes a glomerular disease also interferes with the clearance of waste products by the kidney, so they begin to build up in the blood. Furthermore, loss of blood proteins like albumin in the urine can result in a fall in their level in the bloodstream. In normal blood, albumin acts like a sponge, drawing extra fluid from the body into the bloodstream, where it remains until the kidneys remove it. But when albumin leaks into the urine, the blood loses its capacity to absorb extra fluid from the body. Fluid can accumulate outside the circulatory system in the face, hands, feet, or ankles and cause swelling.

The Symptoms of Glomerular Disease

The signs and symptoms of glomerular disease include the following:

- **proteinuria:** large amounts of protein in the urine
- **hematuria:** blood in the urine
- **reduced glomerular filtration rate:** inefficient filtering of wastes from the blood
- **hypoproteinemia:** low blood protein
- **edema:** swelling in parts of the body

One or more of these symptoms can be the first sign of kidney disease. But how would you know, for example, whether you have proteinuria? Before seeing a doctor, you may not. But some of these symptoms have signs, or visible manifestations:

- Proteinuria may cause foamy urine.
- Blood may cause the urine to be pink or cola-colored.
- Edema may be obvious in hands and ankles, especially at the end of the day, or around the eyes when awakening in the morning, for example.

How Glomerular Disease Is Diagnosed

Patients with glomerular disease have significant amounts of protein in the urine, which may be referred to as "nephrotic range" if levels are very high. Red blood cells in the urine are a frequent finding

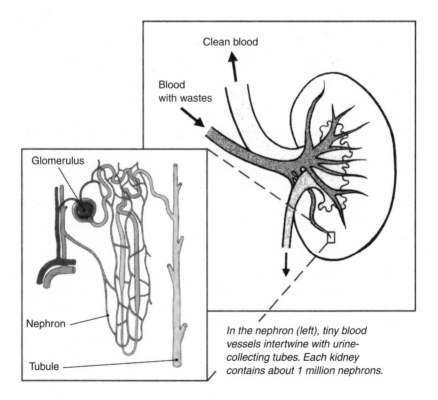

Clean blood

Blood with wastes

Glomerulus

Nephron

Tubule

In the nephron (left), tiny blood vessels intertwine with urine-collecting tubes. Each kidney contains about 1 million nephrons.

Figure 33.1. *In the nephron, tiny blood vessels intertwine with fluid collecting tubes. Each kidney contains about one million nephrons.*

as well, particularly in some forms of glomerular disease. Urinalysis provides information about kidney damage by indicating levels of protein and red blood cells in the urine. Blood tests measure the levels of waste products such as creatinine and urea nitrogen to determine whether the filtering capacity of the kidneys is impaired. If these lab tests indicate kidney damage, the doctor may recommend ultrasound or an x-ray to see whether the shape or size of the kidneys is abnormal. These tests are called renal imaging. But since glomerular disease causes problems at the cellular level, the doctor will probably also recommend a kidney biopsy—a procedure in which a needle is used to extract small pieces of tissue for examination under different types of microscopes, each of which shows a different aspect of the tissue. A biopsy may be helpful in confirming glomerular disease and identifying the cause.

Glomerular Disease Causes

A number of different diseases can result in glomerular disease. It may be the direct result of an infection or a drug toxic to the kidneys, or it may result from a disease that affects the entire body, like diabetes or lupus. Many different kinds of diseases can cause swelling or scarring of the nephron or glomerulus. Sometimes glomerular disease is idiopathic, meaning that it occurs without an apparent associated disease.

The categories presented below can overlap: that is, a disease might belong to two or more of the categories. For example, diabetic nephropathy is a form of glomerular disease that can be placed in two categories: systemic diseases, since diabetes itself is a systemic disease, and sclerotic diseases, because the specific damage done to the kidneys is associated with scarring.

Autoimmune Diseases

When the body's immune system functions properly, it creates protein-like substances called antibodies and immunoglobulins to protect the body against invading organisms. In an autoimmune disease, the immune system creates autoantibodies, which are antibodies or immunoglobulins that attack the body itself. Autoimmune diseases may be systemic and affect many parts of the body, or they may affect only specific organs or regions.

Systemic lupus erythematosus (SLE) affects many parts of the body: primarily the skin and joints, but also the kidneys. Because women are more likely to develop SLE than men, some researchers believe that a sex-linked genetic factor may play a part in making a person susceptible, although viral infection has also been implicated as a triggering factor. Lupus nephritis is the name given to the kidney disease caused by SLE, and it occurs when autoantibodies form or are deposited in the glomeruli, causing inflammation. Ultimately, the inflammation may create scars that keep the kidneys from functioning properly.

Goodpasture syndrome involves an autoantibody that specifically targets the kidneys and the lungs. Often, the first indication that patients have the autoantibody is when they cough up blood. But lung damage in Goodpasture syndrome is usually superficial compared with progressive and permanent damage to the kidneys. Goodpasture syndrome is a rare condition that affects mostly young men but also occurs in women, children, and older adults. Treatments include immunosuppressive drugs and a blood-cleaning therapy called plasmapheresis that removes the autoantibodies.

IgA nephropathy is a form of glomerular disease that results when immunoglobulin A (IgA) forms deposits in the glomeruli, where it creates inflammation. Researchers funded by the National Institute of Diabetes and Digestive and Kidney Diseases (NIDDK) are trying to discover why these deposits in the glomeruli are formed and whether dietary supplements of fish oil can inhibit IgA-induced inflammation and scarring in the kidney. A study is being conducted to compare the effectiveness of therapy involving daily fish oil supplements with that of a therapy involving prednisone, a drug that blocks the body's immune system. The study includes a placebo group. All three groups of patients in the study are receiving medication to control blood pressure. IgA nephropathy was not recognized as a cause of glomerular disease until the late 1960s, when sophisticated biopsy techniques were developed that could identify IgA deposits in kidney tissue.

The most common symptom of IgA nephropathy is blood in the urine, but it is often a silent disease that may go undetected for many years. The silent nature of the disease makes it difficult to determine how many people are in the early stages of IgA nephropathy, when specific medical tests are the only way to detect it. This disease is estimated to be the most common cause of primary glomerulonephritis—that is, glomerular disease not caused by a systemic disease like lupus or diabetes mellitus. It appears to affect men more than women.

375

Although IgA nephropathy is found in all age groups, young people rarely display signs of kidney failure because the disease usually takes several years to progress to the stage where it causes detectable complications.

Hereditary Nephritis: Alport Syndrome

The primary indicator of Alport syndrome is a family history of chronic glomerular disease, although it may also involve hearing or vision impairment. This syndrome affects both men and women, but men are more likely to experience chronic renal failure and sensory loss. Men with Alport syndrome usually first show evidence of renal insufficiency while in their twenties and reach ESRD by age 40. Women rarely have significant renal impairment, and hearing loss may be so slight that it can be detected only through testing with special equipment. Usually men can pass the disease only to their daughters. Women can transmit the disease to either their sons or their daughters.

Infection-Related Glomerular Disease

Glomerular disease sometimes develops rapidly after an infection in other parts of the body.

Acute post-streptococcal glomerulonephritis (PSGN) can occur after an episode of strep throat or, in rare cases, impetigo (a skin infection). The *Streptococcus* bacteria do not attack the kidney directly, but an infection may stimulate the immune system to overproduce antibodies, which are circulated in the blood and finally deposited in the glomeruli, causing damage. PSGN can bring on sudden symptoms of swelling (edema), reduced urine output (oliguria), and blood in the urine (hematuria). Tests will show large amounts of protein in the urine and elevated levels of creatinine and urea nitrogen in the blood, thus indicating reduced kidney function. High blood pressure frequently accompanies reduced kidney function in this disease.

PSGN is most common in children between the ages of three and seven, although it can strike at any age, and it most often affects boys. It lasts only a brief time and usually allows the kidneys to recover. In a few cases, however, kidney damage may be permanent, requiring dialysis or transplantation to replace renal function.

Bacterial endocarditis, infection of the tissues inside the heart, is also associated with subsequent glomerular disease. Researchers are not sure whether the renal lesions that form after a heart infection are caused entirely by the immune response or whether some other disease mechanism contributes to kidney damage. Treating the heart infection is the most effective way of minimizing kidney damage. Chronic renal failure can result from endocarditis, but is not inevitable.

HIV, the virus that leads to AIDS, can also cause glomerular disease. Between five and ten percent of people with HIV experience kidney failure, even before developing full-blown AIDS. HIV-associated nephropathy usually begins with heavy proteinuria and progresses rapidly (within a year of detection) to ESRD. Researchers are looking for therapies that can slow down or reverse this rapid deterioration of renal function, but some possible solutions involving immunosuppression are risky because of the patients' already compromised immune system.

Sclerotic Diseases

Glomerulosclerosis is scarring (sclerosis) of the glomeruli. In several sclerotic conditions, a systemic disease like lupus or diabetes is responsible. Glomerulosclerosis is caused by the activation of glomerular cells to produce scar material. This may be stimulated by molecules called growth factors, which may be made by glomerular cells themselves or may be brought to the glomerulus by the circulating blood that enters the glomerular filter.

Diabetic nephropathy is the leading cause of glomerular disease and of ESRD in the United States. Kidney disease is one of several problems caused by elevated levels of blood glucose, the central feature of diabetes. In addition to scarring the kidney, elevated glucose levels appear to increase the speed of blood flow into the kidney, putting a strain on the filtering glomeruli and raising blood pressure.

Diabetic nephropathy usually takes many years to develop. People with diabetes can slow down damage to their kidneys by controlling their blood glucose through healthy eating with moderate protein intake, physical activity, and medications. People with diabetes should also be careful to keep their blood pressure at a level below 130/85 mm Hg, if possible. Blood pressure medications called angiotensin-converting enzyme (ACE) inhibitors and angiotensin receptor blockers (ARBs) are particularly effective at minimizing kidney damage and are now frequently prescribed to control blood pressure in patients with diabetes and in patients with many forms of kidney disease.

Focal segmental glomerulosclerosis (FSGS) describes scarring in scattered regions of the kidney, typically limited to one part of the glomerulus and to a minority of glomeruli in the affected region. FSGS may result from a systemic disorder or it may develop as an idiopathic kidney disease, without a known cause. Proteinuria is the most common symptom of FSGS, but, since proteinuria is associated with several other kidney conditions, the doctor cannot diagnose FSGS on the basis of proteinuria alone. Biopsy may confirm the presence of glomerular scarring if the tissue is taken from the affected section of the kidney. But finding the affected section is a matter of chance, especially early in the disease process, when lesions may be scattered.

Confirming a diagnosis of FSGS may require repeat kidney biopsies. Arriving at a diagnosis of idiopathic FSGS requires the identification of focal scarring and the elimination of possible systemic causes such as diabetes or an immune response to infection. Since idiopathic FSGS is, by definition, of unknown cause, it is difficult to treat. No universal remedy has been found, and most patients with FSGS progress to ESRD over 5 to 20 years. Some patients with an aggressive form of FSGS reach ESRD in two to three years. Treatments involving steroids or other immunosuppressive drugs appear to help some patients by decreasing proteinuria and improving kidney function. But these treatments are beneficial to only a minority of those in whom they are tried, and some patients experience even poorer kidney function as a result. ACE inhibitors and ARBs may also be used in FSGS to decrease proteinuria. Treatment should focus on controlling blood pressure and blood cholesterol levels, factors that may contribute to kidney scarring.

Other Glomerular Diseases

Membranous nephropathy, also called membranous glomerulopathy, is the second most common cause of the nephrotic syndrome (proteinuria, edema, high cholesterol) in U.S. adults after diabetic nephropathy. Diagnosis of membranous nephropathy requires a kidney biopsy, which reveals unusual deposits of immunoglobulin G and complement C3, substances created by the body's immune system. Fully 75 percent of cases are idiopathic, which means that the cause of the disease is unknown. The remaining 25 percent of cases are the result of other diseases like systemic lupus erythematosus, hepatitis B or C infection, or some forms of cancer. Drug therapies involving penicillamine, gold, or captopril have also been associated with membranous nephropathy. About 20 to 40 percent of patients with membranous nephropathy progress, usually over decades, to ESRD, but most patients experience either complete remission or continued symptoms without progressive kidney failure. Doctors disagree about how aggressively to treat this condition, since about 20 percent of patients recover without treatment. ACE inhibitors and ARBs are generally used to reduce proteinuria. Additional medication to control high blood pressure and edema is frequently required. Some patients benefit from steroids, but this treatment does not work for everyone. Additional immunosuppressive medications are helpful for some patients with progressive disease.

Minimal change disease (MCD) is the diagnosis given when a patient has the nephrotic syndrome and the kidney biopsy reveals little or no change to the structure of glomeruli or surrounding tissues when examined by a light microscope. Tiny drops of a fatty substance called a lipid may be present, but no scarring has taken place within the kidney. MCD may occur at any age, but it is most common in childhood. A small percentage of patients with idiopathic nephrotic syndrome do not respond to steroid therapy. For these patients, the doctor may recommend a low-sodium diet and prescribe a diuretic to control edema. The doctor may recommend the use of nonsteroidal anti-inflammatory drugs to reduce proteinuria. ACE inhibitors and ARBs have also been used to reduce proteinuria in patients with steroid-resistant MCD. These patients may respond to larger doses of steroids, more prolonged use of steroids, or steroids in combination with immunosuppressant drugs, such as chlorambucil, cyclophosphamide, or cyclosporine.

Renal Failure and End-Stage Renal Disease (ESRD)

Renal failure is any acute or chronic loss of kidney function and is the term used when some kidney function remains. ESRD is total, or nearly total, and permanent kidney failure [More information about ESRD can be found in Part VII of this book]. Depending on the form of glomerular disease, renal function may be lost in a matter of days or weeks or may deteriorate slowly and gradually over the course of decades.

Acute Renal Failure

A few forms of glomerular disease cause very rapid deterioration of kidney function. For example, PSGN can cause severe symptoms (hematuria, proteinuria, edema) within two to three weeks after a sore throat or skin infection develops. The patient may temporarily require dialysis to replace renal function. This rapid loss of kidney function is called acute renal failure (ARF). Although ARF can be life-threatening while it lasts, kidney function usually returns after the cause of the kidney failure has been treated. In many patients, ARF is not associated with any permanent damage. However, some patients may recover from ARF and subsequently develop chronic renal failure (CRF).

Chronic Renal Failure

Most forms of glomerular disease develop gradually, often causing no symptoms for many years. CRF is the slow, gradual loss of kidney function. Some forms of CRF can be controlled or slowed down. For example, diabetic nephropathy can be delayed by tightly controlling blood glucose levels and using ACE inhibitors and ARBs to reduce proteinuria and control blood pressure. But CRF cannot be cured. Partial loss of renal function means that some portion of the patient's nephrons has been scarred, and scarred nephrons cannot be repaired. In most cases, CRF leads to ESRD.

Chapter 34

IgA Nephropathy

Introduction to IgA Nephropathy (IgAN)

IgA nephropathy (or Berger disease) is an immune complex disorder (or immune-system mediated disease) which causes IgA immune complexes to be deposited in the glomeruli (the filters in the kidneys), where they cause inflammation (called glomerulonephritis), and eventual scarring of the glomeruli (called glomerulosclerosis).

It is one of a group of kidney diseases which are sometimes referred to as glomerulonephropathies, or simply, nephropathies—hence the name IgA nephropathy. IgAN is thought to be the most common type of glomerulonephritis. Despite this, IgAN is not the most common cause of end-stage renal disease. According to some estimates, IgAN accounts for about ten percent of end-stage renal failure.

A very variable disease, it can present as an acute or a chronic form, and in some cases it can be rapidly progressive. The majority of patients have the less aggressive chronic form, which may or may not progress to end-stage renal disease (ESRD) over many years (10 to 25 years or more). In the small number of patients who have the rapidly progressive form, it can lead to ESRD within five years or less.

IgAN is suspected when protein and blood (visible or not) are found in the urine, and is ultimately diagnosed by biopsy.

From "IgA Nephropathy Notebook," reprinted with permission from the IgA Nephropathy Support Group, © 2004 Pierre Lachaîne. Revised by David A. Cooke, M.D., on May 23, 2005.

IgAN can affect people of all ages, but it is most commonly diagnosed from adolescence until about the age of 40, and it is thought to be three times more frequent in males than in females. Pediatric IgAN may appear in childhood to adolescence (and into the early 20s) in its more acute presentation.

History of IgAN

IgAN was first described and differentiated from other types of glomerulonephritis by Dr. J. Berger, in France, around 1968, when research instrumentation had become available that made it possible to better analyze kidney tissues.

In France particularly, it is more often referred to as "la maladie de Berger," or Berger disease. Before that time, it would have simply been vaguely considered to be glomerulonephritis (primarily what was called focal nephritis at that time, where nephritis means inflammation of the nephrons and focal is a pathology term). Some older people might have been said to have suffered from Bright disease, which was sort of the generic, catch all name for these diseases at one time.

Until the late 1980s and even into the 1990s, IgAN was regarded by many as a mostly benign (harmless) disease, and many doctors, even nephrologists, sometimes didn't pay as much attention to it as they could have—until patients were in a more advanced stage of renal failure. Today, IgAN is specifically diagnosed much sooner after the first symptoms appear or are discovered, and nephrologists are much more active in pre-end stage care of their IgAN patients.

How It Presents

For some patients, IgAN first appears as an acute glomerulonephritis with macroscopic hematuria (visible blood in the urine). In this case patients are visibly sick enough to seek medical attention, and may exhibit any or all the symptoms of acute glomerulonephritis.

For others, especially adults, blood is first detected in the urine on a routine medical examination (often work or insurance-related). There are usually no visible symptoms, and the patient is totally unaware that anything is wrong. The blood in the urine is in the form of microscopic hematuria, which means that it isn't visible in the urine to the naked eye.

In both cases, protein in the urine may be discovered at the same time as the blood is found, or it may gradually appear as time goes by. The acute form is often accompanied by heavy proteinuria which may be treated with oral steroids. Protein in the urine is not visible as such, but unusually foamy urine is often a clue to its presence.

Although other kidney diseases may have similar symptoms, it is common to at least suspect IgAN when protein and blood are found in the urine (especially when occurring in conjunction with an upper respiratory infection.)

Causes of IgAN

General: At this writing, nobody really knows what causes a person to develop IgAN. Our immune system produces a number of different immunoglobulin complexes to fight off infections, allergens, etc. Among these are IgE, IgM, IgG, and IgA. In the case of IgAN, something appears to go wrong with either the form of the IgA immune complex itself, or with their production and clearance within the body, or both. There may also be abnormal deposits of IgM or IgG, although with IgAN, the IgA proteins are the predominant ones.

IgA proteins: IgA stands for immunoglobulin A. We all have IgA proteins circulating in our blood at all times. IgA proteins (also referred to as IgA complexes) are produced at various sites in the body, such as the bone marrow and mucosal tissues in the tonsils, lungs, and the intestines. While it may be logical to think that lowering the amount of these IgA proteins that circulate in the blood might slow the progression of IgAN, research has shown that this is not the case. For one thing, the amount of IgA that somehow sticks in the kidneys is tiny in comparison to the overall number of IgA proteins that are in the circulation, doing their job of fighting infection.

Mechanism of injury: The short explanation for IgAN is that some of these large IgA proteins are deposited in the glomeruli, where they remain to cause inflammation and to eventually choke off (or clog) the glomeruli so that blood cannot flow through them. Commonly, they are deposited and accumulate in the portion of glomeruli called the mesangium, until eventually, the tiny blood vessels which form the glomeruli are deprived of blood flow. When glomeruli become damaged through inflammation and loss of blood flow, they become scarred. This is referred to as glomerulosclerosis. Most adult patients already have some degree of glomerulosclerosis by the time a biopsy is performed. Ultimately, it is the glomerulosclerosis which causes permanent loss of kidney function.

Progressive chronic renal failure: Since there are about a million glomeruli in each kidney, there is an ample reserve of kidney function, and a person can go many years or even decades without feeling the effects of renal failure. However, once a glomerulus is damaged, it cannot be repaired. IgAN progressively destroys these glomeruli. As more and more glomeruli become scarred and non-functional, the remaining ones start working harder (a process called hyperfiltration), and eventually, as more and more of them fail at an increasingly faster rate, the kidneys no longer have enough function left to perform their task of filtering waste products from the blood. When this happens, the person is said to have reached end-stage renal disease (ESRD). At that point, some form of renal replacement therapy is required to sustain life (dialysis or a kidney transplant).

Symptoms of IgAN

Patients with IgAN usually exhibit a few common symptoms (not to be confused with the uremic symptoms of more advanced renal failure). These are as follows:

Hematuria: Blood in the urine, referred to as hematuria, is often the first sign of IgAN. Blood in the urine may originate from elsewhere in the urinary tract, so, at this point, some patients may be referred to a urologist in order to rule out non-renal causes. However, the finding of red blood cell casts and dysmorphic (small deformed, misshapen, sometimes fragmented) red blood cells combined with proteinuria is suggestive of the type of hematuria caused by IgAN and other glomerular diseases, while eumorphic red blood cells (normal sized, biconcavely shaped) are suggestive of a nonglomerular origin not related to IgAN. The color of the urine can give a clue as to the origin of the blood. For example, cola- or tea-colored urine suggests it is coming from the glomeruli (these are the filters in the kidney that are affected by glomerular diseases like IgAN). If it's bright red, especially near the end of urination, this tends to suggest that it is coming from the bladder or urethra, and not from the kidneys. However, these are just very general guidelines. There are many other reasons for blood in the urine, so it always needs to be investigated medically until the reason or source is found. There are two presentations of hematuria, depending on how much blood is being leaked into the urine:

- *Macroscopic hematuria:* This is when the blood is visible. It is usually called macro-hematuria for short, or gross hematuria.

This may be seen as dark, tea- or cola-colored urine which the patient discovers him or herself while in the midst or shortly after an upper respiratory infection (such as a cold or flu). Reddish or pink colored urine is more suggestive of a bleeding site other than the glomeruli. Colored urine will often cause the person to seek a doctor's advice, and this is the more dramatic way that IgAN makes its appearance. While a person's first experience with macro-hematuria can be frightening, it really only takes a tiny amount of blood to color the urine this way. Many people with IgAN have recurring episodes of macro-hematuria every time they get an upper respiratory infection. There is no specific treatment for blood in the urine, and episodes of visible hematuria usually resolve on their own after some time. Whether it's the first time or a recurrence, doctors will usually treat the respiratory infection that gave rise to it. However, some IgAN patients never have episodes of macro-hematuria.

- *Microscopic hematuria:* Usually shortened as micro-hematuria. This is when blood in the urine is not visible to the naked eye. Often, micro-hematuria is first detected in the doctor's office during a routine medical examination, by means of a simple dipstick which is "dipped" in a spot urine sample. It may also be reported after a urinalysis. Such patients are usually unaware that they have anything wrong with them, or they may have gone to see a doctor for another ailment or, as is often the case, for a simple insurance exam. Micro-hematuria is one of the main features of IgAN. For the majority of patients, micro-hematuria is always present.

Proteinuria: A second symptom which may or may not be present initially is protein in the urine. As glomeruli become inflamed or damaged, they begin to allow protein to spill into the urine. Protein in the urine is called "proteinuria." As with hematuria, proteinuria may vary from very mild to heavy. Proteinuria can also be detected in the doctor's office by means of a protein dipstick. If protein is found, more precise urinalysis is usually ordered. Whether proteinuria is present at the first discovery of hematuria or not, it eventually does make its appearance. You cannot see protein in the urine, although very foamy urine is usually a reliable clue that protein is present. Normally, there should be no protein in a person's urine (except trace amounts of albumin), so even trace amounts are usually cause for further investigation. Heavy proteinuria may be treated with oral corticosteroids, as it may cause other symptoms which are independent of the IgAN itself (this is what is referred to as the nephrotic syndrome).

Hypertension: As IgAN progresses, it is common for patients to develop high blood pressure (or hypertension). It is very important to treat hypertension by whatever means are necessary, because hypertension itself greatly increases the risk of progressing to end-stage renal disease.

Fatigue: Many report extreme fatigue, even with mild IgAN. In the absence of anemia, it is not known why this might happen, although it may be a crossover symptom on the continuum between IgAN and HSP [Henoch-Schönlein purpura].

Flank pain: Also referred to as loin pain. Flank pain is also often reported. It is thought to be caused by swelling and stretching of the renal capsule (which is the covering forming the outside of the kidney) during acute episodes of the disease. This flank pain is usually reported as a dull ache. A very small percentage of patients seem to develop persistent, severe attacks of flank pain. Some of these patients may be diagnosed with loin pain hematuria syndrome (LPHS)—a condition which is not exclusive to IgAN (it remains unclear if or how this is associated with IgAN).

Joint pain: May be a crossover symptom on the continuum between IgAN and HSP which a small minority of patients may experience.

Abdominal pain: This especially occurs in conjunction with an episode of macro-hematuria. The reason is unknown, but like fatigue and joint pain, it may be a crossover symptom on the continuum between IgAN and HSP. Only a minority of patients seem to have this. In some cases, it may be associated with pancreatitis, although it is not clear if this can be directly linked to IgAN. Some people with chronic renal insufficiency or with ESRD (end-stage renal disease, i.e., on dialysis) may develop varying degrees of a condition called gastroparesis. This basically means delayed emptying of stomach contents, and delayed movement of food through the digestive tract. This is more common in people who have diabetes, but kidney failure patients are also more prone to it than the general population. This may cause nausea, bloating, early feeling of fullness after eating even small meals, regurgitation, and abdominal pain.

Weakened immune system: While the exact cause of IgAN is not known, it is suspected that it involves a defect in immunoglobulin A (IgA) immune complexes, and some research seems to bear this out. This should not be interpreted as having a defective, weak immune system. There is little evidence that people with IgAN have an immune system that is weaker than other people's. It could be that some medications or some supplements weaken the immune system though. For example, it has been reported that fish oil in large quantities may do this, and, of course, oral steroids (like prednisone) do this also. On the other hand, the more advanced your chronic renal insufficiency is, the more it tends to depress the immune system.

Nephrotic syndrome: If proteinuria is heavy enough, patients will begin to show symptoms of nephrotic syndrome. Nephrotic syndrome is not a disease in itself, but a group of symptoms which are caused by the heavy loss of protein in the urine. Nephrotic syndrome may require aggressive treatment with corticosteroids or, if that fails, other drugs, until the level of proteinuria goes down. A person usually needs to lose more than 3.5 grams per day of protein in the urine before this begins to happen. Patients with nephrotic-range proteinuria may experience the following main symptoms.

- *Edema (severe):* The main symptom is edema, or swelling of the extremities and/or the abdomen. The majority of IgAN patients do not develop nephrotic syndrome, but it is fairly common in pediatric IgAN. As IgAN further progresses, the patient will start to show some of the symptoms of chronic renal failure.

- *Hypoalbuminemia:* Low blood levels of the protein albumin.

- *High cholesterol:* High cholesterol commonly develops when there is heavy loss of protein in the urine.

- *Other symptoms:* In addition to the above three main symptoms that characterize nephrotic syndrome, people who have such heavy proteinuria may also feel ill in various ways, including excessive fatigue, low appetite, facial swelling, abdominal pain along with the abdominal swelling. Also, apparent food intolerances have been reported.

Other symptoms: As you progress into more advanced chronic renal insufficiency (also referred to as chronic renal failure), you may start to experience some symptoms which are common to all, regardless of whether you have IgAN or any other kidney disease.

How IgAN Is Diagnosed

Initial diagnosis: Most IgAN patients are diagnosed before the age of 40—some as children or adolescents, and many, if not the majority, are diagnosed while in their early to mid 20s. IgAN is usually first suspected when blood and/or protein are found in the urine. When this happens, the physician will order blood work, urinalysis and possibly other non-invasive tests like a kidney ultrasound. Some of the findings can help point towards IgAN or another kidney disease.

Biopsy: At this time, the confirmation of an IgAN diagnosis can only be made by examining tissues taken during a biopsy of the kidney. This is usually a needle biopsy of the left kidney, which is performed as day surgery. If there are no complications with bleeding, the patient usually goes home by the end of the day. If the symptoms are very mild, and serum creatinine is in the normal range, your doctor may elect to wait some time before ordering a biopsy. Since IgAN can be a very slowly progressing disease, in some cases, a biopsy might not be done for a number of years. However, in recent years, it has become more and more common to biopsy very early in the course of the disease (some patients still have 100 percent kidney function when they are diagnosed, whereas before, and still today, many patients have already lost about 50 percent of their kidney function by the time anyone notices that something is wrong). Doctors are most likely to order a biopsy when there is both proteinuria and hematuria, but will often do it even in the absence of proteinuria. If your nephrologist does not recommend a kidney biopsy, ask why. However, you should be aware that one school of thought on delaying biopsies is that when the symptoms are very mild, there is nothing to be gained by performing a biopsy, since there would be no treatment anyway.

- *Light microscopy:* In a biopsy sample showing IgAN, the light microscopy portion of the evaluation is usually characterized by mesangial and focal-segmental proliferation, as well as glomerulosclerosis. In severe cases, there may be evidence of crescents, and this is usually a sign of severe damage.

- *Immunofluorescence:* This aspect of the biopsy tissue examination shows IgA deposited in the mesangium (a part of each glomerulus). In addition to the predominance of IgA deposits (which is the distinguishing feature of IgA nephropathy), IgG, IgM, and/or C3 are also often present, but no C4.

Late diagnosis: Another possibility is a late diagnosis. This happens when a person has had undetected symptoms of IgAN for many years, but for some reason, microscopic blood and/or protein in the urine has escaped medical attention. The IgAN may be discovered when the patient presents with symptoms of severe high blood pressure, or of more advanced renal failure. The more the IgAN has advanced into chronic renal failure, the less distinctive the pattern in the glomeruli, and, if late enough, a biopsy may not allow diagnosis of the original kidney disease which caused the renal failure.

Treatment of IgAN

Standard Treatment

Other than treatments which are currently investigational, there is no standard specific treatment for chronic IgAN. Treatment is given in support of specific symptoms, such as hypertension and edema. Some high blood pressure medications appear to have renal-protective effects that go beyond their ability to lower blood pressure, and one of these may be prescribed even if the blood pressure is not yet elevated. Acute episodes with nephrotic-range proteinuria (>3 g/day) often respond to oral corticosteroids (such as prednisone). In this case, the heavy proteinuria which is typical of nephrotic syndrome often abates, and the disease usually remains as a less aggressive chronic condition. Treatment of common slowly progressive IgAN is usually conservative (blood pressure medications), while rapidly progressive IgAN may be treated more aggressively (steroids, immunosuppressants). As chronic IgAN progresses, the patient will eventually start showing symptoms of chronic renal failure. As this begins to happen (sometimes over many years), nephrologists begin providing more frequent follow up and appropriate pre-ESRD care. Additional information on some aspects of treatment is given in the following paragraphs.

High blood pressure medications: One area where there is near complete agreement is on the subject of blood pressure. Impaired kidneys are very good at secreting a hormone which deliberately raises blood pressure. It is imperative that any treatment for controlling high blood pressure be followed rigorously, as high blood pressure itself further adds to the damage being caused in the kidneys, and it is an independent risk factor for ESRD (not to mention other cardiovascular complications). In addition to lowering blood pressure, some specific high blood pressure medications appear to have renal-protective and/or antiproteinuric effects. Generally, this applies to all the medications of a given class, namely, the ACE inhibitors, and also their close cousins, the angiotensin II receptor blockers. Combined use of the two drug types appears to be even more protective, and it is not uncommon for both to be prescribed. You can expect maximum reduction of proteinuria (up to about 40–50 percent) about four weeks after starting an ACE inhibitor.

Dietary restrictions: A low-protein diet is pretty much a given in patients who have more advanced renal failure (often referred to as pre-ESRD). However, the use of a low-protein diet in mild to moderate IgAN is controversial, as there is no solid evidence that it has any value at all, and in some cases, it can actually be harmful. Your nephrologist will tell you if you need to be on a low protein diet (it doesn't hurt to ask though). If you are hypertensive or have edema, you may be asked to reduce sodium intake. An actual renal diet (low protein, low potassium, low sodium, low phosphorus, high calories) is not required until IgAN has progressed to more advanced renal failure. The purpose of such a renal diet is not to delay progression of IgAN, but mainly to minimize the uremic symptoms of chronic renal failure. Unless you are specifically told to restrict something in your diet, there is no need to do so. There is absolutely no evidence that any food causes or affects IgAN, however, some people do believe an antigenic diet may be useful, and some nephrologists can be found who will suggest it (this is not considered mainstream medicine).

Warning: Patients are cautioned that they need instruction from a renal dietitian to be on a low protein renal diet, as there is much more to it than merely cutting back on protein. Also, contrary to what many would assume, a low protein diet is not a synonym for a vegetarian diet. There is always a risk of malnutrition with low protein diets. Malnutrition may be hard to reverse in more advanced renal failure. Whatever you do, do not embark on a low protein diet, vegetarian or otherwise, without checking with your nephrologist first. This is one area where you can actually make things worse for yourself. Patients with nephrotic syndrome may actually need supplementary protein. Lowering your dietary protein does not necessarily have a significant influence on proteinuria.

Fish oil: Fish oil has been commonly "prescribed" to many IgAN patients since the mid-1990s. Fish oil is an over-the-counter product that may have contraindications and precautions attached to it in the context of IgAN, [for further information, you may read about fish oil on the IgA Nephropathy Support Group website at http://www.igan.ca]. To date, studies of fish oil use in IgAN have given conflicting results, with some studies finding benefits and others showing no improvement. When used, it is usually a second-line medication, given in addition to ACE inhibitors and angiotensin II receptor blockers.

Vitamin E: The evidence in favor of vitamin E for kidney diseases in general has never been very strong, but there have been some studies which suggested that the antioxidant effect of vitamin E might be beneficial in chronic kidney disease. The suggested dose has been a 400 unit capsule per day. Until recently, vitamin E was also sometimes suggested for people with more advanced renal failure who experienced leg and foot cramps. The evidence supporting this use was never strong either, but it was commonly used for this purpose. A study published in late 2004, not in the context of kidney disease, suggested that daily vitamin E at 400 IU or more may actually increase the overall risk of dying. So, it may not be just another harmless supplement as was previously thought. It is not clear as yet how this will affect its use, but it already seems to have dampened enthusiasm for megadoses of vitamin E.

Alcohol restriction: Opinions vary on this subject, but generally speaking, patients may be advised to drink alcohol only moderately. Heavy drinking is injurious to the kidneys and may actually worsen IgAN.

Smoking: You will undoubtedly be asked with some insistence to stop smoking. There is steadily increasing evidence that smoking directly contributes to damaging the delicate blood vessels that form the glomeruli, even in people who do not have a chronic kidney disease. Make no mistake, cigarette smoking is an independent risk factor for progression of inflammatory glomerular diseases such as IgA nephropathy.

Exercise: If there are no other medical contraindications to exercise, nephrologists usually recommend a moderate-to-vigorous exercise program that stimulates the cardiovascular system, such as walking, cycling (stationary or otherwise), etc. Because high-impact exercise can worsen proteinuria and/or hematuria, if applicable, you may be advised to avoid those (unlikely unless your proteinuria is heavy or your hematuria is visible). You may be advised against heavy contact sports, due to the possibility of an impact that might cause direct injury to a kidney. For most patients, there will be few restrictions, if any. Even patients on dialysis are expected to exercise if they can, and some people with transplanted kidneys practice competitive sports. The best policy is to ask your nephrologist. If you know that a certain activity causes you to have visible blood in your urine, it may be reasonable to consider a different type of activity.

Other Symptomatic Treatments

Heavy proteinuria: Heavy proteinuria is usually defined as greater than 3.5 grams per day. It's not really very common with most IgAN, but it does happen. If your proteinuria is at that level or approaching it, your nephrologist will almost certainly want to treat that specific problem with oral steroids—usually prednisone, but there are others. This is because heavy proteinuria itself causes symptoms. These are generally grouped under the term "nephrotic syndrome." Treatment with steroids may be initiated even at a lower level of proteinuria if your nephrologist feels it's appropriate for you. Heavy proteinuria that does not respond to steroids may have to be treated with a stronger immunosuppressant such as CellCept. Many nephrologists are beginning to use drugs like prednisone and/or CellCept at lower levels of proteinuria. However, this use may or may not be justified based on current evidence. The side effects of these drugs can be severe, and, at some point, they may be worse than the disease being treated. It's important to note that proteinuria itself causes loss of erythropoietin, iron, and transferrin, and this is one reason why patients with nephrotic syndrome (heavy proteinuria) may become anemic.

Anemia: Anemia means a level of hemoglobin (red blood cells) that is too low. Symptoms of this are generally unusual fatigue and getting easily short of breath on minor exertion. Anemia from IgAN generally happens later on, when chronic renal insufficiency is more advanced. It happens because the kidneys reduce their ability to produce a certain hormone that signals the bone marrow to produce more red blood cells. It is treated with what most people refer to as EPO (short for erythropoietin). Current brands of synthetic EPO are Eprex, Procrit, Epogen, and Aranesp. These drugs are extremely expensive, and their use is usually only justified (and covered by drug plans) when hemoglobin or hematocrit in your blood work reaches down to a certain specified level. It is theoretically possible to restore hemoglobin levels to normal levels, but in practice, this is never done, because it would greatly increase the risk of excessive blood clotting and it causes high blood pressure. As a result, anemia is only treated up to a certain practical level of hemoglobin. These levels vary from country to country and whether you are pre-dialysis or on dialysis. Ask your nephrologist about it if you have advanced chronic renal insufficiency and you are especially tired or easily short of breath. It's important to note that medical science is not perfect. Sometimes, actual treatments may cause anemia. For example, while ACE inhibitors and angiotensin II receptor blockers (ARB) are the most used blood pressure medications at present for the treatment of chronic kidney disease, they may themselves cause anemia (in about five percent of cases, this fall of hemoglobin can be quite profound, so, it's something to watch out for). If the patient also happens to have heavy proteinuria, which itself causes lower hemoglobin, it is easy to see how, in some cases, a patient who has both nephrotic-range proteinuria and who is on an ACE inhibitor or an ARB (or both) could become much more anemic than the degree of chronic renal insufficiency would suggest. Use of low-dose daily aspirin to prevent a heart attack or stroke might also contribute to anemia due to gastrointestinal bleeding. It's very important to correct anemia, as it can eventually add congestive heart failure to your list of health problems. Heart failure itself leads to chronic renal failure. Luckily, anemia can be treated effectively.

Statins for high cholesterol: Statin drugs (like Zocor, Lipitor) are prescribed to treat the high cholesterol that is very common in chronic renal insufficiency patients, and in patients who have heavy proteinuria. As a bonus, there is some evidence emerging that statin drugs may help with proliferative and inflammatory kidney diseases.

Investigational Treatments

These are various treatments that have or are being evaluated in prospective or clinical trials. There have been both positive and negative results. Generally, for common slowly progressive IgAN, any positive results have been marginal at best, and, all things considered, the treatment may be worse than the disease. Follow the advice of your nephrologist about these (but do ask questions, as some are more aggressive in their approach to IgAN than others). Also, be aware that while the risks versus benefits equation of any investigational treatment may favor no treatment for slowly progressive IgAN, the balance may tip the other way in the case of rapidly progressive IgAN.

Also, patients in nephrotic syndrome usually require some of these treatments in order to reduce proteinuria to a more acceptable level (most often corticosteroids, like prednisone).

Corticosteroids: These are oral steroids like prednisone and prednisolone. Current investigational treatment is for alternate day dosing (approximately 50–60 mg) (for the purpose of reducing the sometimes severe side effects that accompany long-term oral steroid use). So far, there have been conflicting results, and no clearly positive results in terms of slowing the progression of IgAN. This is a different matter than using steroids for nephrotic syndrome and for more aggressive rapidly progressing IgAN, which is now considered to be standard practice in these cases. Consult your doctor on whether alternate day steroids might be considered in your case.

Immunosuppressants: These are the same immune system suppressive agents that are used in transplant patients to prevent organ rejection. The main ones being used in the context of IgAN are Imuran (azathioprine), CellCept (mycophenolate mofetil), cyclosporine, as well as Cytoxan (cyclophosphamide). At present, there is no definitive evidence that suppressing the immune system helps to slow down the progression of IgAN. However, some of these drugs are increasingly being used in more aggressive cases of IgAN, especially the rapidly progressive form. As with steroids, the side effects may be worse than the disease when it comes to common, slowly progressing IgAN. Again, this is something you may want to discuss with your nephrologist. Some patients have reported minimal or no side effects with CellCept in particular, while others have not been able to tolerate it at all. In transplant patients (where IgAN recurs to some degree), regular use of immunosuppressants for anti-rejection purposes has not shown any benefits in terms of preventing the recurrence of IgAN in the transplanted kidney.

Tonsillectomy: This remains a very controversial, and sometimes contentious subject among IgAN patients. There was a flurry of interest in tonsillectomy (removal of tonsils) as a treatment for IgAN in the early to mid-1990s.

- *Theory:* The idea behind this is that some IgA proteins originate in the tonsils, therefore, taking them out might reduce the number of circulating IgA complexes that reach the kidneys. One problem with this theory is that many other sites in the body produce

IgA complexes, and there is other evidence that reducing the levels of circulating IgA complexes doesn't appear to have any effect on the long-term progression of IgAN. There have been some observational studies or retrospective studies that have shown some positive results and others no positive results whatsoever.

- *Current status:* The following is quoted from Yuansheng Xie, Xiangmei Chen, Shinichi Nishi, Ichiei Narita, and Fumitake Gejyo, "Relationship between tonsils and IgA nephropathy as well as indications of tonsillectomy," *Kidney International*, Vol. 65 (2004), pp. 1135-1144. "Unfortunately, studies regarding tonsillectomy were performed until now in a retrospective style and little information has been available about the side effects or complications of the operation in IgAN patients. In order to further clarify the clinical efficacy and security of tonsillectomy, randomized prospective controlled trials are necessary because of the high degree of variability of IgAN."

- *Your nephrologist and tonsillectomy:* Since there is no real evidence that having a tonsillectomy improves the long-term outcome of IgAN, and it is not considered an effective treatment, very few nephrologists will agree with patient requests to recommend one. Some patients do manage to have a tonsillectomy performed via a referral to an ear-nose-throat specialist, especially if there are problems with tonsillitis anyway.

Chapter 35

Nephrotic Syndrome

Nephrotic Syndrome in Adults

Nephrotic syndrome is a condition marked by very high levels of protein in the urine (proteinuria); low levels of protein in the blood; swelling, especially around the eyes, feet, and hands; and high cholesterol. Nephrotic syndrome results from damage to the kidneys' glomeruli (the singular form is glomerulus). Glomeruli are tiny blood vessels that filter waste and excess water from the blood and send them to the bladder as urine.

Nephrotic syndrome can occur with many diseases, including the kidney diseases caused by diabetes mellitus, but some causes are unknown. Prevention of nephrotic syndrome relies on controlling these diseases.

Treatment of nephrotic syndrome focuses on identifying the underlying cause if possible and reducing high cholesterol, blood pressure, and protein in urine through diet, medications, or both. One group of blood pressure medications called ACE inhibitors also protects the kidneys by reducing proteinuria.

Nephrotic syndrome may go away once the underlying cause, if known, has been treated. In children, 80 percent of cases of nephrotic

This chapter contains text from "Nephrotic Syndrome in Adults," Pub. No. 03-4624, August 2003, and "Childhood Nephrotic Syndrome," Pub. No. 04-4695, December 2003, National Kidney and Urologic Diseases Information Clearinghouse (NKUDIC), a service of the National Institute of Diabetes and Digestive and Kidney Diseases (NIDDK), National Institutes of Health (NIH).

397

syndrome are caused by minimal change disease, which can be successfully treated with prednisone. However, in adults, most of the time the underlying cause is a kidney disease such as membranous nephropathy or focal segmental glomerulonephritis, and these diseases often persist even with treatment. In these cases, the kidneys may gradually lose their ability to filter wastes and excess water from the blood. If kidney failure occurs, the patient will need dialysis or a kidney transplant.

Childhood Nephrotic Syndrome

Childhood nephrotic syndrome can occur at any age, but is most common between the ages of 1½ and 5 years. It seems to affect boys more often than girls.

A child with the nephrotic syndrome has these signs:

- high levels of protein in the urine

- low levels of protein in the blood

- swelling resulting from buildup of salt and water

The nephrotic syndrome is not itself a disease. But it can be the first sign of a disease that damages the tiny blood-filtering units (glomeruli) in the kidneys, where urine is made.

The kidneys are two bean-shaped organs found in the lower back. They are about the size of a fist. They clean the blood by filtering out excess water and salt and waste products from food. Healthy kidneys keep protein in the blood, which helps the blood soak up water from tissues. But kidneys with damaged filters may let protein leak into the urine. As a result, not enough protein is left in the blood to soak up the water. The water then moves from the blood into body tissues and causes swelling. You may see swelling around your child's eyes, belly, and legs. Your child may urinate less often than usual and may gain weight from the excess water.

To diagnose childhood nephrotic syndrome, the doctor may ask for a urine sample to check for protein. The doctor will dip a strip of chemically treated paper into the urine sample. Too much protein in the urine will make the paper change color. Or the doctor may ask for a 24-hour collection of urine for a more precise measurement of the protein and other substances in the urine.

The doctor may take a blood sample to see how well the kidneys are removing wastes. Healthy kidneys remove creatinine and urea nitrogen from the blood. If the blood contains high levels of these waste products, some kidney damage may have already occurred. But most children with the nephrotic syndrome do not have permanent kidney damage.

In some cases, the doctor may want to examine a small piece of the child's kidney under a microscope to see if something specific is causing the syndrome. The procedure of collecting a small tissue sample from the kidney is called a biopsy, and it is usually performed with a long needle passed through the skin. The child will be awake during the procedure and receive calming drugs and a local painkiller at the site of the needle entry. General anesthesia may be used in some cases. The child will stay overnight in the hospital to rest and allow the health care team to ensure that no problems occur.

Minimal Change Disease

The most common form of the nephrotic syndrome in children is called minimal change disease. Doctors do not know what causes it. The condition is called minimal change disease because children with this form of the nephrotic syndrome have normal or nearly normal biopsies. If your child is diagnosed with minimal change disease, the doctor will probably prescribe prednisone, which belongs to a class of drugs called corticosteroids. Prednisone stops the movement of protein from the blood into the urine, but it does have side effects that the doctor will explain. Following the doctor's directions exactly is essential to protect your child's health. The doctor may also prescribe another type of drug called a diuretic, which reduces the swelling by helping the child urinate.

When protein is no longer present in the urine, the doctor will begin to reduce the dosage of prednisone. This process takes several weeks. Some children never get sick again, but most do develop swelling and protein in the urine again, usually following a viral illness. However, as long as the child continues to respond to prednisone and the urine becomes protein free, he or she has an excellent long-term outlook without kidney damage.

Children who relapse frequently, or who seem to be dependent on prednisone or have side effects from it, may be given a second type of drug called a cytotoxic agent. The agents most frequently used are cyclophosphamide, chlorambucil, and cyclosporine. After reducing protein in the urine with prednisone, the doctor may prescribe the cytotoxic agent for a while. Treatment with cyclophosphamide and chlorambucil usually lasts for 8 to 12 weeks, while treatment with cyclosporine frequently takes longer. The good news is that most children "outgrow" this disease by their late teens with no permanent damage to their kidneys.

Other Conditions that Involve the Childhood Nephrotic Syndrome

In about 20 percent of children with the nephrotic syndrome, the kidney biopsy reveals scarring or deposits in the glomeruli. The two most common diseases that damage these tiny filtering units are focal segmental glomerulosclerosis (FSGS) and membranoproliferative glomerulonephritis (MPGN).

Since prednisone is less effective in treating these diseases than it is in treating minimal change disease, the doctor may use additional therapies, including cytotoxic agents. Recent experience with a class of drugs called ACE inhibitors (a type of blood pressure drug) indicates that these drugs can help to prevent protein from leaking into the urine and keep the kidneys from being damaged in children with the nephrotic syndrome.

Very rarely, a child may be born with a condition that causes the nephrotic syndrome (congenital nephropathy). The most common form of this condition is congenital nephropathy of the Finnish type (CNF), inherited as an autosomal recessive trait. Another condition that causes nephrotic syndrome in the first months of life is diffuse mesangial sclerosis (DMS). The pattern of inheritance for DMS is not as clearly understood as the pattern for CNF, although the condition does appear to be genetic.

Since medicines have little effect on congenital nephropathy, transplantation is usually required by the second or third year of life, when the child has grown sufficiently to receive a kidney. To keep the child healthy, the doctor may recommend infusions of the protein albumin to make up for the protein lost in urine and prescribe a diuretic to help the child eliminate the extra fluid that causes swelling. The child's immune system may be weakened, so antibiotics should be given at the first sign of infection.

Congenital nephropathy can disturb thyroid activity, so the child may need a substitute hormone, thyroxine, to promote growth and help bones mature. A blood thinner like warfarin may be necessary to keep the child's blood from clotting.

A child with congenital nephropathy may need tube feedings to ensure proper nutrition. In some cases, the diseased kidney may need to be removed to eliminate proteinuria. Dialysis will then be required to replace kidney function until the child's body is big enough to receive a transplanted kidney. Peritoneal dialysis is preferable to hemodialysis for young children.

In peritoneal dialysis, a catheter is surgically placed in the child's abdomen and then used to introduce a solution into the abdominal cavity (the peritoneum). The solution draws wastes and extra fluid from the child's blood stream. After a few hours, the solution is drained and replaced with a fresh supply. The drained solution carries the waste and extra fluid out of the child's body.

Hope through Research

The National Institute of Diabetes and Digestive and Kidney Diseases (NIDDK) conducts and supports research to help many kinds of people with kidney disease, including children. NIDDK's Division of Kidney, Urologic, and Hematologic Diseases (DKUHD) maintains the Pediatric Nephrology Program, which supports research into the causes, treatment, and prevention of kidney diseases in children. In 2003, DKUHD initiated the Prospective Study of Chronic Kidney Disease in Children to learn more about the negative effects of pediatric kidney disease, including cardiovascular disease and neurocognitive impairment.

Chapter 36

Amyloidosis and Kidney Disease

Proteins are important building blocks for all body parts, including muscles, bones, hair, and nails. Proteins circulate throughout the body in the blood and are normally harmless. Occasionally, cells produce abnormal proteins that can settle in body tissue, forming deposits and causing disease. When these deposits of abnormal proteins were first discovered, they were called amyloid, and the disease process amyloidosis.

In recent years, researchers have discovered that different kinds of proteins can form amyloid deposits and have identified several types of amyloidosis. Two of these types are closely related to kidney disease. In primary amyloidosis, abnormal protein production occurs as a first step and can lead to kidney disease. Dialysis-related amyloidosis (DRA), on the other hand, is a result of kidney disease.

Primary Amyloidosis

Primary amyloidosis occurs when the body's antibody-producing cells do not function properly and produce abnormal protein fibers made of antibody fragments. Some people with primary amyloidosis have a condition called multiple myeloma. The antibody fragments come together to form amyloid deposits in different organs, including

National Kidney and Urologic Diseases Information Clearinghouse (NKUDIC), a service of the National Institute of Diabetes and Digestive and Kidney Diseases (NIDDK), National Institutes of Health (NIH), Pub. No. 03-4694, September 2003.

the kidneys, where they cause serious damage. Injured kidneys can't function effectively and may be unable to remove urea and other wastes from the blood. Elevated levels of these protein fibers can also damage the heart, lungs, brain, and digestive system.

One common sign of kidney amyloidosis is the presence of abnormally high levels of protein in the urine, a condition known as proteinuria. Healthy kidneys prevent protein from entering the urine, so the presence of protein may be a sign that the kidneys aren't working properly. A physician who finds large amounts of protein in the urine may also perform a biopsy—take a small sample of tissue for examination under a microscope—to confirm amyloidosis.

No effective treatment has been found to reverse the effects of amyloidosis. Combination drug therapy with melphalan (a cancer drug) and prednisone (an anti-inflammatory steroid drug) may improve organ function and survival rates by interrupting the growth of the abnormal cells that produce amyloid protein. These are the same drugs used in chemotherapy to treat certain cancers (such as multiple myeloma), and they may have serious side effects, such as nausea and vomiting, hair loss, and fatigue.

Dialysis-Related Amyloidosis

Normal kidneys filter and remove excess small proteins from the blood, thus keeping blood levels normal. When the kidneys don't work properly, as in patients receiving dialysis, one type of small protein called beta-2-microglobulin builds up in the blood. When this occurs, beta-2-microglobulin molecules may join together, like the links of a chain, forming a few very large molecules from many smaller ones. These large molecules can form deposits and eventually damage the surrounding tissues and cause great discomfort. This condition is called dialysis-related amyloidosis (DRA).

DRA is relatively common in patients who have been on hemodialysis for more than five years, especially among the elderly. Hemodialysis membranes that have been used for many years don't effectively remove the large, complex beta-2-microglobulin proteins from the bloodstream. Newer hemodialysis membranes, as well as peritoneal dialysis, remove beta-2-microglobulin more effectively, but not enough to keep blood levels normal. As a result, blood levels remain elevated, and deposits form in bone, joints, and tendons. DRA may result in pain, stiffness, and fluid in the joints. Patients with DRA may also develop hollow cavities, or cysts, in some of their bones; these may lead to unexpected bone fractures. Amyloid deposits may cause tears in ligaments and tendons (the tissue that connects the muscle to the bone). Most patients with these problems can be helped by surgical intervention.

Half of the people with DRA also develop a condition called carpal tunnel syndrome, which results from the unusual buildup of protein in the wrists. Patients with this disorder may experience numbness or tingling, sometimes associated with muscle weakness, in their fingers and hands. This is a treatable condition.

Unfortunately, no cure for DRA has been found, although a successful kidney transplant may stop the disease from progressing. However, DRA has caught the attention of dialysis engineers, who are attempting to develop new dialysis membranes that can remove larger amounts of beta-2-microglobulin from the blood.

Hope through Research

In recent years, researchers have learned a great deal about kidney disease. The National Institute of Diabetes and Digestive and Kidney Diseases (NIDDK) sponsors several programs aimed at understanding kidney failure and finding treatments to stop its progression.

NIDDK's Division of Kidney, Urologic, and Hematologic Diseases supports basic research into normal kidney function and the diseases that impair normal function at the cellular and molecular levels, including amyloidosis. Recently, NIDDK-sponsored researchers have identified several genes that may contribute to a hereditary form of primary amyloidosis. In 2001, a team of researchers at the Indiana University School of Medicine located a mutation in the *apolipoprotein A-II* gene of a patient with kidney damage caused by amyloidosis. The researchers noted that the patient had reabsorbed most of the amyloid. They theorize that learning how this reabsorption occurs may point the way to possible therapies for all forms of amyloidosis.

Chapter 37

Proteinuria

Proteinuria describes a condition in which urine contains an abnormal amount of protein. Proteins are the building blocks for all body parts, including muscles, bones, hair, and nails. Proteins in your blood also perform a number of important functions. They protect you from infection, help your blood coagulate, and keep the right amount of fluid circulating through your body.

As blood passes through healthy kidneys, they filter the waste products out and leave in the things the body needs, like proteins. Most proteins are too big to pass through the kidneys' filters into the urine unless the kidneys are damaged. The main protein that is most likely to appear in urine is albumin. Albumin is smaller and therefore more likely to escape through the filters of the kidney, called glomeruli. Sometimes the term albuminuria is used when the test detects albumin specifically. Albumin's function in the body includes retention of fluid in the blood. It acts like a sponge, soaking up fluid from body tissues.

Inflammation in the glomeruli is called glomerulonephritis, or simply nephritis. Many diseases can cause this inflammation, which leads to proteinuria. Additional processes that can damage the glomeruli and cause proteinuria include diabetes, hypertension, and other forms of kidney diseases.

National Kidney and Urologic Diseases Information Clearinghouse (NKUDIC), a service of the National Institute of Diabetes and Digestive and Kidney Diseases (NIDDK), National Institutes of Health (NIH), Pub. No. 03-4732, June 2003.

Research shows that the level and type of proteinuria (whether the urinary proteins are albumin only or include other proteins) strongly determine the extent of damage and whether you are at risk for developing progressive kidney failure.

Proteinuria has also been shown to be associated with cardiovascular disease. Damaged blood vessels may lead to heart failure or stroke as well as kidney failure. If your doctor finds that you have proteinuria, you will want to do what you can to protect your health and prevent any of these diseases from developing.

Several health organizations recommend that some people be regularly checked for proteinuria to detect and treat kidney disease before it progresses. A 1996 study sponsored by the National Institutes of Health determined that proteinuria is the best predictor of progressive kidney failure in people with type 2 diabetes. The American Diabetes Association recommends regular urine testing for proteinuria for people with type 1 or type 2 diabetes. The National Kidney Foundation recommends that routine checkups include testing for excess protein in the urine, especially for people in high-risk groups.

Who is at risk?

People with diabetes, hypertension, or certain family backgrounds are at risk for proteinuria. In the United States, diabetes is the leading cause of end-stage renal disease (ESRD), the result of chronic kidney disease. In both type 1 and type 2 diabetes, the first sign of deteriorating kidney function is the presence of small amounts of albumin in the urine, a condition called microalbuminuria. As kidney function declines, the amount of albumin in the urine increases, and microalbuminuria becomes full-fledged proteinuria.

High blood pressure is the second leading cause of ESRD. Proteinuria in people with high blood pressure is an indicator of declining kidney function. If the hypertension is not controlled, the person can progress to full renal failure.

African Americans are more likely than white Americans to have high blood pressure and to develop kidney problems from it, even when their blood pressure is only mildly elevated. In fact, African Americans ages 20 to 49 are 20 times more likely than their white counterparts to develop hypertension-related kidney failure. High blood pressure is the leading cause of kidney failure among African Americans.

Other groups at risk for proteinuria are American Indians, Hispanic Americans, Pacific Islander Americans, older people, and overweight

408

people. People who have a family history of kidney disease should also have their urine tested regularly.

What are the signs of proteinuria and kidney failure?

Large amounts of protein in your urine may cause it to look foamy in the toilet. Also, because the protein has left your body, your blood can no longer soak up enough fluid and you may notice swelling in your hands, feet, abdomen, or face. These are signs of very large protein loss. More commonly, you may have proteinuria without noticing any signs or symptoms. Testing is the only way to find out how much protein you have in your urine.

What are the tests for proteinuria?

To test for proteinuria, you will need to give a urine sample. A strip of chemically treated paper will change color when dipped in urine that has too much protein. More sensitive tests for protein or albumin in the urine are recommended for people at risk for kidney disease, especially those with diabetes. The protein-to-creatinine or albumin-to-creatinine ratio can be measured on a sample of urine to detect smaller amounts of protein, which can indicate kidney disease. If the laboratory test shows high levels of protein, another test should be done one to two weeks later. If the second test also shows high levels of protein, you have persistent proteinuria and should have additional tests to evaluate your kidney function.

Your doctor will also test a sample of your blood for creatinine and urea nitrogen. These are waste products that healthy kidneys remove from the blood. High levels of creatinine and urea nitrogen in your blood indicate that kidney function is impaired.

How is proteinuria treated?

If you have diabetes, hypertension, or both, the first goal of treatment will be to control your blood glucose and blood pressure. If you have diabetes, you should test your blood glucose often, follow a healthy eating plan, take your medicines, and get plenty of exercise. If you have diabetes and high blood pressure, your doctor may prescribe a medicine from a class of drugs called ACE (angiotensin-converting enzyme) inhibitors or angiotensin receptor blockers (ARB). These drugs have been found to protect kidney function even more than other drugs that provide the same level of blood pressure control. The American Diabetes Association recommends that people with diabetes keep their blood pressure below 130/80.

People who have high blood pressure and proteinuria but not diabetes may also benefit from taking an ACE inhibitor or ARB. Their blood pressure should be maintained below 130/80.

In addition to blood glucose and blood pressure control, the National Kidney Foundation recommends restricting dietary salt and protein. Your doctor may refer you to a dietitian to help you follow a healthy eating plan.

Hope through Research

In recent years, researchers have learned much about kidney disease. The National Institute of Diabetes and Digestive and Kidney Diseases (NIDDK) sponsors several programs aimed at understanding kidney failure and finding treatments to stop its progression.

NIDDK's Division of Kidney, Urologic, and Hematologic Diseases (DKUHD) supports basic research into normal kidney function and the diseases that impair normal function at the cellular and molecular levels, including diabetes, high blood pressure, glomerulonephritis, and other diseases marked by proteinuria.

Part Six

Cancers of the Urinary Tract and Kidneys

Chapter 38

Bladder Cancer

Introduction

Each year in the United States, bladder cancer is diagnosed in 38,000 men and 15,000 women. This is the fourth most common type of cancer in men and the eighth most common in women. This chapter discusses possible causes, symptoms, diagnosis, treatment, and rehabilitation. It also has information to help patients cope with bladder cancer.

Research is increasing what we know about bladder cancer. Scientists are learning more about its causes. They are exploring new ways to prevent, detect, diagnose, and treat this disease. Because of research, people with bladder cancer have an improved quality of life and less chance of dying from this disease.

The Bladder

The bladder is a hollow organ in the lower abdomen. It stores urine, the liquid waste produced by the kidneys. Urine passes from each kidney into the bladder through a tube called a ureter.

An outer layer of muscle surrounds the inner lining of the bladder. When the bladder is full, the muscles in the bladder wall can

"What You Need to Know about Bladder Cancer," National Cancer Institute (NCI), U.S. National Institutes of Health (NIH), http://cancer.gov, Pub. No. 01-1559, September 16, 2002.

tighten to allow urination. Urine leaves the bladder through another tube, the urethra.

Understanding Cancer

Cancer is a group of many related diseases. All cancers begin in cells, the body's basic unit of life. Cells make up tissues, and tissues make up the organs of the body. Normally, cells grow and divide to form new cells as the body needs them. When cells grow old and die, new cells take their place.

Sometimes this orderly process goes wrong. New cells form when the body does not need them, and old cells do not die when they should. These extra cells can form a mass of tissue called a growth or tumor. Tumors can be benign or malignant:

- **Benign tumors** are not cancer. Usually, doctors can remove them. Cells from benign tumors do not spread to other parts of the body. In most cases, benign tumors do not come back after they are removed. Most important, benign tumors are rarely a threat to life.

- **Malignant tumors** are cancer. They are generally more serious. Cancer cells can invade and damage nearby tissues and organs. Also, cancer cells can break away from a malignant tumor and enter the bloodstream or the lymphatic system. That is how cancer cells spread from the original (primary) tumor to form new tumors in other organs. The spread of cancer is called metastasis.

The wall of the bladder is lined with cells called transitional cells and squamous cells. More than 90 percent of bladder cancers begin in the transitional cells. This type of bladder cancer is called transitional cell carcinoma. About eight percent of bladder cancer patients have squamous cell carcinomas.

Cancer that is only in cells in the lining of the bladder is called superficial bladder cancer. The doctor might call it carcinoma in situ. This type of bladder cancer often comes back after treatment. If this happens, the disease most often recurs as another superficial cancer in the bladder.

Cancer that begins as a superficial tumor may grow through the lining and into the muscular wall of the bladder. This is known as invasive cancer. Invasive cancer may extend through the bladder wall. It may grow into a nearby organ such as the uterus or vagina (in women) or the prostate gland (in men). It also may invade the wall of the abdomen.

When bladder cancer spreads outside the bladder, cancer cells are often found in nearby lymph nodes. If the cancer has reached these nodes, cancer cells may have spread to other lymph nodes or other organs, such as the lungs, liver, or bones.

When cancer spreads (metastasizes) from its original place to another part of the body, the new tumor has the same kind of abnormal cells and the same name as the primary tumor. For example, if bladder cancer spreads to the lungs, the cancer cells in the lungs are actually bladder cancer cells. The disease is metastatic bladder cancer, not lung cancer. It is treated as bladder cancer, not as lung cancer. Doctors sometimes call the new tumor "distant" disease.

Bladder Cancer Risk Factors

No one knows the exact causes of bladder cancer. However, it is clear that this disease is not contagious. No one can "catch" cancer from another person.

People who get bladder cancer are more likely than other people to have certain risk factors. A risk factor is something that increases a person's chance of developing the disease. Still, most people with known risk factors do not get bladder cancer, and many who do get this disease have none of these factors. Doctors can seldom explain why one person gets this cancer and another does not.

Studies have found the following risk factors for bladder cancer:

- **Age:** The chance of getting bladder cancer goes up as people get older. People under 40 rarely get this disease.

- **Tobacco:** The use of tobacco is a major risk factor. Cigarette smokers are two to three times more likely than non-smokers to get bladder cancer. Pipe and cigar smokers are also at increased risk.

- **Occupation:** Some workers have a higher risk of getting bladder cancer because of carcinogens in the workplace. Workers in the rubber, chemical, and leather industries are at risk. So are hairdressers, machinists, metal workers, printers, painters, textile workers, and truck drivers.

- **Infections:** Being infected with certain parasites increases the risk of bladder cancer. These parasites are common in tropical areas but not in the United States.

- **Treatment with cyclophosphamide or arsenic:** These drugs are used to treat cancer and some other conditions. They raise the risk of bladder cancer.

- **Race:** Whites get bladder cancer twice as often as African Americans and Hispanics. The lowest rates are among Asians.

- **Being a man:** Men are two to three times more likely than women to get bladder cancer.

- **Family history:** People with family members who have bladder cancer are more likely to get the disease. Researchers are studying changes in certain genes that may increase the risk of bladder cancer.

- **Personal history of bladder cancer:** People who have had bladder cancer have an increased chance of getting the disease again.

Chlorine is added to water to make it safe to drink. It kills deadly bacteria. However, chlorine by-products sometimes can form in chlorinated water. Researchers have been studying chlorine by-products for more than 25 years. So far, there is no proof that chlorinated water causes bladder cancer in people. Studies continue to look at this question.

Some studies have found that saccharin, an artificial sweetener, causes bladder cancer in animals. However, research does not show that saccharin causes cancer in people.

People who think they may be at risk for bladder cancer should discuss this concern with their doctor. The doctor may suggest ways to reduce the risk and can plan an appropriate schedule for checkups.

Symptoms

Common symptoms of bladder cancer include:

- Blood in the urine (making the urine slightly rusty to deep red),

- Pain during urination, and

- Frequent urination, or feeling the need to urinate without results.

These symptoms are not sure signs of bladder cancer. Infections, benign tumors, bladder stones, or other problems also can cause these symptoms. Anyone with these symptoms should see a doctor so that the doctor can diagnose and treat any problem as early as possible. People with symptoms like these may see their family doctor or a urologist, a doctor who specializes in diseases of the urinary system.

Diagnosis

If a patient has symptoms that suggest bladder cancer, the doctor may check general signs of health and may order lab tests. The person may have one or more of the following procedures:

- **Physical exam:** The doctor feels the abdomen and pelvis for tumors. The physical exam may include a rectal or vaginal exam.

- **Urine tests:** The laboratory checks the urine for blood, cancer cells, and other signs of disease.

- **Intravenous pyelogram:** The doctor injects dye into a blood vessel. The dye collects in the urine, making the bladder show up on x-rays.

- **Cystoscopy:** The doctor uses a thin, lighted tube (cystoscope) to look directly into the bladder. The doctor inserts the cystoscope into the bladder through the urethra to examine the lining of the bladder. The patient may need anesthesia for this procedure.

The doctor can remove samples of tissue with the cystoscope. A pathologist then examines the tissue under a microscope. The removal of tissue to look for cancer cells is called a biopsy. In many cases, a biopsy is the only sure way to tell whether cancer is present. For a small number of patients, the doctor removes the entire cancerous area during the biopsy. For these patients, bladder cancer is diagnosed and treated in a single procedure.

Staging

If bladder cancer is diagnosed, the doctor needs to know the stage, or extent, of the disease to plan the best treatment. Staging is a careful attempt to find out whether the cancer has invaded the bladder wall, whether the disease has spread, and if so, to what parts of the body.

The doctor may determine the stage of bladder cancer at the time of diagnosis, or may need to give the patient more tests. Such tests may include imaging tests: CT scan, magnetic resonance imaging (MRI), sonogram, intravenous pyelogram, bone scan, or chest x-ray. Sometimes staging is not complete until the patient has surgery.

These are the main features of each stage of the disease:

- **Stage 0:** The cancer cells are found only on the surface of the inner lining of the bladder. The doctor may call this superficial cancer or carcinoma in situ.

- **Stage I:** The cancer cells are found deep in the inner lining of the bladder. They have not spread to the muscle of the bladder.

- **Stage II:** The cancer cells have spread to the muscle of the bladder.

- **Stage III:** The cancer cells have spread through the muscular wall of the bladder to the layer of tissue surrounding the bladder. The cancer cells may have spread to the prostate (in men) or to the uterus or vagina (in women).

- **Stage IV:** The cancer extends to the wall of the abdomen or to the wall of the pelvis. The cancer cells may have spread to lymph nodes and other parts of the body far away from the bladder, such as the lungs.

Treatment

Many people with bladder cancer want to take an active part in decisions about their medical care. They want to learn all they can about their disease and their treatment choices. However, the shock and stress that people often feel after a diagnosis of cancer can make it hard for them to think of everything they want to ask the doctor. Often it helps to make a list of questions before an appointment. To help remember what the doctor says, patients may take notes or ask whether they may use a tape recorder. Some patients also want to have a family member or friend with them when they talk to the doctor—to take part in the discussion, to take notes, or just to listen.

The doctor may refer patients to doctors who specialize in treating cancer, or patients may ask for a referral. Treatment generally begins within a few weeks after the diagnosis. There will be time for patients to talk with the doctor about treatment choices, get a second opinion, and learn more about bladder cancer.

Getting a Second Opinion

Before starting treatment, a patient may want to get a second opinion about the diagnosis, the stage of cancer, and the treatment plan. Some insurance companies require a second opinion; others may cover a second opinion if the patient requests it. Gathering medical records and arranging to see another doctor may take a little time. In most cases, a brief delay does not make treatment less effective. There are a number of ways to find a doctor for a second opinion:

- The doctor may refer patients to one or more specialists. Specialists who treat bladder cancer include surgeons, urologists, medical oncologists, radiation oncologists, and urologic oncologists. At cancer centers, these doctors often work together as a team.

- The Cancer Information Service, at 800-4-CANCER, can tell callers about treatment facilities, including cancer centers and other programs supported by the National Cancer Institute.

- People can get the names of specialists from their local medical society, a nearby hospital, or a medical school.

- The American Board of Medical Specialties (ABMS) has a list of doctors who have met certain education and training requirements and have passed specialty examinations. The *Official ABMS Directory of Board Certified Medical Specialists* lists doctors' names along with their specialty and their educational background. The directory is available in most public libraries. Also, ABMS offers this information on the internet at http://www.abms.org. (Click on "Who's Certified.")

Methods of Treatment

People with bladder cancer have many treatment options. They may have surgery, radiation therapy, chemotherapy, or biological therapy. Some patients get a combination of therapies.

The doctor is the best person to describe treatment choices and discuss the expected results of treatment. A patient may want to talk to the doctor about taking part in a clinical trial, a research study of new treatment methods. Clinical trials are an important option for people with all stages of bladder cancer. [The section, "The Promise of Cancer Research," in this text has more information about clinical trials.]

Surgery is a common treatment for bladder cancer. The type of surgery depends largely on the stage and grade of the tumor. The doctor can explain each type of surgery and discuss which is most suitable for the patient:

- *Transurethral resection:* The doctor may treat early (superficial) bladder cancer with transurethral resection (TUR). During TUR, the doctor inserts a cystoscope into the bladder through the urethra. The doctor then uses a tool with a small wire loop on the end to remove the cancer and to burn away any remaining cancer cells with an electric current. (This is called fulguration.) The patient may need to be in the hospital and may need anesthesia. After TUR, patients may also have chemotherapy or biological therapy.

- *Radical cystectomy:* For invasive bladder cancer, the most common type of surgery is radical cystectomy. The doctor also chooses this type of surgery when superficial cancer involves a large part of the bladder. Radical cystectomy is the removal of the entire bladder, the nearby lymph nodes, part of the urethra, and the nearby organs that may contain cancer cells. In men, the nearby organs that are removed are the prostate, seminal vesicles, and part of the vas deferens. In women, the uterus, ovaries, fallopian tubes, and part of the vagina are removed.

- *Segmental cystectomy:* In some cases, the doctor may remove only part of the bladder in a procedure called segmental cystectomy. The doctor chooses this type of surgery when a patient has a low-grade cancer that has invaded the bladder wall in just one area.

Sometimes, when the cancer has spread outside the bladder and cannot be completely removed, the surgeon removes the bladder but does not try to get rid of all the cancer. Or, the surgeon does not remove the bladder but makes another way for urine to leave the body. The goal of the surgery may be to relieve urinary blockage or other symptoms caused by the cancer.

When the entire bladder is removed, the surgeon makes another way to collect urine. The patient may wear a bag outside the body, or the surgeon may create a pouch inside the body with part of the intestine.

Radiation therapy (also called radiotherapy) uses high-energy rays to kill cancer cells. Like surgery, radiation therapy is local therapy. It affects cancer cells only in the treated area.

A small number of patients may have radiation therapy before surgery to shrink the tumor. Others may have it after surgery to kill cancer cells that may remain in the area. Sometimes, patients who cannot have surgery have radiation therapy instead.

Doctors use two types of radiation therapy to treat bladder cancer:

- *External radiation:* A large machine outside the body aims radiation at the tumor area. Most people receiving external radiation are treated five days a week for five to seven weeks as an outpatient. This schedule helps protect healthy cells and tissues by spreading out the total dose of radiation. Treatment may be shorter when external radiation is given along with radiation implants.

- *Internal radiation:* The doctor places a small container of a radioactive substance into the bladder through the urethra or through an incision in the abdomen. The patient stays in the hospital for several days during this treatment. To protect others from radiation exposure, patients may not be able to have visitors or may have visitors for only a short period of time while the implant is in place. Once the implant is removed, no radioactivity is left in the body.

Some patients with bladder cancer receive both kinds of radiation therapy.

Chemotherapy uses drugs to kill cancer cells. The doctor may use one drug or a combination of drugs.

For patients with superficial bladder cancer, the doctor may use intravesical chemotherapy after removing the cancer with TUR. This is local therapy. The doctor inserts a tube (catheter) through the urethra and puts liquid drugs in the bladder through the catheter. The drugs remain in the bladder for several hours. They mainly affect the cells in the bladder. Usually, the patient has this treatment once a week for several weeks. Sometimes, the treatments continue once or several times a month for up to a year.

If the cancer has deeply invaded the bladder or spread to lymph nodes or other organs, the doctor may give drugs through a vein. This treatment is called intravenous chemotherapy. It is systemic therapy, meaning that the drugs flow through the bloodstream to nearly every part of the body. The drugs are usually given in cycles so that a recovery period follows every treatment period.

The patient may have chemotherapy alone or combined with surgery, radiation therapy, or both. Usually chemotherapy is an outpatient treatment given at the hospital, clinic, or at the doctor's office. However, depending on which drugs are given and the patient's general health, the patient may need a short hospital stay.

Biological therapy (also called immunotherapy) uses the body's natural ability (immune system) to fight cancer. Biological therapy is most often used after TUR for superficial bladder cancer. This helps prevent the cancer from coming back.

The doctor may use intravesical biological therapy with BCG solution. BCG solution contains live, weakened bacteria [*bacille Calmette-Guérin* (BCG)]. The bacteria stimulate the immune system to kill cancer cells in the bladder. The doctor uses a catheter to put the solution in the bladder. The patient must hold the solution in the bladder for about two hours. BCG treatment is usually done once a week for six weeks.

Side Effects of Cancer Treatment

Because cancer treatment may damage healthy cells and tissues, unwanted side effects sometimes occur. These side effects depend on many factors, including the type and extent of the treatment. Side effects may not be the same for each person, and they may even change from one treatment session to the next. Doctors and nurses will explain the possible side effects of treatment and how they will help the patient manage them.

Surgery

For a few days after TUR, patients may have some blood in their urine and difficulty or pain when urinating. Otherwise, TUR generally causes few problems.

After cystectomy, most patients are uncomfortable during the first few days. However, medicine can control the pain. Patients should feel free to discuss pain relief with the doctor or nurse. Also, it is common to feel tired or weak for a while. The length of time it takes to recover from an operation varies for each person.

After segmental cystectomy, patients may not be able to hold as much urine in their bladder as they used to, and they may need to urinate more often. In most cases, this problem is temporary, but some patients may have long-lasting changes in how much urine they can hold.

If the surgeon removes the bladder, the patient needs a new way to store and pass urine. In one common method, the surgeon uses a piece of the person's small intestine to form a new tube through which urine can pass. The surgeon attaches one end of the tube to the ureters and connects the other end to a new opening in the wall of the abdomen. This opening is called a stoma. A flat bag fits over the stoma to collect urine, and a special adhesive holds it in place. The operation to create the stoma is called a urostomy or an ostomy. [The section, "Rehabilitation," has more information about how patients can learn to care for the stoma.]

For some patients, the doctor is able to use a part of the small intestine to make a storage pouch (called a continent reservoir) inside the body. Urine collects in the pouch instead of going into a bag. The surgeon connects the pouch to the urethra or to a stoma. If the surgeon connects the pouch to a stoma, the patient uses a catheter to drain the urine.

Bladder cancer surgery may affect a person's sexual function. Because the surgeon removes the uterus and ovaries in a radical cystectomy, women are not able to get pregnant. Also, menopause occurs at once. Hot flashes and other symptoms of menopause caused by surgery may be more severe than those caused by natural menopause. Many women take hormone replacement therapy (HRT) to relieve these problems. If the surgeon removes part of the vagina during a radical cystectomy, sexual intercourse may be difficult.

In the past, nearly all men were impotent after radical cystectomy, but improvements in surgery have made it possible for some men to avoid this problem. Men who have had their prostate gland and seminal vesicles removed no longer produce semen, so they have dry orgasms. Men who wish to father children may consider sperm banking before surgery or sperm retrieval later on.

It is natural for a patient to worry about the effects of bladder cancer surgery on sexuality. Patients may want to talk with the doctor about possible side effects and how long these side effects are likely to last. Whatever the outlook, it may be helpful for patients and their partners to talk about their feelings and help one another find ways to share intimacy during and after treatment.

Radiation Therapy

The side effects of radiation therapy depend mainly on the treatment dose and the part of the body that is treated. Patients are likely to become very tired during radiation therapy, especially in the later weeks of treatment. Resting is important, but doctors usually advise patients to try to stay as active as they can.

External radiation may permanently darken or "bronze" the skin in the treated area. Patients commonly lose hair in the treated area and their skin may become red, dry, tender, and itchy. These problems are temporary, and the doctor can suggest ways to relieve them.

Radiation therapy to the abdomen may cause nausea, vomiting, diarrhea, or urinary discomfort. The doctor can suggest medicines to ease these problems.

Radiation therapy also may cause a decrease in the number of white blood cells, cells that help protect the body against infection. If the blood counts are low, the doctor or nurse may suggest ways to avoid getting an infection. Also, the patient may not get more radiation therapy until blood counts improve. The doctor will check the patient's blood counts regularly and change the treatment schedule if it is necessary.

For both men and women, radiation treatment for bladder cancer can affect sexuality. Women may experience vaginal dryness, and men may have difficulty with erections.

Although the side effects of radiation therapy can be distressing, the doctor can usually treat or control them. It also helps to know that, in most cases, side effects are not permanent.

Chemotherapy

The side effects of chemotherapy depend mainly on the drugs and the doses the patient receives as well as how the drugs are given. In addition, as with other types of treatment, side effects vary from patient to patient.

Anticancer drugs that are placed in the bladder cause irritation, with some discomfort or bleeding that lasts for a few days after treatment. Some drugs may cause a rash when they come into contact with the skin or genitals.

Systemic chemotherapy affects rapidly dividing cells throughout the body, including blood cells. Blood cells fight infection, help the blood to clot, and carry oxygen to all parts of the body. When anticancer drugs damage blood cells, patients are more likely to get infections, may bruise or bleed easily, and may have less energy. Cells in hair roots and cells that line the digestive tract also divide rapidly. As a result, patients may lose their hair and may have other side effects such as poor appetite, nausea and vomiting, or mouth sores. Usually, these side effects go away gradually during the recovery periods between treatments or after treatment is over.

Certain drugs used in the treatment of bladder cancer also may cause kidney damage. To protect the kidneys, patients need a lot of fluid. The nurse may give the patient fluids by vein before and after treatment. Also, the patient may need to drink a lot of fluids during treatment with these drugs.

Certain anticancer drugs can also cause tingling in the fingers, ringing in the ears, or hearing loss. These problems may go away after treatment stops.

Biological Therapy

BCG therapy can irritate the bladder. Patients may feel an urgent need to urinate, and may need to urinate frequently. Patients also may have pain, especially when urinating. They may feel tired. Some patients may have blood in their urine, nausea, a low-grade fever, or chills.

Nutrition

Patients need to eat well during cancer therapy. They need enough calories to maintain a good weight and protein to keep up strength. Good nutrition often helps people with cancer feel better and have more energy. But eating well can be difficult. Patients may not feel like eating if they are uncomfortable or tired. Also, the side effects of treatment, such as poor appetite, nausea, or vomiting, can be a problem. Foods may taste different. The doctor, dietitian, or other healthcare provider can suggest ways to maintain a healthy diet.

Rehabilitation

Rehabilitation is an important part of cancer care. The healthcare team makes every effort to help the patient return to normal activities as soon as possible.

Patients who have a stoma need to learn to care for it. Enterostomal therapists or nurses can help. These healthcare specialists often visit patients before surgery to discuss what to expect. They teach patients how to care for themselves and their stomas after surgery. They talk with patients about lifestyle issues, including emotional, physical, and sexual concerns. Often they can provide information about resources and support groups.

Follow-Up Care

Follow-up care after treatment for bladder cancer is important. Bladder cancer can return in the bladder or elsewhere in the body.

Therefore, people who have had bladder cancer may wish to discuss the chance of recurrence with the doctor.

If the bladder was not removed, the doctor will perform cystoscopy and remove any new superficial tumors that are found. Patients also may have urine tests to check for signs of cancer. Follow-up care may also include blood tests, x-rays, or other tests.

People should not hesitate to discuss follow-up care with the doctor. Regular follow up ensures that the doctor will notice changes so that any problems can be treated as soon as possible. Between checkups, people who have had bladder cancer should report any health problems as soon as they appear.

Support for People with Bladder Cancer

Living with a serious disease such as cancer is not easy. Some people find they need help coping with the emotional and practical aspects of their disease. Support groups can help. In these groups, patients or their family members get together to share what they have learned about coping with the disease and the effects of treatment. Patients may want to talk with a member of their healthcare team about finding a support group.

People living with cancer may worry about caring for their families, holding on to their jobs, or keeping up with daily activities. Concerns about treatments and managing side effects, hospital stays, and medical bills are also common. Doctors, nurses, and other members of the healthcare team will answer questions about treatment, working, or other activities. Meeting with a social worker, counselor, or member of the clergy can be helpful to those who want to talk about their feelings or discuss their concerns. Often, a social worker can suggest resources for help with rehabilitation, emotional support, financial aid, transportation, or home care.

The Promise of Cancer Research

Doctors all over the country are conducting many types of clinical trials. These are research studies in which people take part voluntarily. Doctors are studying ways to treat bladder cancer and prevent it from coming back. Research already has led to advances in these areas, and researchers continue to search for more effective approaches.

Patients who join clinical trials have the first chance to benefit from new treatments that have shown promise in earlier research. They also make an important contribution to medical science by helping doctors learn more about the disease. Although clinical trials may pose some risks, researchers take many steps to protect their patients.

Patients who are interested in joining a clinical study should talk with their doctor. They may want to read "Taking Part in Clinical Trials: What Cancer Patients Need to Know." This NCI booklet describes how treatment studies are carried out and explains their possible benefits and risks. NCI's website at http://cancer.gov provides general information about clinical trials. It also offers detailed information about specific ongoing studies of bladder cancer by linking to Physician Data Query (PDQ®), NCI's cancer information database. The Cancer Information Service at 800-4-CANCER can answer questions and provide information from the PDQ database.

Doctors are studying surgery, radiation therapy, chemotherapy, biological therapy, and combinations of these types of treatment. Another approach under study is photodynamic therapy, which uses drugs that start to work when exposed to light. After the cancer cells absorb the drug, the doctor shines a special light inside the bladder through a cystoscope. The drug becomes active and kills the cancer cells.

Doctors also are studying whether large doses of vitamins or certain drugs may prevent bladder cancer from coming back after treatment.

Chapter 39

Urethral Cancer

Description: Cancer of the Urethra

Cancer of the urethra, a rare type of cancer, is a disease in which cancer (malignant) cells are found in the urethra. The urethra is the tube that empties urine from the bladder, the hollow organ in the lower abdomen that stores urine. In women, the urethra is about one and one-half inches long and opens to the outside of the body above the vagina. In men, the urethra is about eight inches long and goes through the prostate gland and then through the penis to the outside of the body. Cancer of the urethra affects women more often then men.

There may be no symptoms of early cancer of the urethra. A doctor should be seen if there is a lump or growth on the urethra, or pain, bleeding, or other difficulty during urination

If there are symptoms, a doctor will examine the patient and feel for lumps in the urethra. In men, a thin lighted tube called a cystoscope may be inserted into the penis so the doctor can see inside the urethra. If the doctor finds cells or other signs that are not normal, a small piece of tissue (called a biopsy) may be cut out and looked at under a microscope for cancer cells.

The chance of recovery (prognosis) and choice of treatment depend on the stage of the cancer (whether it is just in one area or has spread to other places) and the patient's general state of health.

PDQ® Cancer Information Summary. National Cancer Institute; Bethesda, MD. Urethral Cancer (PDQ®): Treatment—Patient. Updated 06/2003. Available at: http://cancer.gov. Accessed 12/2004.

Stages of Cancer of the Urethra

Once cancer of the urethra is found, more tests will be done to find out if cancer cells have spread to other parts of the body (staging). A doctor needs to know the stage of the disease to plan treatment. For cancer of the urethra, patients are grouped into stages depending on where the tumor is and whether it has spread to other places. The following stage groupings are used for cancer of the urethra:

Anterior urethral cancer: The part of the urethra that is closest to the outside of the body is called the anterior urethra, and cancers that start here are called anterior urethral cancers.

Posterior urethral cancer: The part of the urethra that connects to the bladder is called the posterior urethra, and cancers that start here are called posterior urethral cancers. Because the posterior urethra is closer to the bladder and other tissues, cancers that start here are more likely to grow through the inner lining of the urethra and affect nearby tissues.

Urethral cancer associated with invasive bladder cancer: Occasionally, patients who have bladder cancer also have cancer of the urethra. This is called urethral cancer associated with invasive bladder cancer.

Recurrent urethral cancer: Recurrent cancer means that the cancer has come back (recurred) after it has been treated. It may come back in the same place, or in another part of the body.

How Cancer of the Urethra Is Treated

There are treatments for all patients with cancer of the urethra. Three kinds of treatment are used:

- Surgery (taking out the cancer in an operation)
- Radiation therapy (using high-dose x-rays or other high-energy rays to kill cancer cells)
- Chemotherapy (using drugs to kill cancer cells)

Surgery is the most common treatment of cancer of the urethra. A doctor may take out the cancer using one of the following operations:

- *Electrofulguration* uses an electric current to remove the cancer. The tumor and the area around it are burned away and then removed with a sharp tool.

- *Laser therapy* uses a narrow beam of intense light to kill cancer cells.

- *Cystourethrectomy* removes the bladder and the urethra.

In men, the part of the penis containing the urethra that has cancer may be removed in an operation called a partial penectomy. Sometimes the entire penis is removed (penectomy). A patient may need plastic surgery to make a new penis if all or part of the penis is removed. The bladder and prostate may also be removed in an operation called cystoprostatectomy. Lymph nodes in the pelvis may also be removed (lymph node dissection). Lymph nodes are small bean-shaped structures that are found throughout the body. They produce and store infection-fighting cells.

In women, surgery to remove the urethra, the bladder, and the vagina (anterior exenteration) may also be done. Lymph nodes in the pelvis may be removed (lymph node dissection). Plastic surgery may be needed to make a new vagina after this operation.

If the urethra is removed, the doctor will need to make a new way for the urine to pass from the body. This is called urinary diversion.

If the bladder is removed, the doctor will need to make a new way for the patient to store and pass urine. There are several ways to do this. Sometimes the doctor will use part of the small intestine to make a tube through which urine can pass out of the body through an opening (stoma) on the outside of the body. This is sometimes called an ostomy or urostomy. If a patient has an ostomy, a special bag will need to be worn to collect urine. This special bag, which sticks to the skin around the stoma with a special glue, can be thrown away after it is used. This bag does not show under clothing, and most people take care of these bags themselves. The doctor may also use part of the small intestine to make a new storage pouch (a continent reservoir) inside the body where the urine can collect. The patient would then need to use a tube (catheter) to drain the urine through a stoma.

Radiation therapy uses x-rays or other high-energy rays to kill cancer cells and shrink tumors. Radiation may come from a machine outside the body (external radiation therapy) or from putting materials that produce radiation (radioisotopes) through thin plastic tubes (internal radiation therapy) in the area where cancer cells are found. Radiation may be used alone or with surgery and/or chemotherapy.

Chemotherapy uses drugs to kill cancer cells. Chemotherapy may be taken by mouth, or it may be put in the body through a needle in a vein or muscle. Chemotherapy is called a systemic treatment because the drug enters the bloodstream, travels through the body and can kill cancer cells outside the urethra.

Treatment by Stage

Treatment depends on where the cancer is found, whether it has spread to other areas in the body, and the patient's sex, age, and overall health.

Standard treatment may be considered because of its effectiveness in patients in past studies, or participation in a clinical trial may be considered. Not all patients are cured with standard therapy and some standard treatments may have more side effects than are desired. For these reasons, clinical trials are designed to find better ways to treat cancer patients and are based on the most up-to-date information. Clinical trials are going on in many parts of the country for patients with cancer of the urethra. To learn more about clinical trials, call the Cancer Information Service at 800-4-CANCER (800-422-6237); TTY at 800-332-8615.

Anterior Urethral Cancer

Treatment is different for men and women.

For women, treatment may be one of the following:

1.   Electrofulguration

2.   Laser therapy

3.   External and/or internal radiation therapy

4.   Radiation therapy followed by surgery or surgery alone to remove the urethra and the organs in the lower pelvis (anterior exenteration), or the tumor only, if it is small (A new way is made for urine to pass out of the body—urinary diversion.)

For men, treatment may be one of the following:

1.   Electrofulguration

2. Laser therapy

3. Surgery to remove a part of the penis (partial penectomy)

4. Radiation therapy

Posterior Urethral Cancer

Treatment is different for men and women.

For women, treatment will probably be radiation therapy followed by surgery or surgery alone to remove the urethra, the organs in the lower pelvis (anterior exenteration), or the tumor only, if it is small. Lymph nodes in the pelvis are usually removed (lymph node dissection), and lymph nodes in the upper thigh may or may not be removed. A new way is made for urine to pass out of the body (urinary diversion).

For men, treatment will probably be radiation therapy followed by surgery or surgery alone to remove the bladder and prostate (cystoprostatectomy) and the penis and urethra (penectomy). Lymph nodes in the pelvis are usually removed (lymph node dissection), and lymph nodes in the upper thigh may or may not be removed. A new way is made for urine to pass out of the body (urinary diversion).

Urethral Cancer Associated with Invasive Bladder Cancer

Because people with bladder cancer sometimes also have cancer of the urethra, the urethra may be removed at the same time the bladder is taken out (cystourethrectomy). If the urethra is not removed during surgery for bladder cancer, the doctor may follow the patient closely so treatment can be started if cancer of the urethra develops.

Recurrent Urethral Cancer

Treatment depends on what treatment the patient received before. If the patient had surgery, treatment may be radiation therapy and surgery to remove the cancer. If the patient had radiation therapy, treatment may be surgery to remove the cancer. Clinical trials are testing chemotherapy for cancer of the urethra that has spread to other parts of the body.

Chapter 40

Prostate Cancer

Chapter Contents

435

Section 40.1

Facts about Prostate Cancer and Prostate Cancer Screening

"Prostate Cancer Screening: A Decision Guide," U.S. Department of Health and Human Services, Centers for Disease Control and Prevention (CDC), December 2004. Reviewed January 20, 2005.

What is the prostate?

The prostate is a walnut-sized gland that only men have. It is part of the reproductive system that makes the fluid that carries sperm. The prostate is located in front of the rectum and just below the bladder. The urethra (the tube that carries urine from the bladder to outside the body) runs through the center of the prostate. As men age, the prostate tends to increase in size. This can cause the urethra to narrow and decrease urine flow.

What is prostate cancer?

Prostate cancer is made up of cells that do not grow normally. The cells divide and create new cells that the body does not need, forming

Table 40.1. Risk of Being Diagnosed with Prostate Cancer by Age

Age	Risk
Age 45	1 in 2,500
Age 50	1 in 476
Age 55	1 in 120
Age 60	1 in 43
Age 65	1 in 21
Age 70	1 in 13
Age 75	1 in 9
Ever	1 in 6

a mass of tissue called a tumor. These abnormal cells sometimes spread to other parts of the body, multiply, and cause death.

What causes prostate cancer?

As with many types of cancers, medical experts do not know what causes prostate cancer. They are studying several possible causes.

Can prostate cancer be prevented?

Medical experts do not know how to prevent prostate cancer. But they are studying many factors. They do know that not smoking, maintaining a healthy diet, staying physically active, and seeing your doctor regularly contribute to overall good health.

How common is prostate cancer?

For the general population, a man in his lifetime has about a 16 percent chance (1 in 6) of being diagnosed with prostate cancer and about a 3 percent chance (1 in 33) of dying from prostate cancer. The older you are, the greater the risk for getting prostate cancer. See Table 40.1.

Who is at increased risk for prostate cancer?

While all men are at risk for prostate cancer, some factors increase risk.

- **Family history:** Men with a father or brother who has had prostate cancer are at greater risk for developing it themselves.

- **Race:** Prostate cancer is more common in some racial and ethnic groups than in others, but medical experts do not know why. Prostate cancer is more common in African American men than in white men. It is less common in Hispanic, Asian, Pacific Islander, and Native American men than in white men.

Is prostate cancer serious?

Some prostate cancers become a serious threat to health by growing quickly, spreading beyond the prostate gland to other parts of the body, and causing death. Yet other prostate cancers grow slowly and never become a serious threat to health or affect how long a man lives. Doctors can't always be sure what type of cancer is present in your particular case.

Among the leading causes of cancer death in men, prostate cancer is second, behind lung cancer. When compared with all causes of death in men over age 45, prostate cancer ranks fifth.

What are the symptoms of prostate cancer?

Many men with prostate cancer often have no symptoms. If symptoms appear, they can include:

- blood in the urine;
- the need to urinate frequently, especially at night;
- weak or interrupted urine flow;
- pain or burning feeling while urinating;
- the inability to urinate;
- constant pain in the lower back, pelvis, or upper thighs.

If you have any of these symptoms, see your doctor as soon as possible. Keep in mind that these symptoms are also caused by other prostate problems that are not cancer, such as an infection or an enlarged prostate.

Is screening right for you?

The decision is yours. Some medical experts believe all men should be offered regular screening tests for prostate cancer. Other medical experts do not recommend screening. To help you decide, let's begin with the basics.

What does "screening" mean?

Screening means looking for signs of disease in people who have no symptoms. So screening for prostate cancer is looking for early-stage disease when treatment may be more effective. The main screening tools for prostate cancer are the digital rectal examination (DRE) and the prostate-specific antigen (PSA) test. The DRE and PSA test cannot tell if you have cancer; they can only suggest the need for further tests.

What is the DRE?

The DRE or digital (finger) rectal examination is a quick exam for checking the health of the prostate. For this test, the doctor inserts a gloved and lubricated finger into the rectum. This allows the doctor to feel the back portion of the prostate for size and any irregular or abnormally firm areas.

What is the PSA test?

PSA stands for "prostate-specific antigen." PSA is a substance produced by cells from the prostate gland and released into the blood. The PSA test measures the PSA level in the blood. A small amount of blood is drawn from the arm. The doctor checks the blood to see if the PSA level is normal. The doctor may also use this test to check for any increase in your PSA level compared to your last PSA test.

As a rule, the higher the PSA level in the blood, the more likely a prostate problem is present. But many factors, such as age and race, can affect PSA levels. Some prostate glands produce more PSA than others. PSA levels can also be affected by:

- certain medical procedures;
- an enlarged prostate;
- a prostate infection.

Because many factors can affect PSA levels, your doctor is the best person to interpret your PSA test results.

Table 40.2. Top Ten Causes of Death in Men over Age 45

Cause of Death	Percentage (%)
Heart Disease	33.2
Lung Cancer	7.8
Stroke	6.4
Emphysema	6.0
Prostate Cancer	3.3
Pneumonia	2.9
Diabetes	2.7
Unintentional Injuries	2.5
Colorectal Cancer	2.5
Liver Disease	1.7

How accurate are the screening tests?

No test is right all the time and that is true of the PSA test and DRE. The PSA test is better at suggesting that small cancers are present, especially those toward the front or sides of the prostate gland, or deep within it. But the DRE can sometimes help suggest cancers in men with normal PSA levels. That is why both the PSA test and the DRE are usually performed.

If 100 men over age 50 take the PSA test, 85 will have a normal PSA (though a small number of these men will have a cancer that was missed by the PSA test). Fifteen will have a higher than normal PSA and require further tests. After further testing, results will show 12 do not have prostate cancer, three have prostate cancer.

What do medical experts say about screening?

Medical experts agree that every man needs balanced information on the pros and cons of prostate cancer screening to help him make an informed decision. Balanced information is important because medical experts disagree about whether men should be screened regularly for prostate cancer.

Medical experts who encourage regular screening believe current scientific evidence shows that finding and treating prostate cancer early, when treatment might be more effective, may save lives. They recommend that all men who have a life expectancy of at least ten years should be offered the PSA test and DRE annually beginning at age 50. They also recommend offering screening tests earlier to African American men, and men who have a father or brother with prostate cancer.

Medical experts who do not recommend regular screening want convincing evidence that finding early-stage prostate cancer, and treating it, saves lives. They believe some of these cancers may never affect a man's health and treating them could cause temporary or long-lasting side effects like impotence (inability to keep an erection) and incontinence (inability to control the urine flow, resulting in leakage or dribbling). Because they believe it is unclear if the potential benefits of screening outweigh the known side effects of treatment, they recommend that all men be given information on the pros and cons of screening before making their own screening decision.

When will medical experts know more?

Medical experts are working together on major research studies to get answers. These studies are called clinical trials. They will help determine whether a man who gets screened regularly is less likely to die of prostate cancer than a man who does not get screened. Clinical trials involve thousands of male volunteers and take a long time. Results are expected in five to ten years. They should help experts know if screening for prostate cancer saves lives.

Should I be screened for prostate cancer?

The decision is up to you and your doctor. Know your risk factors for prostate cancer and the pros and cons of screening.

Pros: "I will take the screening tests because they will give me peace of mind. It could mean finding a problem, taking further tests, and treating a potentially serious prostate cancer. And because there's no way to tell if the prostate cancer will cause problems in the future, I want it found early when treatments might be more effective."

Cons: "I will not take the screening tests until medical experts agree that finding and treating prostate cancer in its early stages reduce the chance of dying from it. Screening tests could lead to further tests and treatment of a prostate cancer that may never cause problems. And treatment can have serious side effects."

What if the results of your screening tests indicate that you might need further testing?

Do not panic. Most men who go for further testing do not have cancer. If your PSA test or DRE suggests a problem, your doctor most likely will refer you to a urologist (a doctor who has special training in prostate-related problems). Additional testing is necessary to determine if the problem is cancer or something else.

The urologist may perform a transrectal ultrasound—a small probe inserted into the rectum that bounces sound waves off the prostate, producing a video image. Transrectal ultrasound does not provide enough specific information to make it a good screening tool by itself, but some doctors find it useful as a follow up to a suspicious DRE or PSA test.

If the urologist suspects cancer, tiny samples of the prostate may be removed with a needle. This is called a biopsy. A biopsy is usually performed in the urologist's office. The samples are examined under a microscope to determine if cancer cells are present.

What happens if prostate cancer is found?

No two men with prostate cancer are the same. Many factors affect the decision whether or not to treat the disease: the patient's age, whether the cancer has spread, the presence of other medical conditions, and the patient's overall health.

When prostate cancer has been found in its early stages and has not spread beyond the prostate, a doctor and his patient may decide upon:

- **Watchful waiting:** Monitoring the patient's prostate cancer by performing the PSA test and DRE regularly, and treating it only if and when the prostate cancer causes symptoms or shows signs of growing;

- **Surgery (radical prostatectomy):** Removing the prostate;

- **External radiation therapy:** Destroying cancer cells by directing radiation at the prostate;

- **Internal radiation therapy (brachytherapy):** Surgically placing small radioactive pellets inside or near the cancer to destroy cancer cells;

- **Hormone therapy:** Giving certain hormones to keep prostate cancer cells from growing;

- **Cryotherapy:** Placing a special probe inside or near the prostate cancer to freeze and destroy the cancer cells.

More advanced prostate cancers that have spread beyond the prostate can be complex to treat and may be incurable. Patients should discuss with their doctor the best course of action.

Do these treatments have side effects?

Side effects from prostate cancer treatment depend mainly on the type of treatment, the patient's age, and his overall health. Men can experience pain, discomfort, and other mild to severe side effects that may be temporary or may last a long time. Two important side effects are impotence and incontinence. When a doctor explains the treatment options, he or she can discuss how mild or severe side effects might be, and how long they might last. Also, a doctor may be able to perform surgery or prescribe drugs to relieve some side effects.

Conclusion and Resources

To decide whether screening is right for you, discuss the pros and cons of screening with your doctor and the people important in your life. For more information on prostate cancer screening, testing, treatments, and studies, talk with a cancer information specialist at 800-4-CANCER (800-422-6237), or visit the website http://www.health finder.gov and type in the words "prostate cancer."

Section 40.2

What You Can Do to Prevent Prostate Cancer

Excerpted from *What You Should Know about Prostate Cancer*. © 2004 Prostate Cancer Research Institute. Reprinted with permission. Updated September 21, 2004.

Basic Facts about Prostate Cancer

Prostate cancer (PC) is the most common male malignancy in the western world. In the U.S. alone, each year there are more than 230,000 new diagnoses, and in 2005 it is estimated that more than 30,000 men will die from PC. This is the bad news.

The good news is that we can dramatically reduce the number of deaths from prostate cancer through:

- Prevention.
- Early diagnosis.
- Appropriate treatment.

Since each man is primarily responsible for his own health, it is important that you and your loved ones become knowledgeable in all three areas. This gives you a start by providing the most current basic information on prevention and early diagnosis. These are areas you can easily influence. For additional information, please refer to

the Prostate Cancer Research Institute (PCRI) website at http://www
.pcri.org or call the PCRI helpline at 800-641-PCRI. The following
steps are ones you can take now.

Step 1: Maintain a Healthy Diet

- Reduce or eliminate red meat, dairy fats, saturated fats, and
  egg yolk in your diet.

- Eat five servings of fruits and vegetables each day. Tomatoes
  and strawberries are particularly beneficial. In one study, men
  who each week ingested ten or more servings of tomatoes in several forms (sauce, juice, raw or on pizza) had a 41 percent reduction in the incidence of PC. And just one weekly 0.5-cup serving
  of strawberries was associated with a 20 percent decreased risk
  of prostate cancer.

- Restrict your daily caloric intake to roughly 500 calories for
  each of three meals per day and 100 calories for each of three
  snacks per day. Adjust this total of 1800 calories per day based
  on your level of activity and body mass. If everyone were to do
  this, we would eliminate most cases of diabetes, hypertension,
  stroke, hypercholesterolemia, heart disease, and a significant
  amount of cancer in the world.

- Avoid excessive carbohydrate intake. Your protein to carbohydrate intake ratio should be 3:4. If you adhere to a 500-calorie-
  per-meal plan, you could be eating 150 calories of protein along
  with 200 calories of carbohydrates (the 3:4 ratio) plus 150 calories of polyunsaturated fat, (ideally from cold water fish, olive
  oil on your salad, etc.).

- Each day, take supplements of 200 mcg of selenium along with
  200 IU of mixed tocopherol (vitamin E).

- Eliminate smoking, reduce alcohol consumption, and exercise
  properly.

Step 2: Initiate Early Detection Tests

Deaths caused by PC can be significantly reduced if a digital rectal exam (DRE) and a simple blood test for prostate-specific antigen
(PSA) are included in your yearly physical exam. Men should initiate
the following program:

- Have a yearly physical that includes a DRE and a PSA test. This should begin at age 35 if you have a family history of PC. Otherwise, regular testing should start at age 40. It is important to note that even elevated PSA levels may indicate the presence of very treatable urinary conditions, such as benign prostatic hyperplasia (BPH) or prostatitis, and do not necessarily indicate that cancer is present in the prostate.

- Maintain a chronological record of your PSA test results. If you maintain a record and monitor your PSA value, it is possible to predict the emergence of PC several years before it would normally be diagnosed. It is during this early phase of PC growth that methods of cancer detection provide the greatest chance of cure.

- Monitor the PSA doubling time in addition to the absolute value of the PSA. A doubling of the PSA value is consistent with a doubling of tumor size. Clinical evidence suggests that the shorter your PSA doubling time, the greater your risk for PC. A doubling time of less than ten years usually indicates tumor growth and should be regarded as an indication that PC is present and growing unless proven otherwise.

Note that in the example (Table 40.3), even with a PSA value of only 1.6 mg/ml (well below the "normal" value of either 2.5 or 4.0), something abnormal is occurring. The PSA doubling time has dropped from 14 years to 1.2 years. This evidence should trigger an alarm demanding further testing and close surveillance.

Table 40.3. PSA Doubling Time

Age	PSA Value	PSA Doubling Time (PSADT)
40	0.8	Unknown
48	1.2	Approximately 14 years
48.5	1.6	Approximately 1.2 years

Step 3: Become Empowered

If you are diagnosed with PC, there are several things that you can do to become an empowered patient:

- Obtain copies of your medical records.

- Learn about prostate cancer, which includes understanding your diagnosis and proper staging.

- Develop your support network.

- Explore and understand your treatment options.

- Maintain a positive attitude.

You owe it to yourself and to your family to maintain a healthy diet, to have an annual physical examination that includes both a DRE and a PSA test, and to keep track of your PSA values. These steps might save your life.

For more information, you may contact the Prostate Cancer Research Institute (PCRI).

Prostate Cancer Research Institute (PCRI)
5777 W Century Blvd., Suite 800
Los Angeles, CA 90045
Toll-Free: 800-641-7274 (Helpline)
Phone: 310-743-2116
Fax: 310-743-2113

Chapter 41

Transitional Cell Cancer of the Renal Pelvis and Ureter

General Information about Transitional Cell Cancer of the Renal Pelvis and Ureter

Transitional cell cancer of the renal pelvis and ureter is a disease in which malignant (cancer) cells form in the renal pelvis and ureter. The renal pelvis is part of the kidney and the ureter connects the kidney to the bladder. There are two kidneys, one on each side of the backbone, above the waist. The kidneys of an adult are about five inches long and three inches wide and are shaped like a kidney bean. The kidneys clean the blood and produce urine to rid the body of waste. The urine collects in the middle of each kidney in a large cavity called the renal pelvis. Urine drains from each kidney through a long tube called the ureter, into the bladder, where it is stored until it is passed from the body through the urethra.

The renal pelvis and ureters are lined with transitional cells. These cells can change shape and stretch without breaking apart. Transitional cell cancer starts in these cells. Transitional cell cancer can form in the renal pelvis or the ureter or both.

Renal cell cancer is a more common type of kidney cancer.

PDQ® Cancer Information Summary. National Cancer Institute; Bethesda, MD. Transitional Cell Cancer of the Renal Pelvis and Ureter (PDQ®): Treatment—Patient. Updated 04/2005. Available at: http://cancer.gov. Accessed December, 2004.

Misuse of certain pain medicines can affect the risk of developing transitional cell cancer of the renal pelvis and ureter. Risk factors include the following:

- Misusing certain pain medicines, including over-the-counter pain medicines, for a long time

- Being exposed to certain dyes and chemicals used in making leather goods, textiles, plastics, and rubber

- Smoking cigarettes

Possible signs of transitional cell cancer of the renal pelvis and ureter include blood in the urine and back pain. These and other symptoms may be caused by transitional cell cancer of the renal pelvis and ureter. Other conditions may cause the same symptoms. There may be no symptoms in the early stages. Symptoms may appear as the tumor grows. A doctor should be consulted if any of the following problems occur:

- Blood in the urine

- A pain in the back that doesn't go away

- Extreme tiredness

- Weight loss with no known reason

- Painful or frequent urination

Tests that examine the abdomen and kidneys are used to detect (find) and diagnose transitional cell cancer of the renal pelvis and ureter. The following tests and procedures may be used:

- *Physical exam and history:* An exam of the body to check general signs of health, including checking for signs of disease, such as lumps or anything else that seems unusual. A history of the patient's health habits and past illnesses and treatments will also be taken.

- *Urinalysis:* A test to check the color of urine and its contents, such as sugar, protein, blood, and bacteria.

- *Ureteroscopy:* A procedure to look inside the ureter and renal pelvis to check for abnormal areas. A ureteroscope (a thin, lighted tube) is inserted through the urethra into the bladder, ureter, and renal pelvis. Tissue samples may be taken for biopsy.

- *Urine cytology:* Examination of urine under a microscope to check for abnormal cells. Cancer in the kidney, bladder, or ureter may shed cancer cells into the urine.

- *Intravenous pyelogram (IVP):* A series of x-rays of the kidneys, ureters, and bladder to check for cancer. A contrast dye is injected into a vein. As the contrast dye moves through the kidneys, ureters, and bladder, x-rays are taken to see if there are any blockages.

- *CT scan (CAT scan):* A procedure that makes a series of detailed pictures of areas inside the body, taken from different angles. The pictures are made by a computer linked to an x-ray machine. A dye may be injected into a vein or swallowed to help the organs or tissues show up more clearly. This procedure is also called computed tomography, computerized tomography, or computerized axial tomography.

- *Ultrasound:* A procedure in which high-energy sound waves (ultrasound) are bounced off internal tissues or organs and make echoes. The echoes form a picture of body tissues called a sonogram. An ultrasound of the abdomen may be done to help diagnose cancer of the renal pelvis and ureter.

Certain factors affect prognosis (chance of recovery) and treatment options. The prognosis (chance of recovery) depends on the stage and grade of the tumor. The treatment options depend on: the stage and grade of the tumor; where the tumor is; whether the patient's other kidney is healthy; and whether the cancer has recurred. Most transitional cell cancer of the renal pelvis and ureter can be cured if found early.

Stages of Transitional Cell Cancer of the Renal Pelvis and Ureter

After transitional cell cancer of the renal pelvis and ureter has been diagnosed, tests are done to find out if cancer cells have spread within the renal pelvis and ureter or to other parts of the body. The process used to find out if cancer has spread within the renal pelvis and ureter or to other parts of the body is called staging. The information gathered from the staging process determines the stage of the disease. It is important to know the stage in order to plan treatment. The following tests and procedures may be used in the staging process: Intravenous pyelogram (IVP); CT scan (CAT scan); ultrasound; ureteroscopy; and surgery.

The following stages are used for transitional cell cancer of the renal pelvis and/or ureter:

Stage 0 (carcinoma in situ): In stage 0, the cancer is found only on tissue lining the inside of the renal pelvis or ureter. Stage 0 is divided into stage 0a and stage 0is, depending on the type of tumor:

- Stage 0a may look like tiny mushrooms growing from the lining. Stage 0a is also called noninvasive papillary carcinoma.

- Stage 0is is a flat tumor on the tissue lining the inside of the renal pelvis or ureter. Stage 0is is also called carcinoma in situ.

Stage I: In stage I, cancer has spread through the cells lining the renal pelvis and/or ureter, into the layer of connective tissue.

Stage II: In stage II, cancer has spread through the layer of connective tissue to the muscle layer of the renal pelvis and/or ureter.

Stage III: In stage III, cancer has spread to the layer of fat outside the renal pelvis and/or ureter; or into the wall of the kidney.

Stage IV: In stage IV, cancer has spread to at least one of the following: a nearby organ; the layer of fat surrounding the kidney; one or more lymph nodes; or other parts of the body.

Transitional cell cancer of the renal pelvis and ureter is also described as localized, regional, or metastatic:

Localized: The cancer is found only in the kidney.

Regional: The cancer has spread to tissues around the kidney and to nearby lymph nodes and blood vessels in the pelvis.

Metastatic: The cancer has spread to other parts of the body.

Recurrent Transitional Cell Cancer of the Renal Pelvis and Ureter

Recurrent transitional cell cancer of the renal pelvis and ureter is cancer that has recurred (come back) after it has been treated. The cancer may come back in the renal pelvis, ureter, or other parts of the body.

Treatment Option Overview

Different types of treatments are available for patients with transitional cell cancer of the renal pelvis and ureter. Some treatments are standard (the currently used treatment), and some are being tested in clinical trials. Before starting treatment, patients may want to think about taking part in a clinical trial. A treatment clinical trial is a research study meant to help improve current treatments or obtain information on new treatments for patients with cancer. When clinical trials show that a new treatment is better than the standard treatment, the new treatment may become the standard treatment.

Clinical trials are taking place in many parts of the country. Information about ongoing clinical trials is available from the National Cancer Institute (NCI) website at http://cancer.gov. Choosing the most appropriate cancer treatment is a decision that ideally involves the patient, family, and healthcare team.

Standard Treatment

One type of standard treatment is used: surgery. One of the following surgical procedures may be used to treat transitional cell cancer of the renal pelvis and ureter:

- **Nephroureterectomy:** Surgery to remove the entire kidney, the ureter, and the bladder cuff (tissue that connects the ureter to the bladder).

- **Segmental resection of the ureter:** A surgical procedure to remove the part of the ureter that contains cancer and some of the healthy tissue around it. The ends of the ureter are then reattached. This treatment is used when the cancer is superficial and in the lower third of the ureter only, near the bladder.

Clinical Trials

Other types of treatment are being tested in clinical trials.

Fulguration: Fulguration is a surgical procedure that destroys tissue using an electric current. A tool with a small wire loop on the end is used to remove the cancer or to burn away the tumor with electricity.

451

Segmental resection of the renal pelvis: This is a surgical procedure to remove localized cancer from the renal pelvis without removing the entire kidney. Segmental resection may be done to save kidney function when the other kidney is damaged or has already been removed.

Laser surgery: A laser beam (narrow beam of intense light) is used as a knife to remove the cancer. A laser beam can also be used to kill the cancer cells. This procedure may be called laser therapy or laser fulguration.

Regional chemotherapy and regional biologic therapy: Chemotherapy is a cancer treatment that uses drugs to stop the growth of cancer cells, either by killing the cells or by stopping the cells from dividing. Biologic therapy is a treatment that uses the patient's immune system to fight cancer; substances made by the body or made in a laboratory are used to boost, direct, or restore the body's natural defenses against cancer. Regional treatment means the anticancer drugs or biologic substances are placed directly into an organ or a body cavity such as the abdomen, so the drugs will affect cancer cells in that area. Clinical trials are studying the effectiveness of chemotherapy or biologic therapy using drugs placed directly into the renal pelvis or the ureter.

This summary section refers to specific treatments under study in clinical trials, but it may not mention every new treatment being studied. Information about ongoing clinical trials is available from the NCI cancer.gov website.

Chapter 42

Kidney (Renal Cell) Cancer

General Information about Renal Cell Cancer

Renal cell cancer is a disease in which malignant (cancer) cells form in tubules of the kidney. There are two kidneys, one on each side of the backbone, above the waist. The tiny tubules in the kidneys filter and clean the blood, taking out waste products and making urine. The urine passes from each kidney into the bladder through a long tube called a ureter. The bladder stores the urine until it is passed from the body.

Cancer that starts in the ureters or the renal pelvis (the part of the kidney that collects urine and drains it to the ureters) is different from renal cell cancer. [Refer to Chapter 41, "Transitional Cell Cancer of the Renal Pelvis and Ureter" for more information.]

Smoking and misuse of certain pain medicines can affect the risk of developing renal cell cancer. Risk factors include: being a smoker; misusing certain pain medicines, including over-the-counter pain medicines, for a long time; and having certain genetic conditions, such as von Hippel-Lindau disease or hereditary papillary renal cell carcinoma.

Possible signs of renal cell cancer include blood in the urine and a lump in the abdomen. These and other symptoms may be caused

PDQ® Cancer Information Summary. National Cancer Institute; Bethesda, MD. Renal Cell Cancer (PDQ®): Treatment—Patient. Updated 05/2004. Available at: http://cancer.gov. Accessed date 12/2004.

by renal cell cancer or by other conditions. There may be no symptoms in the early stages. Symptoms may appear as the tumor grows. A doctor should be consulted if any of the following problems occur: blood in the urine; a lump in the abdomen; a pain in the side that doesn't go away; loss of appetite; weight loss for no known reason; or anemia.

Tests that examine the abdomen and kidneys are used to detect (find) and diagnose renal cell cancer. The following tests and procedures may be used:

- *Physical exam and history:* An exam of the body to check general signs of health, including checking for signs of disease, such as lumps or anything else that seems unusual. A history of the patient's health habits and past illnesses and treatments will also be taken.

- *Blood chemistry studies:* A procedure in which a blood sample is checked to measure the amounts of certain substances released into the blood by organs and tissues in the body. An unusual (higher or lower than normal) amount of a substance can be a sign of disease in the organ or tissue that produces it.

- *Urinalysis:* A test to check the color of urine and its contents, such as sugar, protein, blood, and bacteria.

- *Liver function test:* A procedure in which a sample of blood is checked to measure the amounts of enzymes released into it by the liver. An abnormal amount of an enzyme can be a sign that cancer has spread to the liver. Certain conditions that are not cancer may also increase liver enzyme levels.

- *Intravenous pyelogram (IVP):* A series of x-rays of the kidneys, ureters, and bladder to find out if cancer is present in these organs. A contrast dye is injected into a vein. As the contrast dye moves through the kidneys, ureters, and bladder, x-rays are taken to see if there are any blockages.

- *Ultrasound:* A procedure in which high-energy sound waves (ultrasound) are bounced off internal tissues or organs and make echoes. The echoes form a picture of body tissues called a sonogram.

- *CT scan (CAT scan):* A procedure that makes a series of detailed pictures of areas inside the body, taken from different angles.

The pictures are made by a computer linked to an x-ray machine. A dye may be injected into a vein or swallowed to help the organs or tissues show up more clearly. This procedure is also called computed tomography, computerized tomography, or computerized axial tomography.

- *MRI (magnetic resonance imaging):* A procedure that uses a magnet, radio waves, and a computer to make a series of detailed pictures of areas inside the body. This procedure is also called nuclear magnetic resonance imaging (NMRI).

- *Biopsy:* The removal of cells or tissues so they can be viewed under a microscope to check for signs of cancer. A thin needle is inserted into the tumor and a sample of tissue is withdrawn. A pathologist then views the tissue under a microscope to check for cancer cells.

Certain factors affect prognosis (chance of recovery) and treatment options. The prognosis (chance of recovery) and treatment options depend on the following: the stage of the disease and the patient's age and general health.

Stages of Renal Cell Cancer

After renal cell cancer has been diagnosed, tests are done to find out if cancer cells have spread within the kidney or to other parts of the body. The process used to find out if cancer has spread within the kidney or to other parts of the body is called staging. The information gathered from the staging process determines the stage of the disease. It is important to know the stage in order to plan treatment. Tests and procedures may be used in the staging process include CT scan (CAT scan) and MRI (magnetic resonance imaging), as well as the following:

- **Chest x-ray:** An x-ray of the organs and bones inside the chest. An x-ray is a type of energy beam that can go through the body and onto film, making a picture of areas inside the body.

- **Bone scan:** A procedure to check if there are rapidly dividing cells, such as cancer cells, in the bone. A very small amount of radioactive material is injected into a vein and travels through the bloodstream. The radioactive material collects in the bones and is detected by a scanner.

The following stages are used for renal cell cancer:

Stage I: In stage I, the tumor is no larger than seven centimeters and is found in the kidney only.

Stage II: In stage II, the tumor is larger than seven centimeters and is found in the kidney only.

Stage III: In stage III, cancer is found in the kidney and in one nearby lymph node; or in an adrenal gland or in the layer of fatty tissue around the kidney, and may be found in one nearby lymph node; or in the main blood vessels of the kidney and may be found in one nearby lymph node.

Stage IV: In stage IV, cancer has spread beyond the layer of fatty tissue around the kidney and may be found in one nearby lymph node; or to two or more nearby lymph nodes; or to other organs, such as the bowel, pancreas, or lungs, and may be found in nearby lymph nodes.

Recurrent Renal Cell Cancer

Recurrent renal cell cancer is cancer that has recurred (come back) after it has been treated. The cancer may come back many years after initial treatment, in the kidney or in other parts of the body.

Treatment Option Overview

There are different types of treatment for patients with renal cell cancer. Some treatments are standard (the currently used treatment), and some are being tested in clinical trials. Before starting treatment, patients may want to think about taking part in a clinical trial. A treatment clinical trial is a research study meant to help improve current treatments or obtain information on new treatments for patients with cancer. When clinical trials show that a new treatment is better than the standard treatment, the new treatment may become the standard treatment.

Clinical trials are taking place in many parts of the country. Information about ongoing clinical trials is available from the National Cancer Institute (NCI) website at http://cancer.gov/clinicaltrials. Choosing the most appropriate cancer treatment is a decision that ideally involves the patient, family, and healthcare team.

Four Types of Standard Treatment Are Used

Surgery to remove part or all of the kidney is often used to treat renal cell cancer. The following types of surgery which may be used include:

- *Partial nephrectomy:* A surgical procedure to remove the cancer within the kidney and some of the tissue around it. A partial nephrectomy may be done to prevent loss of kidney function when the other kidney is damaged or has already been removed.

- *Simple nephrectomy:* A surgical procedure to remove the kidney only.

- *Radical nephrectomy:* A surgical procedure to remove the kidney, the adrenal gland, surrounding tissue, and, usually, nearby lymph nodes.

A person can live with part of one working kidney, but if both kidneys are removed or not working, the person will need dialysis (a procedure to clean the blood using a machine outside of the body) or a kidney transplant (replacement with a healthy donated kidney). A kidney transplant may be done when the disease is in the kidney only and a donated kidney can be found. If the patient has to wait for a donated kidney, other treatment is given as needed.

When surgery to remove the cancer is not possible, a treatment called arterial embolization may be used to shrink the tumor. A small incision is made and a catheter (thin tube) is inserted into the main blood vessel that flows to the kidney. Small pieces of a special gelatin sponge are injected through the catheter into the blood vessel. The sponges block the blood flow to the kidney and prevent the cancer cells from getting oxygen and other substances they need to grow.

Even if the doctor removes all the cancer that can be seen at the time of the surgery, some patients may be given chemotherapy or radiation therapy after surgery to kill any cancer cells that are left. Treatment given after the surgery, to increase the chances of a cure, is called adjuvant therapy.

Radiation therapy is a cancer treatment that uses high-energy x-rays or other types of radiation to kill cancer cells. There are two types of radiation therapy. External radiation therapy uses a machine outside the body to send radiation toward the cancer. Internal radiation therapy uses a radioactive substance sealed in needles, seeds, wires, or catheters that are placed directly into or near the cancer. The way the radiation therapy is given depends on the type and stage of the cancer being treated.

Chemotherapy is a cancer treatment that uses drugs to stop the growth of cancer cells, either by killing the cells or by stopping the cells from dividing. When chemotherapy is taken by mouth or injected into a vein or muscle, the drugs enter the bloodstream and can reach cancer cells throughout the body (systemic chemotherapy). When chemotherapy is placed directly into the spinal column, an organ, or a body cavity such as the abdomen, the drugs mainly affect cancer cells in those areas (regional chemotherapy). The way the chemotherapy is given depends on the type and stage of the cancer being treated.

Biologic therapy is a treatment that uses the patient's immune system to fight cancer. Substances made by the body or made in a laboratory are used to boost, direct, or restore the body's natural defenses against cancer. This type of cancer treatment is also called biotherapy or immunotherapy.

Other types of treatment are being tested in clinical trials. These include stem cell transplantation. Stem cells (immature blood cells) are removed from the blood or bone marrow of a donor and given to the patient through an infusion. These reinfused stem cells grow into (and restore) the body's blood cells.

This summary section refers to specific treatments under study in clinical trials, but it may not mention every new treatment being studied. Information about ongoing clinical trials is available from the NCI cancer.gov website.

Treatment Options by Stage

Stage I Renal Cell Cancer

Standard treatment of stage I renal cell cancer may include the following:

- Surgery (radical nephrectomy, simple nephrectomy, or partial nephrectomy)

- Radiation therapy as palliative therapy to relieve symptoms in patients who cannot have surgery

- Arterial embolization as palliative therapy

New treatments for stage I renal cell cancer are being studied in clinical trials. Information about these and other ongoing clinical trials is available from the NCI website.

Stage II Renal Cell Cancer

Standard treatment of stage II renal cell cancer may include the following:

- Surgery (radical nephrectomy or partial nephrectomy)
- Surgery (nephrectomy), before or after radiation therapy
- Radiation therapy as palliative therapy to relieve symptoms in patients who cannot have surgery
- Arterial embolization as palliative therapy

New treatments for stage II renal cell cancer are being studied in clinical trials. Information about these and other ongoing clinical trials is available from the NCI website.

Stage III Renal Cell Cancer

Standard treatment of stage III renal cell cancer may include the following:

- Surgery (radical nephrectomy). Blood vessels of the kidney and some lymph nodes may also be removed.
- Arterial embolization followed by surgery (radical nephrectomy)
- Radiation therapy as palliative therapy to relieve symptoms and improve the quality of life
- Arterial embolization as palliative therapy
- Surgery (nephrectomy) as palliative therapy
- Radiation therapy before or after surgery (radical nephrectomy)

One of the treatments being studied in clinical trials for stage III renal cell cancer is biologic therapy following surgery. Information about this and other ongoing clinical trials is available from the NCI website.

Stage IV Renal Cell Cancer

Standard treatment of stage IV renal cell cancer may include biologic therapy; radiation therapy as palliative therapy to relieve symptoms and improve the quality of life; surgery (nephrectomy) as palliative therapy; or surgery (radical nephrectomy, with or without removal of cancer from other areas where it has spread).

New treatments for stage IV renal cell cancer are being studied in clinical trials. Information about these and other ongoing clinical trials is available from the NCI website (www.cancer.gov).

Treatment Options for Recurrent Renal Cell Cancer

Standard treatment of recurrent renal cell cancer may include biologic therapy, radiation therapy as palliative therapy to relieve symptoms and improve the quality of life, or chemotherapy.

Some of the treatments being studied in clinical trials for recurrent renal cell cancer include chemotherapy, biologic therapy, and stem cell transplant. Information about these and other ongoing clinical trials is available from the NCI website.

Chapter 43

Wilms Tumor and Other Childhood Kidney Tumors

What is Wilms tumor?

Wilms tumor is a disease in which cancer (malignant) cells are found in certain parts of the kidney. The kidneys are a "matched" pair of organs found on either side of the backbone. The kidneys are shaped like a kidney bean. Inside each kidney are tiny tubes that filter and clean the blood, taking out unneeded products, and making urine. The urine made by the kidneys passes through a tube called a ureter into the bladder where it is held until it is passed from the body.

Wilms tumor is curable in the majority of affected children. If your child has symptoms, your child's doctor will usually feel your child's abdomen for lumps and run blood and urine tests. The doctor may order a special x-ray called an intravenous pyelogram. During this test, a dye containing iodine is injected into your child's bloodstream. This allows your child's doctor to see the kidney more clearly on the x-ray. Your child's doctor may also do an ultrasound, which uses sound waves to make a picture, or a special x-ray called a computed tomographic scan to look for lumps in the kidney. A special scan called magnetic resonance imaging, which uses magnetic waves to make a picture, may also be done. Chest and bone x-rays may also be taken.

PDQ® Cancer Information Summary. National Cancer Institute; Bethesda, MD. Wilms' Tumor and Other Childhood Kidney Tumors (PDQ®): Treatment—Patient. Updated 12/2004. Available at: http://cancer.gov. Accessed 12/2004.

If abnormal tissue is found, your child's doctor will need to cut out a small piece and look at it under the microscope to see if there are any cancer cells. This is called a biopsy.

In Wilms tumor, how the cancer cells look under a microscope (histology) is also very important. The cancer cells can be of favorable histology or anaplastic histology. Anaplastic means the cancer cells divide rapidly and look very different from normal cells. Anaplastic tumors may be focal (in one area) or diffuse (spread widely throughout an area).

Your child's chance of recovery (prognosis) and choice of treatment depend on the stage of your child's cancer (whether it is just in the kidney only or has spread to other places in the body), how the cancer cells look under a microscope (histology), tumor size, and your child's age and general health.

What are other childhood kidney tumors?

Clear cell sarcoma of the kidney, rhabdoid tumor of the kidney, and neuroepithelial tumor of the kidney are childhood kidney tumors unrelated to Wilms tumor. The treatment of these tumors is different from that of Wilms tumor but because of their location near the kidneys, they have been treated on clinical trials developed by the National Wilms Tumor Study Group.

What are the stages of Wilms tumor?

Once Wilms tumor has been found, more tests will be done to find out if cancer cells have spread from the kidney to other parts of the body. This is called staging. Your child's doctor needs to know the stage of the disease to plan treatment. The following stages are used for Wilms tumor:

Stage I: Cancer is found only in the kidney and can be completely removed by surgery.

Stage II: Cancer has spread beyond the kidney, to fat or soft tissue or blood vessels. The cancer can be completely removed by surgery.

Stage III: Cancer has spread within the abdomen and cannot be completely removed by surgery. The cancer may have spread to the lymph nodes (small bean-shaped structures found throughout the body that produce and store infection-fighting cells) near the kidney, blood vessels, or the peritoneum (tissue that lines the abdomen and covers most organs in the abdomen).

Stage IV: Cancer has spread to the lungs, liver, bone, or brain, or to lymph nodes outside of the abdomen and pelvis.

Stage V: Cancer cells are found in both kidneys when the disease is first diagnosed.

Recurrent: Recurrent disease means that the cancer has come back (recurred) after it has been treated. It may come back where it started or in another part of the body.

How are Wilms tumor and other childhood kidney tumors treated?

There are treatments for all patients with Wilms tumor. Three kinds of treatment are used:

- Surgery (taking out the cancer in an operation)

- Chemotherapy (using drugs to kill cancer cells)

- Radiation therapy (using high-dose x-rays or other high-energy x-rays to kill cancer cells)

Surgery is a common treatment for Wilms tumor. Your doctor may take out the cancer using one of the following:

- *Partial nephrectomy* removes the cancer and part of the kidney around the cancer. This operation is usually used only in special cases, such as when the other kidney is damaged or has already been removed.

- *Simple nephrectomy* removes the whole kidney. The kidney on the other side of the body can take over filtering blood.

- *Radical nephrectomy* removes the whole kidney with the tissues around it. Some lymph nodes in the area may also be removed.

Chemotherapy uses drugs to kill cancer cells. Chemotherapy may be taken by pill, or it may be put into the body by a needle in a vein or muscle. Chemotherapy is called a systemic treatment because the drugs enter the bloodstream, travel through the body, and can kill cancer cells throughout the body. Chemotherapy given after an operation to remove the tumor is called adjuvant therapy.

When very high doses of chemotherapy are used to kill cancer cells, these high doses can destroy the blood-forming tissue in the bones (the bone marrow). If very high doses of chemotherapy are needed to treat the cancer, bone marrow may be taken from the bones before therapy and frozen until it is needed. Following chemotherapy, the bone marrow is given back through a needle in a vein. This is called autologous bone marrow reinfusion.

Radiation therapy uses x-rays or other high-energy rays to kill cancer cells and shrink tumors. Radiation for Wilms tumor usually comes from a machine outside the body (external radiation therapy). Radiation may be used before or after surgery and/or chemotherapy.

Some cancer treatments cause side effects that continue or appear years after cancer treatment has ended. These are called late effects. It is important that parents of children who are treated for cancer know about the possible late effects caused by certain treatments. After several years, some patients develop another form of cancer as a result of their treatment with chemotherapy and radiation. Clinical trials are ongoing to determine if lower doses of chemotherapy and radiation can be used.

Which treatments will be used for each stage of Wilms tumor?

Treatments for Wilms tumor depend on the stage of your child's disease, the histology (cell type), and your child's age and general health.

Your child may receive treatment that is considered standard based on its effectiveness in a number of patients in past studies, or you may choose to have your child take part in a clinical trial. Not all patients are cured with standard therapy and some standard treatments may have more side effects than are desired. For these reasons, clinical trials are designed to test new treatments and to find better ways to treat cancer patients. Clinical trials are ongoing in most parts of the country for most stages of Wilms tumor. If you want more information, call the Cancer Information Service at 800-4- CANCER (800-422-6237); TTY at 800-332-8615.

Stage I Wilms tumor: Treatment for stage I Wilms tumor will probably be surgery to remove the kidney and some of the lymph nodes near the kidney, followed by chemotherapy.

Stage II Wilms tumor: Treatment for stage II Wilms tumor depends on the histology of the cancer.

If your child has a favorable histology tumor, treatment will probably be surgery to remove the kidney and some of the lymph nodes near the kidney, followed by chemotherapy.

If your child has an anaplastic histology tumor, treatment will probably be surgery to remove the kidney followed by radiation therapy plus chemotherapy.

Stage III Wilms tumor: Treatment of both favorable and anaplastic stage III Wilms tumors will probably be surgery to remove the kidney and some of the lymph nodes near the kidney, followed by radiation therapy to the abdomen, and chemotherapy.

Stage IV Wilms tumor: Treatment of both favorable and anaplastic stage IV Wilms tumors will probably be surgery to remove the kidney and some of the lymph nodes near the kidney, followed by radiation therapy to the abdomen, and chemotherapy. Patients whose cancer has spread to the lungs will also receive radiation therapy to the lungs.

Stage V Wilms tumor: Your child's doctor will probably do a biopsy of the cancer by taking out a piece of the cancer in both kidneys and removing some of the lymph nodes around the kidney to see whether they contain cancer. Following the biopsy, chemotherapy will be given to shrink the cancer. A second surgery will remove as much of the cancer as possible, while leaving as much of the kidneys as possible. Surgery may be followed by more chemotherapy and/or radiation therapy.

Inoperable Wilms tumors: Sometimes the cancer is inoperable (cannot be removed during surgery) because it is too close to important organs or blood vessels or because it is too large to remove. In this case, the doctor may perform a biopsy only and then give chemotherapy with or without radiation therapy. Once the cancer has become smaller, surgery to remove part or all of the tumor may be done, followed by more chemotherapy and radiation therapy.

Clear cell sarcoma of the kidney: Clear cell sarcoma of the kidney is a primary kidney tumor. It is not a type of Wilms tumor. This tumor can spread to the lung, bone, brain, and soft tissue. If your child has clear cell sarcoma of the kidney, he or she may be treated with surgery to remove the kidney followed by radiation therapy to the abdomen and lung (if cancer has spread to the lung) followed by chemotherapy.

Rhabdoid tumor of the kidney: Rhabdoid tumor of the kidney is a type of cancer that grows and spreads quickly. At diagnosis, children are usually younger than one year and may have fever, blood in the urine, and advanced cancer. This tumor type tends to spread to the lungs and the brain. Treatment is usually a clinical trial.

Neuroepithelial tumor of the kidney: Neuroepithelial tumors of the kidney are tumors that grow and spread quickly. At diagnosis, these tumors have often spread to the outer layer of the kidney, the veins of the kidney, and to other parts of the body. If your child has neuroepithelial tumors of the kidney, treatment on an Ewing/primitive neuroectodermal tumors (PNET) clinical trial should be considered.

Recurrent Wilms tumor and other childhood kidney tumors: If your child's cancer comes back (recurs), treatment depends on the treatment he or she received before, how much time has passed since the first cancer was treated, the histology of the cancer, and where the cancer came back.

Clinical trials are evaluating new treatments, such as new chemotherapy drugs and combinations, and very high doses of chemotherapy followed by bone marrow reinfusion.

Clinical Trials

In the United States, about two-thirds of children with cancer are treated in a clinical trial at some point in their illness. A clinical trial is a study to answer a scientific question, such as whether one treatment is better than another. Trials are based on past studies and what has been learned in the laboratory. Each trial answers certain scientific questions in order to find new and better ways to help cancer patients. During treatment clinical trials, information is collected about new treatments, the risks involved, and how well they do or do not work. If a clinical trial shows that a new treatment is better than one currently being used, the new treatment may become "standard."

Listings of clinical trials are available online at the National Cancer Institute (NCI) website. Descriptions of the trials are available in health professional and patient versions. For additional help in locating a childhood cancer clinical trial, call the Cancer Information Service at 800-4-CANCER (800-422-6237), TTY at 800-332-8615.

Physician Data Query (PDQ®) is the NCI's comprehensive cancer information database. Most of the information contained in PDQ is available online at NCI's website, http://cancer.gov. PDQ is provided as a service of the NCI. The NCI is part of the National Institutes of Health (NIH), the federal government's focal point for biomedical research.

The PDQ database contains listings of groups specializing in clinical trials. The Children's Oncology Group (COG) is the major group that organizes clinical trials for childhood cancers in the United States. Information about contacting COG is available on the NCI website or from the Cancer Information Service at 800-4-CANCER (800-422-6237), TTY at 800-332-8615.

The PDQ database contains listings of cancer health professionals and hospitals with cancer programs. Because cancer in children and adolescents is rare, the majority of children with cancer are treated by health professionals specializing in childhood cancers, at hospitals or cancer centers with special facilities to treat them. The PDQ database contains listings of health professionals who specialize in childhood cancer and listings of hospitals with cancer programs. For help locating childhood cancer health professionals or a hospital with cancer programs, call the Cancer Information Service at 800-4-CANCER (800-422-6237), TTY at 800-332-8615.

Part Seven

Kidney Failure:
End-Stage Renal Disease

Chapter 44

Kidney Failure: Choosing a Treatment That's Right for You

Your kidneys filter wastes from your blood and regulate other functions of your body. When your kidneys fail, you need treatment to replace the work of healthy kidneys to survive.

Developing kidney failure means that you have some decisions to make about your treatment. If you choose to receive treatment, your choices are hemodialysis, peritoneal dialysis, and kidney transplantation. Each of them has advantages and disadvantages. You may also choose to forgo treatment. By learning about your choices, you can work with your doctor to decide what's best for you. No matter which treatment you choose, you'll need to make some changes in your life, including how you eat and plan your activities. But with the help of your healthcare team, family, and friends, you can lead a full, active life.

Treatment Choice: Hemodialysis

Purpose: Hemodialysis cleans and filters your blood using a machine to temporarily rid your body of harmful wastes, extra salt, and extra water. Hemodialysis helps control blood pressure and helps your

National Kidney and Urologic Diseases Information Clearinghouse (NKUDIC), a service of the National Institute of Diabetes and Digestive and Kidney Diseases (NIDDK), National Institutes of Health (NIH), Excerpted from Pub. No. 03-2412, April 2003. The complete text of this document is available online at http://kidney.niddk.nih.gov/kudiseases/pubs/choosingtreatment/index.htm.

body keep the proper balance of important chemicals such as potassium, sodium, calcium, and bicarbonate.

How It Works: Hemodialysis uses a special filter called a dialyzer that functions as an artificial kidney to clean your blood. During treatment, your blood travels through tubes into the dialyzer, which filters out wastes and extra water. Then the cleaned blood flows through another set of tubes back into your body. The dialyzer is connected to a machine that monitors blood flow and removes wastes from the blood. [For more detailed information about how hemodialysis is performed, see chapter 46.]

Pros and Cons: Each person responds differently to similar situations. What may be a negative factor for one person may be positive

Table 44.1. Pros and Cons of In-Center and Home Hemodialysis

In-Center Hemodialysis

Pros

+ Facilities are widely available.

+ You have trained professionals with you at all times.

+ You can get to know other patients.

Cons

- Treatments are scheduled by the center and are relatively fixed.

- You must travel to the center for treatment.

Home Hemodialysis

Pros

+ You can do it at the times you choose (but you still must do it as often as your doctor orders).

+ You don't have to travel to a center.

+ You gain a sense of independence and control over your treatment.

Cons

- You must have a helper.

- Helping with treatments may be stressful to your family.

- You and your helper need training.

- You need space for storing the machine and supplies at home.

for another. See Table 44.1 for a list of the general advantages and disadvantages of in-center and home hemodialysis.

Working with Your Healthcare Team

Questions you may want to ask include the following:

- Is hemodialysis the best treatment choice for me? Why?
- If I'm treated at a center, can I go to the center of my choice?
- What should I look for in a dialysis center?
- Will my kidney doctor see me at dialysis?
- What does hemodialysis feel like?
- What is self-care dialysis?
- Is home hemodialysis available in my area? How long does it take to learn? Who will train my partner and me?
- What kind of blood access is best for me?
- As a hemodialysis patient, will I be able to keep working? Can I have treatments at night?
- How much should I exercise?
- Who will be on my healthcare team? How can these people help me?
- Whom can I talk with about finances, sexuality, or family concerns?
- How/where can I talk to other people who have faced this decision?

Treatment Choice: Peritoneal Dialysis

Purpose: Peritoneal dialysis is another procedure that removes extra water, wastes, and chemicals from your body. This type of dialysis uses the lining of your abdomen to filter your blood. This lining is called the peritoneal membrane and acts as the artificial kidney.

How It Works: A mixture of minerals and sugar dissolved in water, called dialysis solution, travels through a soft tube into your abdomen. The sugar, called dextrose, draws wastes, chemicals, and extra water from the tiny blood vessels in your peritoneal membrane into the dialysis solution. After several hours, the used solution is drained from your abdomen through the tube, taking the wastes from your blood with it. Then you fill your abdomen with fresh dialysis solution, and the cycle is repeated. Each cycle is called an exchange. [For more detailed information about how peritoneal dialysis is performed, see chapter 47.]

Pros and Cons: Each type of peritoneal dialysis has advantages and disadvantages. See Table 44.2 for a list of advantages and disadvantages of each type.

Working with Your Healthcare Team

You may want to ask the following questions:

• Is peritoneal dialysis the best treatment choice for me? Why? If yes, which type is best?

Table 44.2. Pros and Cons of Types of Peritoneal Dialysis

CAPD

Pros

+ You can do it alone.

+ You can do it at times you choose as long as you perform the required number of exchanges each day.

+ You can do it in many locations.

+ You don't need a machine.

Cons

- It can disrupt your daily schedule.

- This is a continuous treatment, and all exchanges must be performed seven days a week.

CCPD

Pros

+ You can do it at night, mainly while you sleep.

Cons

- You need a machine.

- How long will it take me to learn how to do peritoneal dialysis?
- What does peritoneal dialysis feel like?
- How will peritoneal dialysis affect my blood pressure?
- How will I know if I have peritonitis? How is it treated?
- As a peritoneal dialysis patient, will I be able to continue working?
- How much should I exercise?
- Where do I store supplies?
- How often do I see my doctor?
- Who will be on my healthcare team? How can these people help me?
- Whom do I contact with problems?
- Whom can I talk with about finances, sexuality, or family concerns?
- How/where can I talk to other people who have faced this decision?

Dialysis Is Not a Cure

Hemodialysis and peritoneal dialysis are treatments that help replace the work your kidneys did. These treatments help you feel better and live longer, but they don't cure kidney failure. Although patients with kidney failure are now living longer than ever, over the years kidney disease can cause problems such as heart disease, bone disease, arthritis, nerve damage, infertility, and malnutrition. These problems won't go away with dialysis, but doctors now have new and better ways to prevent or treat them. You should discuss these complications and treatments with your doctor.

Treatment Choice: Kidney Transplantation

Purpose: Kidney transplantation surgically places a healthy kidney from another person into your body. The donated kidney does the work that your two failed kidneys used to do.

How It Works: A surgeon places the new kidney inside your lower abdomen and connects the artery and vein of the new kidney to your artery and vein. Your blood flows through the donated kidney, which makes urine, just like your own kidneys did when they were healthy. The new kidney may start working right away or may take up to a few weeks to make urine. Unless your own kidneys are causing infection or high blood pressure, they are left in place. [For more detailed information about kidney transplantation, see chapter 48.]

Pros and Cons: Kidney transplantation has advantages and disadvantages. See Table 44.3 for a list of pros and cons.

Working with Your Healthcare Team

Questions you may want to ask include the following:

• Is transplantation the best treatment choice for me? Why?

• What are my chances of having a successful transplant?

• How do I find out whether a family member or friend can donate?

• What are the risks to a family member or friend who donates?

• If a family member or friend doesn't donate, how do I get placed on a waiting list for a kidney? How long will I have to wait?

Table 44.3. Kidney Transplantation

Pros

+ A transplanted kidney works like a normal kidney.

+ You may feel healthier or "more normal."

+ You have fewer diet restrictions.

+ You won't need dialysis.

+ Patients who successfully go through the selection process have a higher chance of living a longer life.

Cons

- It requires major surgery.

- You may need to wait for a donor.

- Your body may reject the new kidney, so one transplant may not last a lifetime.

- You'll need to take immunosuppressants, which may cause complications.

- What symptoms does rejection cause?

- How long does a transplant work?

- What side effects do immunosuppressants cause?

- Who will be on my healthcare team? How can these people help me?

- Whom can I talk to about finances, sexuality, or family concerns?

- How or where can I talk to other people who have faced this decision?

Treatment Choice: Refusing or Withdrawing from Treatment

For many people, dialysis and transplantation not only extend life but also improve quality of life. For others who have serious ailments in addition to kidney failure, dialysis may seem a burden that only prolongs suffering. You have the right to refuse or withdraw from dialysis if you feel you have no hope of leading a life with dignity and meaning. You may want to speak with your spouse, family, religious counselor, or social worker as you make this decision.

If you withdraw from dialysis treatments or refuse to begin them, you may live for a few days or for several weeks, depending on your health and your remaining kidney function. Your doctor can give you medicines to make you more comfortable during this period. Should you change your mind about refusing dialysis, you may start or resume your treatments at any time.

Even if you're satisfied with your quality of life on dialysis, you should think about circumstances that might make you want to stop dialysis treatments. At some point in a medical crisis, you might lose the ability to express your wishes to your doctor. An advance directive is a statement or document in which you give instructions either to withhold treatment or to provide it, depending on your wishes and the specific circumstances.

An advance directive may be a living will, a document that details the conditions under which you would want to refuse treatment. You may state that you want your healthcare team to use all available means to sustain your life. Or you may direct that you be withdrawn from dialysis if you become permanently unresponsive or fall into a coma from which you won't awake. In addition to dialysis, other life-sustaining treatments that you may choose or refuse include the following:

- cardiopulmonary resuscitation (CPR)
- tube feedings
- mechanical or artificial respiration
- antibiotics
- surgery
- blood transfusions

Another form of advance directive is called a durable power of attorney for healthcare decisions or a healthcare proxy. In this type of advance directive, you assign a person to make healthcare decisions for you if you become unable to make them for yourself. Make sure the person you name understands your values and is willing to follow through on your instructions.

Each state has its own laws governing advance directives. You can obtain a form for an advance medical directive that's valid in your state from Partnership for Caring. [For contact information, see the listing for Partnership for Caring in Chapter 53, "Directory of Urinary and Kidney Disorders Organizations."]

Paying for Treatment

Treatment for kidney failure is expensive, but federal health insurance plans pay much of the cost, usually up to 80 percent. Often, private insurance or state programs pay the rest. [For more information, see Chapter 50, "Financial Information for Dialysis and Transplant Patients."]

Conclusion

Deciding which type of treatment is best for you isn't easy. Your decision depends on your medical condition, lifestyle, and personal likes and dislikes. Discuss the pros and cons of each treatment with your healthcare team and family. You can switch between treatment methods during the course of your therapy. If you start one form of treatment and decide you'd like to try another, talk to your doctor. The key is to learn as much as you can about your choices first. With that knowledge, you and your doctor will choose the treatment that suits you best.

Chapter 45

Treatment Methods for Kidney Failure in Children

Kidneys play an important part in a child's growth and health.

- They remove wastes and extra water from the blood.

- They regulate blood pressure.

- They balance chemicals like sodium and potassium.

- They make a hormone that signals bone marrow to make red blood cells.

- They make a hormone to help bones grow and keep them strong.

Kidney failure can lead directly to more health problems, like swelling of the body, bone deformities, and growth failure. A successful kidney transplant can give a child with chronic kidney failure the best chance to grow normally and lead a full, active life. Dialysis can help a child to survive an acute episode of kidney failure or to stay healthy until a donated kidney becomes available.

Families caring for a child with kidney disease often need help—not just from doctors and nurses, but from a whole team of pediatric specialists, including dietitians, social workers, and family counselors. Learning about treatments for kidney disease and getting to know

National Kidney and Urologic Diseases Information Clearinghouse (NKUDIC), a service of the National Institute of Diabetes and Digestive and Kidney Diseases (NIDDK), National Institutes of Health (NIH), Pub. No. 04-5082, December 2003.

the entire team can make life easier for your child and your entire family.

Problems Specific to Children

Everyone who has kidney failure, adults and children alike, will experience medical complications, which may include extreme fatigue, inability to concentrate, weak bones, nerve damage, depression, and sleep problems. Additional problems for children can include effects on their growth and development. Children may fall behind on the growth chart and in school.

The isolation people feel because of kidney failure is especially a problem in children and adolescents because of the importance of making friends and fitting in at this age. Finding the best treatment for a child takes on special significance to ensure that the child with kidney failure can become an active, productive, well-adjusted adult.

Treatment Choices for Kidney Failure in Children

Children usually have a range of treatment options for kidney failure. In most cases, the goal is to have a successful transplant that allows your child to lead the most normal life possible. But viable kidneys are not always readily available, and not all children can have a transplant. Many children begin with dialysis to stay healthy until a suitable kidney becomes available. Sometimes, a transplant itself may stop working, and the child may need to return to dialysis. Knowing about transplantation and dialysis will prepare you and your child for any circumstance.

Transplantation

Transplantation means that a healthy kidney from a donor is placed inside a child's body to take over the job of filtering wastes and extra fluid from the blood. The donor may be a stranger who has just died or a living family member or friend.

Once kidneys fail because of chronic kidney disease, function cannot be restored, so transplantation is the closest thing to a cure we have. A child with a transplant will still need to take medicines every day, follow a restricted diet, and get regular checkups to make sure the new kidney is accepted and functioning in the body.

In adults, most transplanted kidneys come from people who have just died. However, about half of the kidney transplants in children come from a living donor, usually a parent or other close family member.

Deceased donor kidneys: To receive a deceased donor kidney, your child will be placed on a waiting list. Every person who needs an organ from a deceased donor is registered with the United Network for Organ Sharing (UNOS), which maintains a centralized computer network linking all regional organ gathering organizations and transplant centers. [For contact information for the UNOS, see Chapter 53, "Directory of Urinary and Kidney Disorders Organizations."]

How long your child will have to wait for a transplant depends on many things but is determined primarily by how good the match is between your child and a donor. When a kidney becomes available, the hospital that has obtained the kidney reports to UNOS, where the central computer generates a list of compatible recipients. Candidates' ages and length of time they have waited are factors in the point system. Children 18 and under get extra points compared with adults because they are likely to receive the greatest benefit from a donated kidney.

While your child is on the waiting list, notify the transplant center of any changes in health status, address, or phone number. The center will need to find you immediately when a kidney becomes available.

Living donor kidneys: About half of the kidneys transplanted into children are donated by family members—usually a parent—or a family friend. Potential donors need to be tested for matching factors and to make sure that donating a kidney will not endanger their health. Most people can donate a kidney with little risk.

A kidney from a living donor often has advantages over a kidney from a person who has just died.

- A kidney from a parent is guaranteed to match on at least three of six proteins; mismatched proteins may cause rejection.

- Living donation allows for greater preparation and for the operation to be scheduled.

- A kidney from a living donor may be in better condition because it does not have to be transported from one site to another.

Preemptive transplantation: Preemptive transplantation means that the child receives a donated kidney before dialysis is needed. Some studies indicate that preemptive transplantation reduces the chances of rejecting the new kidney and improves the chances that it will function for a long time. Other studies show little or no survival advantage in preemptive transplants, although some families may feel that avoiding dialysis is an advantage in itself.

Keeping a healthy kidney: Health professionals use the term "non-compliance" or "non-adherence" to describe a patient's failure or refusal to take prescribed medicines or follow a doctor's directions. Teenagers with transplanted organs are often non-compliant because the immunosuppressive drugs they must take change their appearance in unflattering ways. A child psychologist may be able to suggest techniques that reinforce desired behaviors. But communicating clearly about the reasons for treatment and the importance of following the regimen is an important part of helping all patients, including children. Children who understand that their decisions can affect their health are more likely to take responsibility for their actions.

Dialysis

The kidneys remove waste products and extra water from the blood. If the kidneys fail before transplantation is possible, your child may need some form of dialysis to do this job. Each type of dialysis will affect your family's lifestyle. Your doctor will help you choose the one that is best for your child. Each situation is different.

Peritoneal dialysis: Peritoneal dialysis uses the lining of your child's abdomen, called the peritoneal membrane, to filter blood. A mixture of minerals and sugar dissolved in water, called dialysis solution, is inserted into your child's abdomen through a soft tube. The sugar, called dextrose, draws wastes, chemicals, and extra water from the tiny blood vessels in the peritoneal membrane into the dialysis solution. After some time, the used solution—now loaded with the wastes and extra fluid that the kidneys would have filtered out—is drained from your child's abdomen through the tube. The period that dialysis solution is in the abdomen is called the dwell time. The abdomen is filled again with fresh dialysis solution, and the cycle repeats. The process of emptying and refilling the abdomen is called an exchange and takes about 30 to 40 minutes. [See chapter 47 for more information about peritoneal dialysis.]

Hemodialysis: In hemodialysis, a machine cleans and filters your child's blood to remove harmful wastes, extra salt, and extra water. Hemodialysis helps control blood pressure and keep the proper balance of potassium, sodium, calcium, and bicarbonate.

Hemodialysis uses a special filter called a dialyzer. During treatment, blood travels from the child's body through tubes into the dialyzer, which filters out wastes and extra water. Then the cleaned blood flows through another set of tubes back into the child's body. The dialyzer is connected to a machine that monitors blood flow and disposes of the wastes.

When a child starts hemodialysis, problems can be caused by rapid changes in the body's water and chemical balance during treatment. Muscle cramps and a sudden drop in blood pressure are two common side effects. Low blood pressure, called hypotension, can make a child feel weak, dizzy, or nauseated.

Most children need a few months to adjust to hemodialysis. Side effects can often be treated quickly and easily, so you should always report them to your doctor and dialysis staff. You can avoid many side effects by making sure your child gets a proper diet, limits liquid intake, and takes all medicines as directed. [See chapter 46 for more information about hemodialysis.]

Role of the Healthcare Team

Because the treatments for kidney failure involve complicated procedures with a number of steps, many skilled professionals must work together to ensure that your child gets the best possible care. As a parent or guardian, you are the most important member of your child's team. You may need to speak for your child or ask questions when instructions are not clear. Knowing the roles of the different team members can help you ask the right questions and contribute to your child's care.

Pediatrician: A pediatrician is a doctor who treats children. Your child's pediatrician is likely to be the first to recognize a kidney problem—either during a routine physical exam or while treating an ailment. Depending on how well the kidneys are working, the doctor may decide to monitor your child or advise you to see a specialist. (Your health insurance plan may require a written referral from the pediatrician in order for you to make an appointment with a specialist.) As your child's regular doctor, the pediatrician should talk with any specialists who become involved. A referral for consultation should optimally occur soon after chronic kidney disease is diagnosed, even if dialysis and transplantation are still a long way off.

Nephrologist: A nephrologist is a doctor who treats kidney diseases and kidney failure. If possible, your child should see a pediatric nephrologist because they are specifically trained to take care of kidney problems in children. In many areas of the country, pediatric nephrologists are in short supply, so you and your child may need to travel. If traveling is not possible, some nephrologists who treat adults can also treat children in consultation with a pediatric nephrologist.

The nephrologist may prescribe treatments to slow disease progression and will determine when referral to a transplant center or to a dialysis clinic is appropriate.

Dialysis nurse: If your child needs dialysis, a nurse with special training will make sure all procedures are followed carefully. If you and your child choose peritoneal dialysis, the dialysis nurse will train you so you feel comfortable doing the exchanges at home. For hemodialysis in a clinic, the dialysis nurse will make sure that all needles are placed correctly and watch for any problems. The dialysis nurse can talk to you about the advantages and disadvantages of the different types of dialysis and explain the laboratory reports that indicate how well the treatments are working.

Transplant coordinator: A coordinator at the transplantation center will be your main contact. He or she will schedule any required examinations and procedures and make sure your child's medical information is complete and properly placed on the UNOS national waiting list. The transplant coordinator will make sure that every member of the child's healthcare team has all the necessary information and paperwork.

Social worker: Every dialysis clinic and transplant center has a social worker who can help you locate financial assistance and social services like transportation or family counseling and help with applications for Medicare. The social worker can tell you about support groups in your community and ways to reduce the stress that caring for a child with a chronic illness can cause.

Psychologist, psychiatrist, or counselor: Kidney disease can disrupt a child's life and create emotional turmoil. A psychologist or counselor can help your child find ways to express emotions constructively. Adults and siblings may also find that counseling helps them with the conflicts and stresses they face. For example, medical bills can strain family finances. A parent or guardian may need to give up work to care for the child full-time. Siblings may feel resentment over the huge amount of attention given to their sibling and guilt over thinking bad thoughts about the sick child. Couples sometimes report increased tension in their marriage when a child is sick. A counselor can help families deal with conflicts that may arise, and social workers or financial counselors can help families meet the financial obligations that chronic illness creates.

Dietitian: When the kidneys stop working, wastes and excess fluid build up in the body and create chemical and hormonal imbalances. In children, however, these problems are especially troublesome because they can interfere with physical growth and mental development. Avoiding certain foods can help minimize the build-up of wastes and prevent chemical imbalance, but it can also lead to nutritional deficiencies. The buildup of wastes often makes children lose their appetite, causing further nutritional problems. These complications are the reason your clinic's dietitian is so important.

Proper nutrition is extremely important for children with chronic kidney disease. Every dialysis clinic has a dietitian to help patients understand how the food they eat affects their health. The dietitian can help you develop meal plans that will fit your child's restricted diet and will talk with you about laboratory reports that may show nutritional deficiencies caused by your child's kidney disease. They may recommend special dietary supplements or formulas so that your child receives the best nutrition possible.

You can also ask your dietitian for recipes and titles of cookbooks for patients with kidney disease. Following the restrictions of a kidney disease diet might be hard at first, but with a little creativity, you can make tasty and satisfying meals. Reading "Eat Right to Feel Right on Hemodialysis," reprinted from a booklet by the National Institute of Diabetes and Digestive and Kidney Diseases (NIDDK) in Chapter 48, can help you get started.

Vaccinations and Immunosuppression

The wastes and toxins that build up in the bloodstream of a child with kidney disease can weaken the immune system and make the child vulnerable to infections and the kinds of diseases that vaccines are designed to prevent. Children with kidney failure should receive the standard vaccinations recommended for all children, plus additional vaccinations for pneumonia and influenza.

Children who take immunosuppressive medication to treat an autoimmune disease or to prevent rejection of a transplanted kidney, however, should not receive vaccines containing live viruses, that is, the oral polio vaccine, the measles, mumps, and rubella (MMR) vaccine, or the varicella (chicken pox) vaccine. Children who are likely to need a transplant may benefit from early immunization with these vaccines before immunosuppressive drugs are needed.

The body's immune system protects against foreign substances like bacteria and viruses that can cause disease. But the immune system also attacks transplanted organs, and the medicines that recipients must take to prevent rejection leave them vulnerable to infections. Children need relatively higher doses of immunosuppressive drugs than adults because their immune systems are more active. But these high doses can slow down growth and development. Over a long period of time, immunosuppression may lead to malignant growths. Immunosuppressive drugs can also have side effects such as weight gain, unusual hair growth, and acne. Children, especially teenagers, cite these side effects as the reason they do not take their pills, a problem that contributes to the high rate of organ rejection in children.

Medical Complications of Kidney Failure

The kidneys not only clean waste and extra fluid from the blood, they also help make red blood cells and balance nutrients needed for strong bones and growth. In addition, the kidneys may play a role in the metabolism of growth hormone (somatotropin). Chronic kidney disease can make children feel more tired, limit physical growth, and interfere with their ability to concentrate in school.

Anemia

Diseased kidneys do not make enough of a hormone called erythropoietin, or EPO, which stimulates the bone marrow to produce the red blood cells needed to carry oxygen to vital organs. Anemia is a shortage of red blood cells, and it is common in children with kidney disease. A child with anemia may tire easily and look pale. Anemia may also contribute to heart problems. A genetically engineered form of EPO injected under the skin one or more times a week can treat this form of anemia.

Bone Problems and Growth Failure

The kidneys help keep bones healthy by balancing phosphorus and calcium levels in the blood. When the kidneys stop working normally, phosphorus levels in the blood can become high and interfere with bone formation and normal growth.

Your child's doctor may recommend dietary changes and food supplements to treat growth failure. Dietary changes may include limiting foods that contain large amounts of phosphorus, such as milk and cheese, cola, dried beans, peas, and nuts. Since avoiding all of these foods is impossible, caregivers will need to work with a dietitian to find a healthy way to limit the phosphorus in the child's diet while maintaining a desirable intake of the calories, protein, and other nutrients necessary to maintain growth and general health. In addition to dietary restrictions, most children will need to take specific medications called phosphate binders to lower their blood phosphorus levels.

For more information, see the fact sheet "Growth Failure in Children with Kidney Disease" available from NIDDK at their website http://kidney.niddk.nih.gov.

Financial Help for Treatment of Kidney Failure

No matter what treatment method your family chooses, medical expenses will be high. Fortunately, the federal government and many other organizations offer programs to help with the cost of treatments.

Medicare

In 1972, Congress passed legislation making people with permanent kidney failure, no matter what their age, eligible for Medicare, a program that helps people over 65 and people with disabilities pay for medical care.

Role of the Social Worker

Your child's dialysis or transplant center has a social worker who can help you apply for Medicare and locate other sources of financial assistance. [For more information about Medicare and other organizations that can help, see Chapter 50, "Financial Information for Dialysis and Transplant Patients."]

Chapter 46

What You Should Know about Hemodialysis

Hemodialysis is the most common method used to treat advanced and permanent kidney failure. Since the 1960s, when hemodialysis first became a practical treatment for kidney failure, we've learned much about how to make hemodialysis treatments more effective and minimize side effects. But even with better procedures and equipment, hemodialysis is still a complicated and inconvenient therapy that requires a coordinated effort from your whole healthcare team, including your nephrologist, dialysis nurse, dialysis technician, dietitian, and social worker. But the most important members of your healthcare team are you and your family. By learning about your treatment, you can work with your healthcare team to give yourself the best possible results, and you can lead a full, active life.

When Your Kidneys Fail

Healthy kidneys clean your blood by removing excess fluid, minerals, and wastes. They also make hormones that keep your bones strong and your blood healthy. When your kidneys fail, harmful wastes build up in your body, your blood pressure may rise, and your body may retain excess fluid and not make enough red blood cells. When this happens, you need treatment to replace the work of your failed kidneys.

"Treatment Methods for Kidney Failure: Hemodialysis," National Kidney and Urologic Diseases Information Clearinghouse (NKUDIC), a service of the National Institute of Diabetes and Digestive and Kidney Diseases (NIDDK), National Institutes of Health (NIH), Pub. No. 03-4666, September 2003.

How Hemodialysis Works

In hemodialysis, your blood is allowed to flow, a few ounces at a time, through a machine with a special filter that removes wastes and extra fluids. The clean blood is then returned to your body. Removing the harmful wastes and extra salt and fluids helps control your blood pressure and keep the proper balance of chemicals like potassium and sodium in your body.

One of the biggest adjustments you must make when you start hemodialysis treatments is following a rigid schedule. Most patients go to a clinic—a dialysis center—three times a week for three to five or more hours each visit. For example, you may be on a Monday-Wednesday-Friday schedule or a Tuesday-Thursday-Saturday schedule. You may be asked to choose a morning, afternoon, or evening shift, depending on availability and capacity at the dialysis unit. Your dialysis center will explain your options for scheduling regular treatments.

A few centers teach people how to perform their own hemodialysis treatments at home. A family member or friend who will be your helper must also take the training, which usually takes at least four to six weeks. Home dialysis gives you a little more flexibility in your

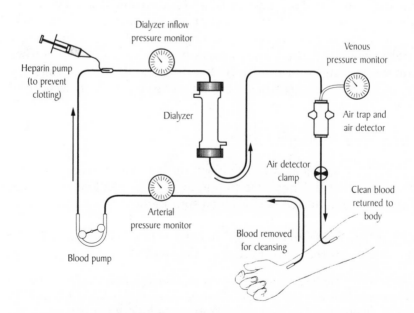

Figure 46.1. *Hemodialysis.*

dialysis schedule, but a regular schedule is still important. With home hemodialysis, the time for each session and the number of sessions per week may vary.

Adjusting to Changes

Even in the best situations, adjusting to the effects of kidney failure and the time you spend on dialysis can be difficult. Aside from the "lost time," you may have less energy. You may need to make changes in your work or home life, giving up some activities and responsibilities. Keeping the same schedule you kept when your kidneys were working can be very difficult now that your kidneys have failed. Accepting this new reality can be very hard on you and your family. A counselor or social worker can help you cope.

Many patients feel depressed when starting dialysis, or after several months of treatment. If you feel depressed, you should talk with your social worker, nurse, or doctor because this is a common problem that can often be treated effectively.

Getting Your Vascular Access Ready

One important step before starting hemodialysis is preparing a vascular access, a site on your body from which your blood is removed and returned. A vascular access should be prepared weeks or months before you start dialysis. It will allow easier and more efficient removal and replacement of your blood with fewer complications. For more information about the different kinds of vascular accesses and how to care for them, see the National Institute of Diabetes and Digestive and Kidney Diseases (NIDDK) fact sheet "Vascular Access for Hemodialysis" available at the NIDDK website http://kidney.niddk.nih.gov/kudiseases/pubs/vascularaccess/index.htm.

Equipment and Procedures

When you first visit a hemodialysis center, it may seem like a complicated mix of machines and people. But once you learn how the procedure works and become familiar with the equipment, you'll be more comfortable.

Dialysis Machine

The dialysis machine is about the size of a large television. This machine has three main jobs:

- pump blood and monitor flow for safety
- clean wastes from blood
- monitor your blood pressure and the rate of fluid removal from your body

Dialyzer

The dialyzer is a large canister containing thousands of small fibers through which your blood is passed. Dialysis solution, the cleansing fluid, is pumped around these fibers. The fibers allow wastes and extra fluids to pass from your blood into the solution, which carries them away. The dialyzer is sometimes called an artificial kidney.

Your dialysis center may use the same dialyzer more than once for your treatments. Reuse is considered safe as long as the dialyzer is cleaned and disinfected before each use. The dialyzer is tested each time to make sure it's still working, and it should never be used for

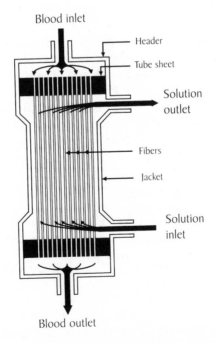

Figure 46.2. Structure of a typical hollow fiber dialyzer.

anyone but you. Before each session, you should be sure that the dialyzer is labeled with your name and check to see that it has been cleaned, disinfected, and tested.

Dialysis Solution

Dialysis solution, also known as dialysate, is the fluid in the dialyzer that helps remove wastes and extra fluid from your blood. It contains chemicals that make it act like a sponge. Your doctor will prescribe a specific dialysate for your treatments. This formula can be adjusted based on how well you tolerate the treatments and on your blood tests.

Needles

Many people find the needle sticks to be one of the most unpleasant parts of hemodialysis treatments. Most people, however, report getting used to them after a few sessions. If you find the needle insertion painful, an anesthetic cream or spray can be applied to the skin.

Most dialysis centers use two needles—one to carry blood to the dialyzer and one to return the cleaned blood to your body. Some specialized needles are designed with two openings for two-way flow of blood, but these needles are less efficient and require longer sessions. Needles for high-flux or high-efficiency dialysis need to be a little larger than those used with regular dialyzers.

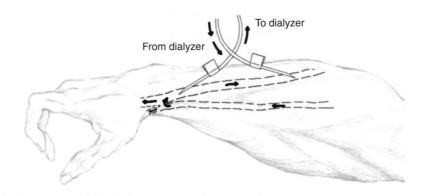

From dialyzer   To dialyzer

Figure 46.3. Arterial and venous needles.

Some people prefer to insert their own needles. You'll need insertion training to learn how to prevent infection and protect your vascular access. You may also learn a "ladder" strategy for needle placement in which you "climb" up the entire length of the access session by session so that you don't weaken an area with a grouping of needle sticks. An alternative approach is the "buttonhole" strategy in which you use a limited number of sites but insert the needle precisely into the same hole made by the previous needle stick. Whether you insert your own needles or not, you should know these techniques to better care for your access.

Tests to See How Well Your Dialysis Is Working

About once a month, your dialysis care team will test your blood by using one of two formulas—URR [urea reduction ratio] or Kt/V [a mathematical formula where k = clearance, t = time, and v = volume)—to see whether your treatments are removing enough wastes. Both tests look at one specific waste product, called blood urea nitrogen (BUN), as an indicator for the overall level of waste products in your system. For more information about these measurements, see the National Institute of Diabetes and Digestive and Kidney Diseases (NIDDK) fact sheet "Hemodialysis Dose and Adequacy," available at http://www.kidney.niddk.nih.gov/kudiseases/pubs/hemodialysisdose/index.htm.

Conditions Related to Kidney Failure and Their Treatments

Your kidneys do much more than remove wastes and extra fluid. They also make hormones and balance chemicals in your system. When your kidneys stop working, you may have problems with anemia and conditions that affect your bones, nerves, and skin. Some of the more common conditions caused by kidney failure are fatigue, bone problems, joint problems, itching, and "restless legs."

Anemia and Erythropoietin (EPO)

Anemia is a condition in which the volume of red blood cells is low. Red blood cells carry oxygen to cells throughout the body. Without oxygen, cells can't use the energy from food, so someone with anemia may tire easily and look pale. Anemia can also contribute to heart problems.

Anemia is common in people with kidney disease because the kidneys produce the hormone erythropoietin, or EPO, which stimulates the bone marrow to produce red blood cells. Diseased kidneys often don't make enough EPO, and so the bone marrow makes fewer red blood cells. EPO is available commercially and is commonly given to patients on dialysis. [For more information about the causes of and treatments for anemia in kidney failure, see Chapter 48, "Health Maintenance for Dialysis Patients."]

Renal Osteodystrophy

The term "renal" describes things related to the kidneys. Renal osteodystrophy, or bone disease of kidney failure, affects 90 percent of dialysis patients. It causes bones to become thin and weak or malformed and affects both children and adults. Symptoms can be seen in growing children with kidney disease even before they start dialysis. Older patients and women who have gone through menopause are at greater risk for this disease. [For more information about the causes of this bone disease and its treatment in dialysis patients, see Chapter 48, "Health Maintenance for Dialysis Patients."]

Itching (Pruritus)

Many people treated with hemodialysis complain of itchy skin, which is often worse during or just after treatment. Itching is common even in people who don't have kidney disease; in kidney failure, however, itching can be made worse by uremic toxins that current dialyzer membranes can't remove from the blood. The problem can also be related to high levels of parathyroid hormone (PTH). Some people have found dramatic relief after having their parathyroid glands removed. But a cure that works for everyone has not been found. Phosphate binders seem to help some people; others find relief after exposure to ultraviolet light. Still others improve with EPO shots. A few antihistamines (Benadryl, Atarax, Vistaril) have been found to help; also, capsaicin cream applied to the skin may relieve itching by deadening nerve impulses. In any case, taking care of dry skin is important. Applying creams with lanolin or camphor may help.

Sleep Disorders

Patients on dialysis often have insomnia, and some people have a specific problem called the sleep apnea syndrome. Episodes of apnea are breaks in breathing during sleep. Over time, these sleep disturbances can lead to "day-night reversal" (insomnia at night, sleepiness during the day), headache, depression, and decreased alertness. The apnea may be related to the effects of advanced kidney failure on the control of breathing. Treatments that work with people who have sleep apnea, whether they have kidney failure or not, include losing weight, changing sleeping position, and wearing a mask that gently pumps air continuously into the nose (nasal continuous positive airway pressure, or CPAP).

Many people on dialysis have trouble sleeping at night because of aching, uncomfortable, jittery, or "restless" legs. You may feel a strong impulse to kick or thrash your legs. Kicking may occur during sleep and disturb a bed partner throughout the night. Theories about the causes of this syndrome include nerve damage and chemical imbalances.

Moderate exercise during the day may help, but exercising a few hours before bedtime can make it worse. People with restless leg syndrome should reduce or avoid caffeine, alcohol, and tobacco; some people also find relief with massages or warm baths. A class of drugs called benzodiazepines, often used to treat insomnia or anxiety, may help as well. These prescription drugs include Klonopin, Librium, Valium, and Halcion. A newer and sometimes more effective therapy is levodopa (Sinemet), a drug used to treat Parkinson disease.

Sleep disorders may seem unimportant, but they can impair your quality of life. Don't hesitate to raise these problems with your nurse, doctor, or social worker.

Amyloidosis

Dialysis-related amyloidosis (DRA) is common in people who have been on dialysis for more than five years. DRA develops when proteins in the blood deposit on joints and tendons, causing pain, stiffness, and fluid in the joints, as is the case with arthritis. Working kidneys filter out these proteins, but dialysis filters are not as effective. [For more information, see Chapter 36, "Amyloidosis and Kidney Disease."]

How Diet Can Help

Eating the right foods can help improve your dialysis and your health. Your clinic has a dietitian to help you plan meals. Follow the dietitian's advice closely to get the most from your hemodialysis treatments. Here are a few general guidelines.

Fluids: Your dietitian will help you determine how much fluid to drink each day. Extra fluid can raise your blood pressure, make your heart work harder, and increase the stress of dialysis treatments. Remember that many foods—such as soup, ice cream, and fruits—contain plenty of water. Ask your dietitian for tips on controlling your thirst.

Potassium: The mineral potassium is found in many foods, especially fruits and vegetables. Potassium affects how steadily your heart beats, so eating foods with too much of it can be very dangerous to your heart. To control potassium levels in your blood, avoid foods like oranges, bananas, tomatoes, potatoes, and dried fruits. You can remove some of the potassium from potatoes and other vegetables by peeling and soaking them in a large container of water for several hours, then cooking them in fresh water.

Phosphorus: The mineral phosphorus can weaken your bones and make your skin itch if you consume too much. Control of phosphorus may be even more important than calcium itself in preventing bone disease and related complications. Foods like milk and cheese, dried beans, peas, colas, nuts, and peanut butter are high in phosphorus and should be avoided. You'll probably need to take a phosphate binder with your food to control the phosphorus in your blood between dialysis sessions.

Salt (sodium chloride): Most canned foods and frozen dinners contain high amounts of sodium. Too much of it makes you thirsty, and when you drink more fluid, your heart has to work harder to pump the fluid through your body. Over time, this can cause high blood pressure and congestive heart failure. Try to eat fresh foods that are naturally low in sodium, and look for products labeled "low sodium."

Protein: Before you were on dialysis, your doctor may have told you to follow a low-protein diet to preserve kidney function. But now you have different nutritional priorities. Most people on dialysis are encouraged to eat as much high-quality protein as they can. Protein helps you keep muscle and repair tissue, but protein breaks down into urea (blood urea nitrogen, or BUN) in your body. Some sources of protein, called high-quality proteins, produce less waste than others. High-quality proteins come from meat, fish, poultry, and eggs. Getting most of your protein from these sources can reduce the amount of urea in your blood.

Calories: Calories provide your body with energy. Some people on dialysis need to gain weight. You may need to find ways to add calories to your diet. Vegetable oils—like olive, canola, and safflower oils—are good sources of calories and do not contribute to problems controlling your cholesterol. Hard candy, sugar, honey, jam, and jelly also provide calories and energy. If you have diabetes, however, be very careful about eating sweets. A dietitian's guidance is especially important for people with diabetes.

Supplements: Vitamins and minerals may be missing from your diet because you have to avoid so many foods. Dialysis also removes some vitamins from your body. Your doctor may prescribe a vitamin and mineral supplement designed specifically for people with kidney failure. Take your prescribed supplement after treatment on the days you have hemodialysis. Never take vitamins that you can buy off the store shelf, since they may contain vitamins or minerals that are harmful to you.

You can also ask your dietitian for recipes and titles of cookbooks for patients with kidney disease. Following the restrictions of a diet for kidney disease might be hard at first, but with a little creativity, you can make tasty and satisfying meals.

Financial Issues

Treatment for kidney failure is expensive, but federal health insurance plans pay much of the cost, usually up to 80 percent. Often, private insurance or state programs pay the rest. Your social worker can help you locate resources for financial assistance.

Hope through Research

NIDDK, through its Division of Kidney, Urologic, and Hematologic Diseases, supports several programs and studies devoted to improving treatment for patients with progressive kidney disease and permanent kidney failure, including patients on hemodialysis.

The End-Stage Renal Disease Program promotes research to reduce medical problems from bone, blood, nervous system, metabolic, gastrointestinal, cardiovascular, and endocrine abnormalities in kidney failure and to improve the effectiveness of dialysis and transplantation. The research focuses on reusing hemodialysis membranes and on using alternative dialyzer sterilization methods; on devising more efficient, biocompatible membranes; and on developing criteria for dialysis adequacy. The program also seeks to increase kidney graft and patient survival and to maximize quality of life.

The HEMO Study, completed in 2002, tested the theory that a higher dialysis dose and/or high-flux membranes would reduce patient mortality (death) and morbidity (medical problems). Doctors at 15 medical centers recruited more than 1,800 hemodialysis patients and randomly assigned them to high or standard dialysis doses and high- or low-flux filters. The study found no increase in the health or survival of patients who had a higher dialysis dose, who dialyzed with high-flux filters, or who did both.

The U.S. Renal Data System (USRDS) collects, analyzes, and distributes information about the use of dialysis and transplantation to treat kidney failure in the United States. The USRDS is funded directly by NIDDK in conjunction with the Centers for Medicare and Medicaid Services. The USRDS publishes an Annual Data Report, which characterizes the total population of people being treated for kidney failure; reports on incidence, prevalence, mortality rates, and trends over time; and develops data on the effects of various treatment modalities. The report also helps identify problems and opportunities for more focused special studies of renal research issues.

The Hemodialysis Vascular Access Clinical Trials Consortium will conduct a series of multicenter, randomized, placebo-controlled clinical trials of drug therapies to reduce the failure and complication rate of arteriovenous grafts and fistulas in hemodialysis. Recently developed antithrombotic agents and drugs to inhibit cytokines may be evaluated in these large clinical trials.

Chapter 47

What You Should Know about Peritoneal Dialysis

With peritoneal dialysis (PD), you have some choices in treating advanced and permanent kidney failure. Since the 1980s, when PD first became a practical and widespread treatment for kidney failure, we've learned much about how to make PD more effective and minimize side effects. Since you don't have to schedule dialysis sessions at a center, PD gives you more control. You can give yourself treatments at home, at work, or on trips. But this independence makes it especially important that you work closely with your healthcare team: your nephrologist, dialysis nurse, dialysis technician, dietitian, and social worker. But the most important members of your healthcare team are you and your family. By learning about your treatment, you can work with your healthcare team to give yourself the best possible results, and you can lead a full, active life.

When Your Kidneys Fail

Healthy kidneys clean your blood by removing excess fluid, minerals, and wastes. They also make hormones that keep your bones strong and your blood healthy. When your kidneys fail, harmful wastes build up in your body, your blood pressure may rise, and your body

"Treatment Methods for Kidney Failure: Peritoneal Dialysis," National Kidney and Urologic Diseases Information Clearinghouse (NKUDIC), a service of the National Institute of Diabetes and Digestive and Kidney Diseases (NIDDK), National Institutes of Health (NIH), Pub. No. 01-4688, May 2001.

may retain excess fluid and not make enough red blood cells. When this happens, you need treatment to replace the work of your failed kidneys.

How PD Works

In PD, a soft tube called a catheter is used to fill your abdomen with a cleansing liquid called dialysis solution. The walls of your abdominal cavity are lined with a membrane called the peritoneum, which allows waste products and extra fluid to pass from your blood into the dialysis solution. The solution contains a sugar called dextrose that will pull wastes and extra fluid into the abdominal cavity. These wastes and fluid then leave your body when the dialysis solution is drained. The used solution, containing wastes and extra fluid, is then thrown away. The process of draining and filling is called an exchange and takes about 30 to 40 minutes. The period the dialysis solution is in your abdomen is called the dwell time. A typical

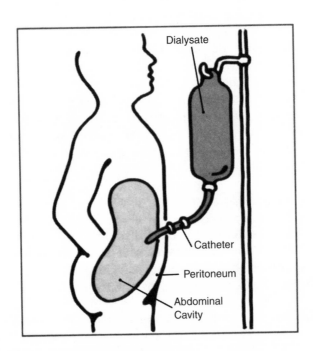

Figure 47.1. *Peritoneal dialysis.*

schedule calls for four exchanges a day, each with a dwell time of four to six hours. Different types of PD have different schedules of daily exchanges.

The most common form of PD, continuous ambulatory peritoneal dialysis (CAPD), doesn't require a machine. As the word ambulatory suggests, you can walk around with the dialysis solution in your abdomen. Other forms of PD require a machine called a cycler to fill and drain your abdomen, usually while you sleep. The different types of cycler-assisted PD are sometimes called automated peritoneal dialysis, or APD.

Getting Ready for PD

Whether you choose an ambulatory or automated form of PD, you'll need to have a soft catheter placed in your abdomen. The catheter is the tube that carries the dialysis solution into and out of your abdomen. After giving you a local anesthetic to minimize any pain, your doctor will make a small cut, often below and a little to the side of your navel (belly button), and then guide the catheter through the slit into the peritoneal cavity. As soon as the catheter is in place, you can

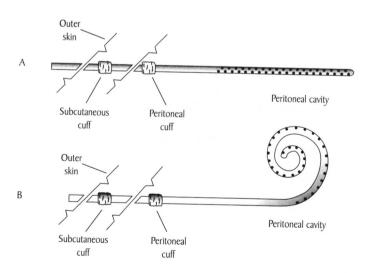

Figure 47.2. Two double-cuff Tenckhoff chronic peritoneal catheters: standard (A), curled (B).

start to receive solution through it, although you probably won't begin a full schedule of exchanges for two to three weeks. This break-in period lets you build up scar tissue that will hold the catheter in place.

The standard catheter for PD is made of soft tubing for comfort. It has Dacron cuffs that merge with your scar tissue to keep it in place. (Dacron is a polyester fabric.) The end of the tubing that is inside your abdomen has many holes to allow the free flow of solution in and out.

Types of PD

The type of PD you choose will depend on the schedule of exchanges you would like to follow, as well as other factors. You may start with one type of PD and switch to another, or you may find that a combination of automated and non-automated exchanges suits you best. Work with your healthcare team to find the best schedule and techniques to meet your lifestyle and health needs.

Continuous Ambulatory Peritoneal Dialysis (CAPD)

If you choose CAPD, you'll drain a fresh bag of dialysis solution into your abdomen. After four to six or more hours of dwell time, you'll drain the solution, which now contains wastes, into the bag. You then repeat the cycle with a fresh bag of solution. You don't need a machine for CAPD; all you need is gravity to fill and empty your abdomen. Your doctor will prescribe the number of exchanges you'll need, typically three or four exchanges during the day and one evening exchange with a long overnight dwell time while you sleep.

Continuous Cycler-Assisted Peritoneal Dialysis (CCPD)

CCPD uses an automated cycler to perform three to five exchanges during the night while you sleep. In the morning, you begin one exchange with a dwell time that lasts the entire day.

Nocturnal Intermittent Peritoneal Dialysis (NIPD)

NIPD is like CCPD, only the number of overnight exchanges is greater (six or more), and you don't perform an exchange during the day. NIPD is usually reserved for patients whose peritoneum is able to transport waste products very rapidly or for patients who still have substantial remaining kidney function.

Customizing Your PD

If you've chosen CAPD, you may have a problem with the long overnight dwell time. It's normal for some of the dextrose in the solution to cross into your body and become glucose. The absorbed dextrose doesn't create a problem during short dwell times. But overnight, some people absorb so much dextrose that it starts to draw fluid from the peritoneal cavity back into the body, reducing the efficiency of the exchange. If you have this problem, you may be able to use a mini-cycler (a small version of a machine that automatically fills and drains your abdomen) to exchange your solution once or several times overnight while you sleep. These additional, shorter exchanges will minimize solution absorption and give you added clearance of wastes and excess fluid.

If you've chosen CCPD, you may have a solution absorption problem with the daytime exchange, which has a long dwell time. You may find you need an additional exchange in the mid-afternoon to increase the amount of waste removed and to prevent excessive absorption of solution.

Preventing Problems

Infection is the most common problem for people on PD. Your healthcare team will show you how to keep your catheter bacteria-free to avoid peritonitis, which is an infection of the peritoneum. Improved catheter designs protect against the spread of bacteria, but peritonitis is still a common problem that sometimes makes continuing PD impossible. You should follow your healthcare team's instructions carefully, but here are some general rules:

- Store supplies in a cool, clean, dry place.

- Inspect each bag of solution for signs of contamination before you use it.

- Find a clean, dry, well-lit space to perform your exchanges.

- Wear sterile gloves to perform exchanges.

- Wash your hands every time you need to handle your catheter.

- Clean the exit site with antiseptic every day.

- Wear a surgical mask when performing exchanges if you have a cold.

Keep a close watch for any signs of infection and report them so they can be treated promptly. Here are some signs to watch for:

- Fever

- Nausea or vomiting

- Redness or pain around the catheter

- Unusual color or cloudiness in used dialysis solution

- A catheter cuff that has been pushed out

Equipment and Supplies for PD

Transfer Set

A transfer set is tubing that connects the bag of dialysis solution to the catheter. Two types of transfer sets are available.

A **straight transfer set** is a straight piece of tubing that stays connected to your catheter. To begin each exchange, you connect the free end to a fresh bag of solution and hang the bag higher than the catheter, usually attaching it to a special stand, so that gravity pulls the solution into your abdomen. While the solution is in your abdomen, you can roll up the bag and wear it under your clothes. When you've finished your dwell time, you take the bag out and place it near the floor so that gravity pushes the used solution down into the bag. When the bag is full, you disconnect it from the straight transfer set and connect a fresh bag of solution to start the next exchange.

A **Y-set** is a Y-shaped piece of tubing that can be disconnected between exchanges. To start, you connect the base of the Y to your catheter. You then connect one branch of the Y to a fresh bag of solution and the other to an empty bag. To flush away any bacteria that might be in the transfer set, you close off the base of the Y and drain a small amount of solution from the full bag into the empty one. Then you close the branch that leads to the empty bag and let the solution flow into your abdomen. Once the bag has emptied, you can disconnect the Y-set from your catheter so you won't need to conceal a bag or extra tubing under your clothes. When it's time to empty the used solution, you reconnect the catheter to the Y-set and drain the solution into an empty bag to discard. Then you connect a fresh bag and begin the process again.

The Y-set is filled with disinfectant when not in use. This disinfectant is flushed out with the used dialysis solution. These procedures make the Y-set more effective at protecting against peritonitis. A Y-set can be reused for several months.

Dialysis Solution

Dialysis solution comes in 1.5-, 2-, 2.5-, or 3-liter bags. A liter is slightly more than one quart. The dialysis dose can be increased by using a larger bag, but only within the limit of the amount your abdomen can hold. The solution contains a sugar called dextrose, which pulls extra fluid from your blood. Your doctor will prescribe a formula that fits your needs.

You'll need a clean space to store your bags of solution and other supplies. You may also need a special heating device to warm each

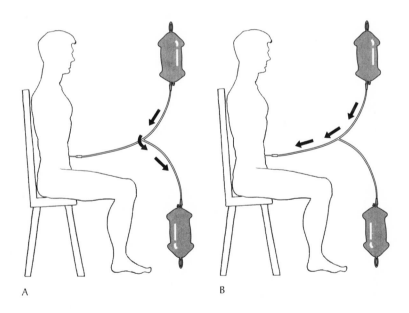

A   B

Figure 47.3. *Flush-before-fill strategy used with Y transfer sets. (A) A small volume of fresh dialysis solution is drained directly into the drainage container (either before or just after drainage of the abdomen). This acts to wash away any bacteria that may have been introduced in the limb of the Y leading to the new bag at the time of connection. (B) Fresh solution is introduced through the rinsed connector.*

bag of solution to body temperature before use. Manufacturers do not recommend using microwave ovens to warm solution because they change its chemical makeup.

Cycler

The cycler—which automatically fills and drains your abdomen, usually at night while you sleep—can be programmed to deliver specified volumes of dialysis solution on a specified schedule. Most systems include the following components:

- **Solution storage:** At the beginning of the session, you connect bags of dialysis solution to tubing that feeds the cycler. Most systems include a separate tube for the last bag because this solution may have a higher dextrose content so that it can work for a day-long dwell time.

- **Pump:** The pump sends the solution from the storage bags to the heater bag before it enters the body and then sends it from the weigh bag to the disposal container after it's been used. The pump doesn't fill and drain your abdomen; gravity performs that job more safely.

- **Heater bag:** Before the solution enters your abdomen, a measured dose is warmed to body temperature. Once the solution is the right temperature and the previous exchange has been drained, a clamp is released to allow the warmed solution to flow into your abdomen.

- **Weigh bag:** The cycler's timer releases a clamp to let the used dialysis solution drain from your abdomen into a weigh bag that measures and records how much solution has been removed. Some systems compare the amount of solution inserted with the amount drained and display the net difference between the two volumes. This lets you know whether the treatment is removing enough fluid from your body.

- **Disposal container:** After the used solution is weighed, it's pumped to a disposal container that you can throw away in the morning.

- **Alarms:** Sensors will trigger an alarm and shut off the machine if there's a problem with inflow or outflow.

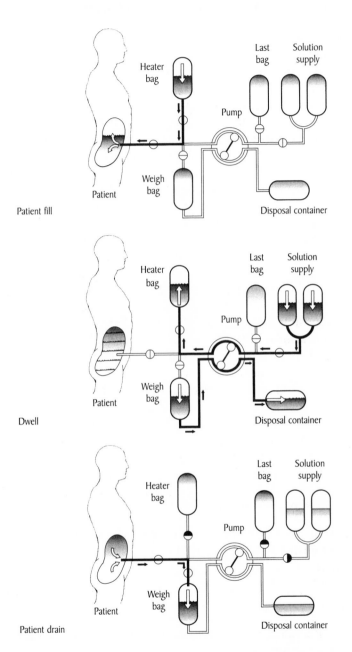

Figure 47.4. *An example of a system used for cycler-assisted peritoneal dialysis. Solution is heated before use and weighed after use. The last bag of solution may have a different concentration to last throughout the day.*

Testing the Effectiveness of Your Dialysis

To see if the exchanges are removing enough waste products, such as urea, your healthcare team must perform several tests. These tests are especially important during the first weeks of dialysis to determine whether you're receiving an adequate amount, or dose, of dialysis.

The peritoneal equilibration test (often called the PET) measures how much sugar has been absorbed from a bag of infused dialysis solution and how much urea and creatinine have entered into the solution during a four-hour exchange. The peritoneal transport rate varies from person to person. If you have a high rate of transport, you absorb sugar from the dialysis solution quickly and should avoid exchanges with a very long dwell time because you're likely to absorb too much solution from such exchanges.

In the clearance test, samples of used solution drained over a 24-hour period are collected, and a blood sample is obtained during the day when the used solution is collected. The amount of urea in the used solution is compared with the amount in the blood, to see how effective the PD schedule is in removing urea from the blood. For the first months or even years of PD treatment, you may still produce small amounts of urine. If your urine output is more than several hundred milliliters per day, urine is also collected during this period to measure its urea concentration.

From the used solution, urine, and blood measurements, your healthcare team can compute a urea clearance, called Kt/V, and a creatinine clearance rate (adjusted to body surface area). The residual clearance of the kidneys is also considered. These measurements will show whether the PD prescription is adequate.

If the laboratory results show that the dialysis schedule is not removing enough urea and creatinine, the doctor may change the prescription by doing the following:

- increasing the number of exchanges per day for patients treated with CAPD or per night for patients treated with CCPD or NIPD

- increasing the volume of each exchange (amount of solution in the bag) in CAPD

- adding an extra, automated middle-of-the-night exchange to the CAPD schedule

- adding an extra middle-of-the-day exchange to the CCPD schedule

For more information about testing the effectiveness of your dialysis, see the National Institute of Diabetes and Digestive and Kidney Diseases (NIDDK) fact sheet "Peritoneal Dialysis Dose and Adequacy" available at http://kidney.niddk.nih.gov/kudiseases/pubs/peritoneal dose/index.htm.

Compliance

One of the big problems with PD is that patients sometimes don't perform all of the exchanges prescribed by their medical team. They either skip exchanges or sometimes skip entire treatment days when using CCPD or NIPD. Skipping PD treatments has been shown to increase the risk of hospitalization and death.

Remaining Kidney Function

Normally the PD prescription factors in the amount of residual, or remaining, kidney function. Residual kidney function typically falls, although slowly, over months or even years of PD. This means that more often than not, the number of exchanges prescribed, or the volume of exchanges, needs to increase as residual kidney function falls.

The doctor should determine your PD dose on the basis of practice standards established by the National Kidney Foundation Dialysis Outcomes Quality Initiative (NKF-DOQI). Work closely with your healthcare team to ensure that you get the proper dose, and follow instructions carefully to make sure you get the most out of your dialysis exchanges.

Conditions Related to Kidney Failure and Their Treatments

Your kidneys do much more than remove wastes and extra fluid. They also make hormones and balance chemicals in your system. When your kidneys stop working, you may have problems with anemia and conditions that affect your bones, nerves, and skin. Some of the more common conditions caused by kidney failure are fatigue, bone problems, joint problems, itching, and "restless legs."

Anemia and Erythropoietin (EPO)

Anemia is a condition in which the volume of red blood cells is low. Red blood cells carry oxygen to cells throughout the body. Without oxygen, cells can't use the energy from food, so someone with anemia may tire easily and look pale. Anemia can also contribute to heart problems.

Anemia is common in people with kidney disease because the kidneys produce the hormone erythropoietin, or EPO, which stimulates the bone marrow to produce red blood cells. Diseased kidneys often don't make enough EPO, and so the bone marrow makes fewer red blood cells. EPO is available commercially and is commonly given to patients on dialysis.

Renal Osteodystrophy

The term "renal" describes things related to the kidneys. Renal osteodystrophy, or bone disease of kidney failure, affects up to 90 percent of dialysis patients. It causes bones to become thin and weak or malformed and affects both children and adults. Symptoms can be seen in growing children with kidney disease even before they start dialysis. Older patients and women who have gone through menopause are at greater risk for this disease.

Itching (Pruritus)

Many people treated with peritoneal dialysis complain of itchy skin, which is often worse during or just after treatment. Itching is common even in people who don't have kidney disease; in kidney failure, however, itching can be made worse by uremic toxins in the blood that dialysis doesn't adequately remove. The problem can also be related to high levels of parathyroid hormone (PTH). Some people have found dramatic relief after having their parathyroid glands removed. But a cure that works for everyone has not been found. Phosphate binders seem to help some people; others find relief after exposure to ultraviolet light. Still others improve with EPO shots. A few antihistamines (Benadryl, Atarax, Vistaril) have been found to help; also, capsaicin cream applied to the skin may relieve itching by deadening nerve impulses. In any case, taking care of dry skin is important. Applying creams with lanolin or camphor may help.

Sleep Disorders

Patients on dialysis often have insomnia, and some people have a specific problem called the sleep apnea syndrome. Episodes of apnea are breaks in breathing during sleep. Over time, these sleep disturbances can lead to "day-night reversal" (insomnia at night, sleepiness during the day), headache, depression, and decreased alertness. The apnea may be related to the effects of advanced kidney failure on the control of breathing. Treatments that work with people who have sleep apnea, whether they have kidney failure or not, include losing weight, changing sleeping position, and wearing a mask that gently pumps air continuously into the nose (nasal continuous positive airway pressure, or CPAP).

Many people on dialysis have trouble sleeping at night because of aching, uncomfortable, jittery, or "restless" legs. You may feel a strong impulse to kick or thrash your legs. Kicking may occur during sleep and disturb a bed partner throughout the night. Theories about the causes of this syndrome include nerve damage and chemical imbalances.

Moderate exercise during the day may help, but exercising a few hours before bedtime can make it worse. People with restless leg syndrome should reduce or avoid caffeine, alcohol, and tobacco; some people also find relief with massages or warm baths. A class of drugs called benzodiazepines, often used to treat insomnia or anxiety, may help as well. These prescription drugs include Klonopin, Librium, Valium, and Halcion. A newer and sometimes more effective therapy is Sinemet (levodopa), a drug used to treat Parkinson disease.

Sleep disorders may seem unimportant, but they can impair your quality of life. Don't hesitate to raise these problems with your nurse, doctor, or social worker.

Amyloidosis

Dialysis-related amyloidosis (DRA) is common in people who have been on dialysis for more than five years. DRA develops when proteins in the blood deposit on joints and tendons, causing pain, stiffness, and fluid in the joints, as is the case with arthritis. Working kidneys filter out these proteins, but dialysis is not as effective.

Adjusting to Changes

You can do your exchanges in any clean space, and you can take part in many activities with solution in your abdomen. Even though PD gives you more flexibility and freedom than hemodialysis, which requires being connected to a machine for three to five hours three times a week, you must still stick to a strict schedule of exchanges and keep track of supplies. You may have to cut back on some responsibilities at work or in your home life. Accepting this new reality can be very hard on you and your family. A counselor or social worker can help you cope.

Many patients feel depressed when starting dialysis, or after several months of treatment. Some people can't get used to the fact that the solution makes their body look larger. If you feel depressed, you should talk with your social worker, nurse, or doctor because depression is a common problem that can often be treated effectively.

How Diet Can Help

Eating the right foods can help improve your dialysis and your health. You may have chosen PD over hemodialysis because the diet is less restrictive. With PD, you're removing wastes from your body slowly but constantly, while in hemodialysis, wastes may build up for two to three days between treatments. You still need to be very careful about the foods you eat, however, because PD is much less efficient than working kidneys. Your clinic has a dietitian to help you plan meals. Follow the dietitian's advice closely to get the most from your dialysis treatments. You can also ask your dietitian for recipes and titles of cookbooks for patients with kidney disease. Following the restrictions of a diet for kidney failure might be hard at first, but with a little creativity, you can make tasty and satisfying meals.

Financial Issues

Treatment for kidney failure is expensive, but federal health insurance programs pay much of the cost, usually up to 80 percent. Often, private insurance or state programs pay the rest. Your social worker can help you locate resources for financial assistance.

Hope through Research

NIDDK, through its Division of Kidney, Urologic, and Hematologic Diseases, supports several programs and studies devoted to improving treatment for patients with progressive kidney disease and permanent kidney failure, including patients on PD.

The End-Stage Renal Disease Program promotes research to reduce medical problems from bone, blood, nervous system, metabolic, gastrointestinal, cardiovascular, and endocrine abnormalities in kidney failure and to improve the effectiveness of dialysis and transplantation. The research focuses on reusing hemodialysis membranes and on using alternative dialyzer sterilization methods; on devising more efficient, biocompatible membranes; on refining high-flux hemodialysis; and on developing criteria for dialysis adequacy. The program also seeks to increase kidney graft and patient survival and to maximize quality of life.

The U.S. Renal Data System (USRDS) collects, analyzes, and distributes information about the use of dialysis and transplantation to treat kidney failure in the United States. The USRDS is funded directly by NIDDK in conjunction with the Healthcare Financing Administration. The USRDS publishes an Annual Data Report, which characterizes the total population of people being treated for kidney failure; reports on incidence, prevalence, mortality rates, and trends over time; and develops data on the effects of various treatment modalities. The report also helps identify problems and opportunities for more focused special studies of renal research issues.

Chapter 48

Health Maintenance for Dialysis Patients

Chapter Contents

Section 48.1

What You Can Do about Chronic Kidney Disease

"Chronic Kidney Disease Information: What You Can Do," is reprinted with permission from the Medical Education Institute (MEI) website of the Life Options Rehabilitation Program (www.lifeoptions.org). The text is intended to serve as a general resource; the MEI and its Licensors are not engaged in rendering medical advice and this information is not intended to replace medical advice offered by a physician. Additionally, the MEI and its Licensors disclaim any liability for any direct, indirect, incidental, consequential, or special damages arising out of or in any way connected with access to or use of this text. This information is copyrighted to the MEI. All rights reserved. Publication date: October 15, 2003.

Most chronic kidney disease (CKD) is not curable. The good news is that if your doctor finds out that you have a kidney problem, there may be a number of ways to help slow down the disease, help you feel better, and help you make better medical decisions. What can you do?

1. **Know your lab tests.** Know the names of the lab tests your doctor orders and what the results mean. Kidney disease is often diagnosed, and always monitored, by measuring levels of substances in the blood or urine. Knowing—and tracking—your lab tests is an important way for you to be involved in your care. Normal lab test ranges vary slightly from one laboratory to another. When you get your results, be sure to ask what the laboratory's normal range is.

2. **Control your blood pressure.** Keep your blood pressure below 130/85 (adults) with weight loss and exercise, a low sodium/low fat diet, reducing stress, and taking your blood pressure medication correctly. For some patients, the target blood pressure is lower (125/75). Controlling high blood pressure may delay the progression of kidney disease by slowing damage to the kidneys.

3. **Ask your doctor about certain medications that may help treat kidney disease.** ACE (angiotensin-converting enzyme) inhibitors are a class of blood pressure medicines that can protect kidney function in some cases (generic names include ramipril, captopril, and enalapril). In some people, ACE inhibitors cause a persistent cough, which stops when the drug is discontinued. This is not a serious side effect of the drug. ARBs (angiotensin receptor blockers) may sometimes be used along with or instead of ACE inhibitors. Calcium channel blockers and beta blockers are other drugs that may help to control blood pressure and protect kidney function.

4. **Ask your doctor about anemia.** Anemia—a shortage of red blood cells—starts very early in kidney failure. Anemia can cause you to feel tired and worn out, and can damage your heart. Heart disease is the leading cause of death in people with kidney problems. Ask your doctor about medications such as epoetin (EPO) and iron to treat anemia.

5. **Ask your doctor about a low protein diet.** Some doctors believe a diet lower in some proteins can help slow kidney disease. Ask your doctor to refer you to a dietitian who specializes in treating those with chronic kidney disease. A dietitian can help you learn how to keep your kidneys healthy longer by eating the right foods. It is important not to adjust your protein intake until you have discussed this with your doctor or dietitian.

6. **Control your blood sugar levels.** If you have diabetes, stay at a healthy weight, exercise, and take medications as prescribed to keep your blood glucose in the "normal" range. Tight control of blood sugar can help slow the progression of kidney disease. Your HbA1c [hemoglobin A1c] levels, which measure your blood sugar control over a period of three months, should be less than 6.5 percent.

7. **Quit smoking.** In people with kidney disease, smoking is linked to an increase in the amount of protein spilled in the urine. In smokers with diabetes, kidney disease may progress twice as fast. Scientists are not sure why this is the case, but if you have kidney disease and you smoke, quitting may help slow down the damage.

8. **Avoid certain pain medications.** Ask your doctor or healthcare specialist about certain pain medications. Some over-the-counter pain pills containing ibuprofen, naproxen, and ketoprofen (e.g., Motrin® and Advil® and Aleve®) can affect kidney function. This is especially true if you have kidney, heart, or liver disease or take diuretics (water pills). Avoid using combinations of these pain medications and caffeine because these combinations can further damage your kidneys.

9. **Exercise.** With your doctor's permission, start a regular exercise program to control weight and keep your heart healthy and blood vessels working as well as possible. It is very important to keep your muscles and joints in good working order. Although written for people on dialysis, "Exercise: A Guide for People on Dialysis" has useful information to help anyone with a chronic illness increase physical activity. [You may obtain the guide by calling the Life Options Rehabilitation Resource Center at 800-468-7777 or going to their website at http://www .lifeoptions.org/catalog/pdfs/booklets/exercise.pdf.]

Section 48.2

Staying Fit with Kidney Disease

Physical fitness is very important in today's world. Everyone is enjoying the benefits of greater strength and feeling better. Exercise keeps your body strong and healthy.

Can I take part in vigorous physical activity?

Yes. In the past, it was thought that people with kidney disease would not be able to join in vigorous activity. We know now that patients who decide to follow an exercise program are stronger and have more energy.

How does exercise benefit me?

With exercise, it becomes easier to get around, do your necessary tasks, and still have some energy left over for other activities you enjoy. In addition to increased energy, other benefits from exercise may include the following:

- improved muscle physical functioning
- better blood pressure control
- improved muscle strength
- lowered level of blood fats (cholesterol and triglycerides)
- better sleep
- better control of body weight

Do I need to see my doctor before starting exercise?

Yes. Before beginning any exercise program, be sure to check with your doctor. When planning a directed exercise program, you need to look at four things:

521

- type of exercise
- length of time you spend exercising
- how often you exercise
- how hard you work while exercising

Here are some tips on each.

Type of exercise: Choose continuous activity such as walking, swimming, bicycling (indoors or out), skiing, aerobic dancing or any other activities in which you need to move large muscle groups continuously.

Low-level strengthening exercises may also be beneficial as part of your program. Design your program to use low weights and high repetitions, and avoid heavy lifting.

How long to exercise: Work toward 30 minutes a session. You should build up gradually to this level.

There is nothing magical about 30 minutes. If you feel like walking 45 to 60 minutes, go ahead. Just be sure to follow the advice listed under "When should I stop exercising?" in this text.

How often to exercise: Exercise at least three days a week. These should be non-consecutive days, for example, Monday, Wednesday and Friday. Three days a week is the minimum requirement to achieve the benefits of your exercise.

How hard to work while exercising: This is the most difficult to talk about without knowing your own exercise capacity. Usually, the following ideas are helpful:

- Your breathing should not be so hard that you cannot talk with someone exercising with you. (Try to get an exercise partner such as a family member or a friend.) You should feel completely normal within one hour after exercising. (If not, slow down next time.)
- You should not feel so much muscle soreness that it keeps you from exercising the next session.
- The intensity should be a "comfortable push" level.
- Start out slowly each session to warm up, then pick up your pace, then slow down again when you are about to finish.

The most important thing is to start slowly and progress gradually, allowing your body to adapt to the increased levels of activity.

When should I exercise?

Try to schedule your exercise into your normal day. Here are some ideas about when to exercise:

- Wait one hour after a large meal.
- Avoid the very hot times of the day.
- Morning or evening seems to be the best time for exercising.
- Do not exercise less than an hour before bedtime.

When should I stop exercising?

- If you feel very tired
- If you are short of breath
- If you feel chest pain
- If you feel irregular or rapid heart beats
- If you feel sick to your stomach
- If you get leg cramps
- If you feel dizzy or light-headed

Are there any times when I should not exercise?

Yes. You should not exercise without talking with your doctor if any of the following occurs:

- You have a fever.
- You have changed your dialysis schedule.
- You have changed your medicine schedule.
- Your physical condition has changed.
- You have eaten too much.
- The weather is very hot and humid, unless you exercise in an air-conditioned place.
- You have joint or bone problems that become worse with exercise.

If you stop exercising for any of these reasons, speak to your doctor before beginning again.

Section 48.3

Eat Right to Feel Right on Hemodialysis

National Kidney and Urologic Diseases Information Clearinghouse (NKUDIC), a service of the National Institute of Diabetes and Digestive and Kidney Diseases (NIDDK), National Institutes of Health (NIH), Pub. No. 03-4274, April 2003.

When you start hemodialysis, you must make many changes in your life. Watching the foods you eat will make you healthier. This text will help you choose the right foods.

Use this text with a dietitian to help you learn how to eat right to feel right on hemodialysis. Read one portion at a time. Then go through the exercise with your dietitian. Once you have completed every exercise, keep a copy of this text to remind yourself of foods you can eat and foods you need to avoid.

[See Chapter 52, "Further Reading about Urinary and Kidney Diseases and Disorders," for a list of cookbooks and other publications for dialysis patients.]

How does food affect my hemodialysis?

Food gives you energy and helps your body repair itself. Food is broken down in your stomach and intestines. Your blood picks up nutrients from the digested food and carries them to all your body cells. These cells take nutrients from your blood and put waste products back into the bloodstream. When your kidneys were healthy, they worked around the clock to remove wastes from your blood. The wastes left your body when you urinated. Other wastes are removed in bowel movements.

Now your kidneys have stopped working. Hemodialysis removes wastes from your blood. But between sessions, wastes can build up in your blood and make you sick. You can reduce the amount of wastes by watching what you eat and drink. A good meal plan can improve your dialysis and your health.

Your clinic has a dietitian to help you plan meals. A dietitian specializes in food and nutrition. A dietitian with special training in care for kidney health is called a renal dietitian.

Use a copy of Form 48.1 (on page 526) with your dietitian's help to learn what to eat and what foods to avoid in order to feel right while you are on hemodialysis.

What do I need to know about fluids?

You already know you need to watch how much you drink. Any food that is liquid at room temperature also contains water. These foods include soup, Jell-O, and ice cream. Many fruits and vegetables contain lots of water, too. They include melons, grapes, apples, oranges, tomatoes, lettuce, and celery. All these foods add to your fluid intake.

Fluid can build up between dialysis sessions, causing swelling and weight gain. The extra fluid affects your blood pressure and can make your heart work harder. You could get serious heart trouble from overloading your system with fluid.

Control your thirst: You can keep your fluids down by drinking from smaller cups or glasses. Freeze juice in an ice cube tray and eat it like a popsicle. (Remember to count the popsicle in your fluid allowance!) The dietitian will be able to give you other tips for managing your thirst.

Your dry weight is your weight after a dialysis session when all of the extra fluid in your body has been removed. If you let too much fluid build up between sessions, it is harder to get down to your proper dry weight. Your dry weight may change over a period of three to six weeks. Talk to your doctor regularly about what your dry weight should be.

Talk to a dietitian: Even though you are on hemodialysis, your kidneys may still be able to remove some fluid. Or your kidneys may not remove any fluid at all. That is why every patient has a different daily allowance for fluid. Talk to your dietitian about how much fluid you can have each day.

What do I need to know about potassium?

Potassium is a mineral found in many foods, especially milk, fruits, and vegetables. It affects how steadily your heart beats. Healthy kidneys keep the right amount of potassium in the blood to keep the heart

Talk to a Dietitian

My dietitian's name is _____.

Phone _____.

Daily Fluid Allowance

I can have _____ ounces of fluid each day.

I can have _____ ounce(s) of _____ with breakfast.

I can have _____ ounce(s) of _____ in the morning.

I can have _____ ounce(s) of _____ with lunch.

I can have _____ ounce(s) of _____ in the afternoon.

I can have _____ ounce(s) of _____ with supper.

I can have _____ ounce(s) of _____ in the evening.

TOTAL _____ ounces (should equal the allowance written above)

Foods I Can Eat Instead of High-Potassium Foods

Instead of _____, I will eat _____.

Instead of _____, I will eat _____.

Instead of _____, I will eat _____.

Instead of _____, I will eat _____.

High-Quality Protein Foods I Can Eat

I will eat _____ servings of meat each day.

I (will) (will not) drink milk. I will drink _____ cup(s) of milk a day.

Spices and Other Healthy Foods I Can Use to Flavor My Diet

Spice: _____

Spice: _____

Spice: _____

Food: _____

Food: _____

Form 48.1. Learn what to eat and what foods to avoid.

beating at a steady pace. Potassium levels can rise between dialysis sessions and affect your heartbeat. Eating too much potassium can be very dangerous to your heart. It may even cause death.

To control potassium levels in your blood, avoid foods like avocados, bananas, kiwis, and dried fruit, which are very high in potassium. Also, eat smaller portions of other high-potassium foods. For example, eat half a pear instead of a whole pear. Eat only very small portions of oranges and melons.

Dialyzing potatoes and other vegetables: You can remove some of the potassium from potatoes and other vegetables by peeling them, then soaking them in a large amount of water for several hours. Drain and rinse before cooking. Your dietitian will give you more specific information about the potassium content of foods.

Talk to a dietitian: Make a food plan that reduces the potassium in your diet. Start by noting the high-potassium foods (from the following list) that you now eat. A dietitian can help you add other foods to the list.

- apricots
- avocados
- bananas
- beets
- brussel sprouts
- cantaloupe
- clams
- dates
- figs
- kiwi fruit
- lima beans
- melons
- milk
- nectarines
- orange juice
- oranges
- peanuts
- pears (fresh)
- potatoes
- prune juice
- prunes
- raisins
- sardines
- spinach
- tomatoes
- winter squash
- yogurt
- others:_____

Changes: Talk to a dietitian about foods you can eat instead of high-potassium foods.

What do I need to know about phosphorus?

Phosphorus is a mineral found in many foods. If you have too much phosphorus in your blood, it pulls calcium from your bones. Losing calcium will make your bones weak and likely to break. Also, too much phosphorus may make your skin itch. Foods like milk and cheese, dried beans, peas, colas, nuts, and peanut butter are high in phosphorus. Usually, people on dialysis are limited to ½ cup of milk per day. The renal dietitian will give you more specific information regarding phosphorus.

You probably will need to take a phosphate binder like Renagel, PhosLo, Tums, or calcium carbonate to control the phosphorus in your blood between dialysis sessions. These medications act like sponges to soak up, or bind, phosphorus while it is in the stomach. Because it is bound, the phosphorus does not get into the blood. Instead, it is passed out of the body in the stool.

What do I need to know about protein?

Before you were on dialysis, your doctor may have told you to follow a low-protein diet. Being on dialysis changes this. Most people on dialysis are encouraged to eat as much high-quality protein as they can. The better nourished you are, the healthier you will be. You will also have greater resistance to infection and recover from surgery more quickly.

Protein helps you keep muscle and repair tissue. In your body, protein breaks down into a waste product called urea. If urea builds up in your blood, you can become very sick. Some sources of protein produce less waste than others. These are called high-quality proteins. High-quality proteins come from meat, fish, poultry, and eggs (especially egg whites). Getting most of your protein from these sources can reduce the amount of urea in your blood.

Talk to a dietitian: Meat, fish, and chicken are good sources of protein. Talk to a dietitian about the meats you eat. A regular serving size is three ounces. This is about the size of the palm of your hand or a deck of cards.

Try to choose lean (low-fat) meats that are also low in phosphorus. If you are a vegetarian, ask about other ways to get your protein.

Low-fat milk is a good source of protein. But milk is high in phosphorus and potassium. And milk adds to your fluid intake. Talk to a dietitian to see if milk fits into your food plan.

What do I need to know about sodium?

Sodium is found in salt and other foods. Most canned foods and frozen dinners contain large amounts of sodium. Too much sodium makes you thirsty. But if you drink more fluid, your heart has to work harder to pump the fluid through your body. Over time, this can cause high blood pressure and congestive heart failure.

Try to eat fresh foods that are naturally low in sodium. Look for products labeled low sodium.

Do not use salt substitutes because they contain potassium. Talk to a dietitian about spices you can use to flavor your food. The dietitian can help you find spice blends without sodium or potassium.

Talk to a dietitian: Talk to a dietitian about spices and other healthy foods you can use to flavor your diet.

What do I need to know about calories?

Calories provide energy for your body. If your doctor recommends it, you may need to cut down on the calories you eat. A dietitian can help you plan ways to cut calories in the best possible way.

But some people on dialysis need to gain weight. You may need to find ways to add calories to your diet. Vegetable oils—like olive oil, canola oil, and safflower oil—are good sources of calories. Use them generously on breads, rice, and noodles.

Butter and margarines are rich in calories. But these fatty foods can also clog your arteries. Use them less often. Soft margarine that comes in tubs is better than stick margarine. Vegetable oils are the healthiest way to add fat to your diet if you need to gain weight.

Hard candy, sugar, honey, jam, and jelly provide calories and energy without clogging arteries or adding other things that your body does not need. If you have diabetes, be very careful about eating sweets. A dietitian's guidance is very important for people with diabetes.

Should I take vitamins and minerals?

Vitamins and minerals may be missing from your diet because you have to avoid so many foods. Your doctor may prescribe a vitamin and mineral supplement like Nephrocaps.

Warning: Do not take vitamins that you can buy off the store shelf. They may contain vitamins or minerals that are harmful to you.

Section 48.4

Nutrition and Peritoneal Dialysis

As a patient beginning peritoneal dialysis treatments, you are adjusting to many changes in your daily life. Your doctor has probably told you that some changes in your diet will be necessary.

Why will you have to follow a special diet?

You will have to follow a special diet because your kidneys are not able to get rid of enough waste products and fluids from your body.

It is important that you have the right amounts of protein, calories, vitamins, and minerals in your diet. Your dietitian will help you plan your meals to make sure that you get the proper balance. Here are some general guidelines:

Protein: Your body needs protein for growth, building muscles, and repairing tissue.

After your body uses the protein in the foods you eat, a waste product called urea is left. Since your kidneys are not able to get rid of this urea, you may have too much in your blood. Dialysis and your diet are important to keep the urea level down.

Along with the clearing of urea, your body loses proteins that are normally retained in your blood. You will need to eat more protein to replace what is lost. The type of protein you eat is also very important. High quality protein should be eaten at each meal. It comes from animal sources such as eggs, fish, chicken and meat. Low quality protein needs to be limited in your diet. It comes from plant sources such as vegetables and grains.

Calories: Calories give your body energy. One source of calories is the food you eat. Another source is the sugar in dialysate solution that can affect you because:

- It takes extra fluid out of the body.
- It is taken in by your body.
- It can cause unwanted weight gain.

Potassium: Potassium is a mineral found naturally in foods that is dangerous when you have too much or too little. It is plentiful in dried fruits, dried beans and peas, nuts, meat, milk, fruits and vegetables, and also in salt substitutes. Since both high and low levels of potassium in your body are dangerous to your heart, your potassium level will be watched closely.

Fluid and sodium: Sodium is a mineral that is found naturally in foods and can affect your blood pressure. It is found in large amounts in table salt and in canned foods and processed meats (cold cuts).

With continuous ambulatory peritoneal dialysis (CAPD), you may be able to follow your usual diet. Watching your sodium can help to control your thirst and your weight gain. It may also lower your use of high-sugar solutions. Your doctor will choose the right dialysate for you to control your blood pressure and fluid level.

Phosphorus: Phosphorus is a mineral present in all foods. It is found in large amounts in milk, cheese, nuts, dried beans, and peas.

Eating foods high in phosphorus will raise the phosphorus in your blood and this can cause calcium to be pulled from your bones. This will make your bones weak and cause them to break easily. To help control the phosphorus in your blood, you may need to take medicine called a phosphate binder. It should be taken with your meals and snacks as ordered by your doctor. Your renal dietitian can also tell you about protein foods that are lower in phosphorus.

Vitamins and minerals: The dialysis treatment washes some water-soluble vitamins out of your body. If you are not getting all the vitamins and minerals you need from the foods you eat, vitamin and mineral supplements may be recommended. It is important to take only what is ordered for you. Certain vitamins and minerals can be harmful to persons on dialysis.

Section 48.5

Anemia and Dialysis

"Anemia in Kidney Disease and Dialysis," National Kidney and Urologic Diseases Information Clearinghouse (NKUDIC), a service of the National Institute of Diabetes and Digestive and Kidney Disease (NIDDK), National Institutes of Health (NIH), Pub. No. 05-4619, January 2005.

If your blood is low in red blood cells, you have anemia. Red blood cells carry oxygen (O_2) to tissues and organs throughout your body and enable them to use the energy from food. Without oxygen, these tissues and organs—particularly the heart and brain—may not do their jobs as well as they should. For this reason, if you have anemia, you may tire easily and look pale. Anemia may also contribute to heart problems.

Anemia is common in people with kidney disease. Healthy kidneys produce a hormone called erythropoietin, or EPO, which stimulates the bone marrow to produce the proper number of red blood cells needed to carry oxygen to vital organs. Diseased kidneys, however, often don't make enough EPO. As a result, the bone marrow makes fewer red blood cells. Other common causes of anemia include loss of blood from hemodialysis and low levels of iron and folic acid. These nutrients from food help young red blood cells make hemoglobin (Hgb), their main oxygen-carrying protein.

Laboratory Tests

A complete blood count (CBC), a laboratory test performed on a sample of your blood, includes a determination of your hematocrit (Hct), the percentage of the blood that consists of red blood cells. The CBC also measures the amount of Hgb in your blood. The range of normal Hct and Hgb in women who menstruate is slightly lower than for healthy men or healthy postmenopausal women. The Hgb is usually about one-third the value of the Hct.

When Anemia Begins

Anemia may begin to develop in the early stages of kidney disease, when you still have 20 percent to 50 percent of your normal kidney function. This partial loss of kidney function is often called chronic renal insufficiency. Anemia tends to worsen as kidney disease progresses. End-stage kidney failure, the point at which dialysis or kidney transplantation becomes necessary, doesn't occur until you have only about 10 percent of your kidney function remaining. Nearly everyone with end-stage kidney failure has anemia.

Diagnosis

If you have lost at least half of normal kidney function (based on your glomerular filtration rate calculated using your serum creatinine measurement) and have a low Hct, the most likely cause of anemia is decreased EPO production. The National Kidney Foundation's Dialysis Outcomes Quality Initiative (DOQI) recommends that doctors begin a detailed evaluation of anemia in men and postmenopausal women on dialysis when the Hct value falls below 37 percent. For women of childbearing age, evaluation should begin when the Hct falls below 33 percent. The evaluation will include tests for iron deficiency and blood loss in the stool to be certain there are no other reasons for the anemia.

Treatment

EPO: If no other cause for EPO deficiency is found, it can be treated with a genetically engineered form of the hormone, which is usually injected under the skin two or three times a week. Hemodialysis patients who can't tolerate EPO shots may receive the hormone intravenously during treatment, but this method requires a larger, more expensive dose and may not be as effective. DOQI recommends that patients treated with EPO therapy should achieve a target Hgb of 11 to 12 g/dL.

Iron: Many people with kidney disease need both EPO and iron supplements to raise their Hct to a satisfactory level. If your iron levels are too low, EPO won't help and you'll continue to experience the effects of anemia. You may be able to take an iron pill, but many studies show that iron pills don't work as well in people with kidney failure as iron given intravenously. Iron is injected directly into an arm or into the tube that returns blood to your body during hemodialysis.

A nurse or doctor will give you a test dose because a very small number of people (less than one percent) have a bad reaction to iron injections. If you begin to wheeze or have trouble breathing, your healthcare provider can administer epinephrine or corticosteroids to counter the reaction. Even though the risk is small, you'll be asked to sign a form stating that you understand the possible reaction and that you agree to have the treatment. Talk with your healthcare provider if you have any questions.

In addition to measuring your Hct and Hgb, your tests will also include two measurements to show whether you have enough iron.

- Your ferritin level indicates the amount of iron stored in your body. According to DOQI guidelines, your ferritin score should be no less than 100 micrograms per liter (mcg/L) and no more than 800 mcg/L.

- TSAT stands for transferrin saturation, a score that indicates how much iron is available to make red blood cells. DOQI guidelines call for a TSAT score between 20 percent and 50 percent.

Other Causes of Anemia

In addition to EPO and iron, a few people may also need vitamin B_{12} and folic acid supplements.

If EPO, iron, vitamin B_{12}, and folic acid all fail, your doctor should look for other causes such as sickle cell disease or an inflammatory problem. At one time, aluminum poisoning contributed to anemia in people with kidney failure because many phosphate binders used to treat bone disease caused by kidney failure were antacids that contained aluminum. But aluminum-free alternatives are now widely available. Be sure your phosphate binder and your other drugs are free of aluminum.

Anemia keeps many people with kidney disease from feeling their best. But EPO treatments help most patients raise their Hgb, feel better, live longer, and have more energy.

Section 48.6

Renal Osteodystrophy

National Kidney and Urologic Diseases Information Clearinghouse (NKUDIC), a service of the National Institute of Diabetes and Digestive and Kidney Diseases (NIDDK), National Institutes of Health (NIH), Pub. No. 05-4630, January 2005.

The medical term "renal" describes things related to the kidneys. Renal osteodystrophy is a bone disease that occurs when your kidneys fail to maintain the proper levels of calcium and phosphorus in your blood. It's a common problem in people with kidney disease and affects 90 percent of dialysis patients.

Renal osteodystrophy is most serious in children because their bones are still growing. The condition slows bone growth and causes deformities. One such deformity occurs when the legs bend inward or outward (toward or away from the body); this deformity is referred to as "renal rickets." Another important consequence is short stature. Symptoms can be seen in growing children with renal disease even before they start dialysis.

The bone changes from renal osteodystrophy can begin many years before symptoms appear in adults with kidney disease. For this reason, it's called the "silent crippler." The symptoms of renal osteodystrophy aren't usually seen in adults until they have been on dialysis for several years. Older patients and women who have gone through menopause are at greater risk for this disease because they're already vulnerable to osteoporosis, another bone disease, even without kidney disease. If left untreated, the bones gradually become thin and weak, and a person with renal osteodystrophy may begin to feel bone and joint pain. There's also an increased risk of bone fractures.

Hormones and Minerals

In healthy adults, bone tissue is continually being remodeled and rebuilt. The kidneys play an important role in maintaining healthy bone mass and structure because one of their jobs is to balance calcium and phosphorus levels in the blood.

Calcium is a mineral that builds and strengthens bones. It's found in many foods, particularly milk and other dairy products. If calcium levels in the blood become too low, four small glands in the neck called the parathyroid glands release a hormone called parathyroid hormone (PTH). This hormone draws calcium from the bones to raise blood calcium levels. Too much PTH in the blood will remove too much calcium from the bones; over time, the constant removal of calcium weakens the bones.

Phosphorus, which is found in most foods, also helps regulate calcium levels in the bones. Healthy kidneys remove excess phosphorus from the blood. When the kidneys stop working normally, phosphorus levels in the blood can become too high, leading to lower levels of calcium in the blood and resulting in the loss of calcium from the bones.

Healthy kidneys produce calcitriol, a form of vitamin D, to help the body absorb dietary calcium into the blood and the bones. If calcitriol levels drop too low, PTH levels increase, and calcium is removed from the bones. Calcitriol and PTH work together to keep calcium balance normal and bones healthy. In a patient with kidney failure, the kidneys stop making calcitriol. The body then can't absorb calcium from food and starts removing it from the bones.

Diagnosis

To diagnose renal osteodystrophy, your doctor may take a sample of your blood to measure levels of calcium, phosphorus, PTH, and calcitriol. The doctor may perform a bone biopsy to see how dense your bones are. A bone biopsy is done under local anesthesia and involves removing a small sample of bone from the hip and analyzing it under a microscope. Determining the cause of renal osteodystrophy helps the doctor decide on a course of treatment.

Treatment

Controlling PTH levels prevents calcium from being withdrawn from the bones. Usually, overactive parathyroid glands are controllable with a change in diet, dialysis treatment, or medication. The drug cinacalcet hydrochloride (Sensipar), approved by the Food and Drug Administration in 2004, lowers PTH levels by imitating calcium. If PTH levels can't be controlled, the parathyroid glands may need to be removed surgically.

If your kidneys aren't making adequate amounts of calcitriol, you can take synthetic calcitriol as a pill or in an injectable form. Your doctor may prescribe a calcium supplement in addition to calcitriol.

Renal osteodystrophy can also be treated with changes in diet. Reducing dietary intake of phosphorus is one of the most important steps in preventing bone disease. Almost all foods contain phosphorus, but it's especially high in milk, cheese, dried beans, peas, nuts, and peanut butter. Limit drinks such as cocoa, dark sodas, and beer. Often, medications such as calcium carbonate (Tums), calcium acetate (PhosLo), sevelamer hydrochloride (Renagel), or lanthanum carbonate (Fosrenol) are prescribed with meals and snacks to bind phosphorus in the bowel. These decrease the absorption of phosphorus into the blood. Be sure your phosphate binder is aluminum-free because aluminum can be toxic and cause anemia. A renal dietitian can help develop a dietary plan to control phosphorus levels in the blood.

Exercise has been found to increase bone strength in some patients. It's important, however, to consult a doctor or healthcare professional before beginning any exercise program.

A good treatment program, including proper attention to dialysis, diet, and medications, can improve your body's ability to repair bones damaged by renal osteodystrophy.

Chapter 49

Facts about Kidney Transplants

If you have advanced and permanent kidney failure, kidney transplantation may be the treatment option that allows you to live much like you lived before your kidneys failed. Since the 1950s, when the first kidney transplants were performed, we've learned much about how to prevent rejection and minimize the side effects of medicines.

But transplantation is not a cure; it's an ongoing treatment that requires you to take medicines for the rest of your life. And the wait for a donated kidney can be years long.

A successful transplant takes a coordinated effort from your whole healthcare team, including your nephrologist, transplant surgeon, transplant coordinator, pharmacist, dietitian, and social worker. But the most important members of your healthcare team are you and your family. By learning about your treatment, you can work with your healthcare team to give yourself the best possible results, and you can lead a full, active life.

When Your Kidneys Fail

Healthy kidneys clean your blood by removing excess fluid, minerals, and wastes. They also make hormones that keep your bones strong and your blood healthy. When your kidneys fail, harmful wastes build

"Treatment Methods for Kidney Failure: Transplantation," National Kidney and Urologic Diseases Information Clearinghouse (NKUDIC), a service of the National Institute of Diabetes and Digestive and Kidney Diseases (NIDDK), National Institutes of Health (NIH), Pub. No. 03-4687, September 2003.

up in your body, your blood pressure may rise, and your body may retain excess fluid and not make enough red blood cells. When this happens, you need treatment to replace the work of your failed kidneys.

How Transplantation Works

Kidney transplantation is a procedure that places a healthy kidney from another person into your body. This one new kidney takes over the work of your two failed kidneys.

A surgeon places the new kidney inside your lower abdomen and connects the artery and vein of the new kidney to your artery and vein. Your blood flows through the new kidney, which makes urine, just like your own kidneys did when they were healthy. Unless they are causing infection or high blood pressure, your own kidneys are left in place.

The Transplant Process

Your Doctor's Recommendation

The transplantation process begins when you learn that your kidneys are failing and you must start to consider your treatment options. Whether transplantation is to be among your options will depend on your specific situation. Transplantation isn't for everyone. Your doctor may tell you that you have a condition that would make transplantation dangerous or unlikely to succeed.

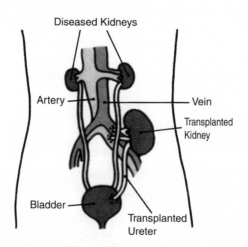

Figure 49.1. *Kidney Transplantation.*

Medical Evaluation at a Transplant Center

If your doctor sees transplantation as an option, the next step is a thorough medical evaluation at a transplant hospital. The pre-transplant evaluation may require several visits over the course of several weeks or even months. You'll need to have blood drawn and x-rays taken. You'll be tested for blood type and other matching factors that determine whether your body will accept an available kidney.

The medical team will want to see whether you're healthy enough for surgery. Cancer, a serious infection, or significant cardiovascular disease would make transplantation unlikely to succeed. In addition, the medical team will want to make sure that you can understand and follow the schedule for taking medicines.

If a family member or friend wants to donate a kidney, he or she will need to be evaluated for general health and to see whether the kidney is a good match. (See the "Organ Donation" section.)

Placement on the Waiting List

If the medical evaluation shows that you're a good candidate for a transplant but you don't have a family member or friend who can donate a kidney, you'll be put on the transplant program's waiting list to receive a kidney from someone who has just died. You may hear your healthcare team refer to this as a cadaveric kidney.

Every person waiting for a cadaveric organ is registered with the Organ Procurement and Transplantation Network (OPTN), which maintains a centralized computer network linking all regional organ gathering organizations (known as organ procurement organizations, or OPOs) and transplant centers. The United Network for Organ Sharing (UNOS), a private nonprofit organization, administers OPTN under a contract with the federal government. (See the "Resources" section.)

UNOS rules allow patients to register with multiple transplant centers. Each transplant center will probably require a separate medical evaluation, even if a patient is already registered at another center.

Some observers of OPTN operations have raised the concern that people in some parts of the country have to wait longer than others because allocation policies for some organs give preference to patients within the donor's region. Kidneys, however, are assigned to the best match regardless of geographic region. The federal government continues to monitor policies and regulations to ensure that every person waiting for an organ has a fair chance. Everyone agrees that the key to making waiting times shorter is to increase the number of donated organs.

Waiting Period

How long you'll have to wait depends on many things, but is primarily determined by the degree of matching between you and the donor. Some people wait several years for a good match, while others get matched within a few months.

While you're on the waiting list, notify the transplant center of any changes in your health. Also, let the transplant center know if you move or change telephone numbers. The center will need to find you immediately when a kidney becomes available.

OPOs are responsible for identifying potential organs for transplant and coordinating with the national network. The 69 regional OPOs are all UNOS members. When a cadaveric kidney becomes available, the OPO notifies UNOS, and a computer-generated list of suitable recipients is created. Suitability is initially based on two factors:

- **Blood type:** Your blood type (A, B, AB, or O) must be compatible with the donor's blood type.

- **HLA factors:** HLA stands for human leukocyte antigen, a genetic marker located on the surface of your white blood cells. You inherit a set of three antigens from your mother and three from your father. A higher number of matching antigens increases the chances that your new kidney will last for a long time.

If you're selected on the basis of the first two factors, a third is evaluated:

- **Antibodies:** Your immune system may produce antibodies that act specifically against something in the donor's tissues. To see whether this is the case, a small sample of your blood will be mixed with a small sample of the donor's blood in a tube. If no reaction occurs, you should be able to accept the kidney. Your transplant team might use the term negative cross-match to describe this lack of reaction.

Transplant Operation

If you have a living donor, you'll schedule the operation in advance. You and your donor will be operated on at the same time, usually in side-by-side rooms. One team of surgeons will perform the nephrectomy—that is, the removal of the kidney from the donor—while another prepares the recipient for placement of the donated kidney.

If you're on a waiting list for a cadaveric kidney, you must be ready to hurry to the hospital as soon as a kidney becomes available. Once there, you'll give a blood sample for the antibody cross-match test. If you have a negative cross-match, it means that your antibodies don't react and the transplantation can proceed.

You'll be given a general anesthetic to make you sleep during the operation, which usually takes three or four hours. The surgeon will make a small cut in your lower abdomen. The artery and vein from the new kidney will be attached to your artery and vein. The ureter from the new kidney will be connected to your bladder.

Often, the new kidney will start making urine as soon as your blood starts flowing through it, but sometimes a few weeks pass before it starts working.

Recovery from Surgery

As after any major surgery, you'll probably feel sore and groggy when you wake up. However, many transplant recipients report feeling much better immediately after surgery. Even if you wake up feeling great, you'll need to stay in the hospital for about a week to recover from surgery, and longer if you have any complications.

Post-Transplant Care

Your body's immune system is designed to keep you healthy by sensing "foreign invaders," such as bacteria, and rejecting them. But your immune system will also sense that your new kidney is foreign. To keep your body from rejecting it, you'll have to take drugs that turn off, or suppress, your immune response. You may have to take two or more of these immunosuppressant medicines, as well as other medications to treat other health problems. Your healthcare team will help you learn what each pill is for and when to take it. Be sure that you understand the instructions for taking your medicines before you leave the hospital.

If you've been on hemodialysis, you'll find that your post-transplant diet is much less restrictive. You can drink more fluids and eat many of the fruits and vegetables you were previously told to avoid. You may even need to gain a little weight, but be careful not to gain too much weight too quickly and avoid salty foods that can lead to high blood pressure. Work with your clinic's dietitian to make sure you're following a healthy eating plan.

Rejection

You can help prevent rejection by taking your medicines and following your diet, but watching for signs of rejection—like fever or soreness in the area of the new kidney or a change in the amount of urine you make—is important. Report any such changes to your healthcare team.

Even if you do everything you're supposed to do, your body may still reject the new kidney and you may need to go back on dialysis. Unless your healthcare team determines that you're no longer a good candidate for transplantation, you can go back on the waiting list for another kidney.

Side Effects of Immunosuppressants

Immunosuppressants can weaken your immune system, which can lead to infections. Some drugs may also change your appearance. Your face may get fuller; you may gain weight or develop acne or facial hair. Not all patients have these problems, though, and diet and makeup can help.

Immunosuppressants work by diminishing the ability of immune cells to function. In some patients, over long periods of time, this diminished immunity can increase the risk of developing cancer. Some immunosuppressants cause cataracts, diabetes, extra stomach acid, high blood pressure, and bone disease. When used over time, these drugs may also cause liver or kidney damage in a few patients.

Financial Issues

Treatment for kidney failure is expensive, but federal health insurance plans pay much of the cost, usually up to 80 percent. Often, private insurance or state programs pay the rest. Your social worker can help you locate resources for financial assistance. [For more information, see Chapter 50, "Financial Information for Dialysis and Transplant Patients," which is a reprint of the National Institute of Diabetes and Digestive and Kidney Diseases (NIDDK) fact sheet.]

Patient Assistance Programs from Prescription Drug Companies

The immunosuppressants and other drugs you must take after your transplant will be a large part of your medical expenses. Most drug manufacturers have patient assistance programs giving discounts to patients who can show that they can't afford the cost of their prescribed medications. The Pharmaceutical Research and Manufacturers of America (PhRMA) publishes the *Directory of PhRMA Member Company Patient Assistance Programs*, which is available for download at https://www.pparx.org/PPA_Directory.pdf on the internet. To request a directory through the mail, contact PhRMA.

Pharmaceutical Research and Manufacturers of America
1100 Fifteenth Street NW
Washington, DC 20005
Phone: 202-835-3400
Fax: 202-835-3414
Website: http://www.phrma.org

An organization called the Medicine Program offers help in finding and applying for free medicines supplied by pharmaceutical companies. To request assistance, obtain an application form, available on the website or through the mail, and list the medicines you need. Send the application back with a $5 processing fee for each medicine you request. If the Medicine Program fails to qualify you to receive the medicine, your processing fee will be returned.

The Medicine Program
P.O. Box 1089
Poplar Bluff, MO 63901-1089
Toll-Free: 866-694-3893
Website: http://www.themedicineprogram.com

Additional Patient Assistance Programs

UNOS maintains a website called Transplant Living to help patients learn about their treatment and find resources. The website includes a page that lists organizations that provide financial assistance. That page can be found at http://www.transplantliving.org/beforethetransplant/finance/funding.aspx on the internet.

Organ Donation

Deceased Donor

Most transplanted kidneys come from people who have died. However, the number of people waiting for kidneys has increased in recent years, while the number of kidneys available from deceased donors has remained constant. The result is a shortage of kidneys and a longer waiting time for people with kidney failure.

Many suitable kidneys go unused because family members of potential donors don't know their loved one's wishes. People who wish to donate their organs should talk about this issue with their families. Several organizations, including UNOS and the National Kidney Foundation (see the "Resources" section), provide organ donor cards for people who wish to make this life-preserving gift when they die. A properly completed organ donor card notifies medical officials that you've decided to donate your organs. In most states, you can indicate your desire to be an organ donor on your driver's license.

Living Donor

A growing number of transplanted kidneys are donated by living family members or friends. Potential donors need to be tested to make sure that donating a kidney won't endanger their health, as well as for matching factors. Most people, however, can donate a kidney with little risk.

A kidney from a living donor often has advantages over a deceased donor kidney:

- People who receive a kidney from a family member or friend don't have to wait until a kidney becomes available. Living donation allows for greater preparation and for the operation to be scheduled at a convenient time.

- Kidneys from family members are more likely to be good matches, although there's no guarantee.

- Kidneys from living donors don't need to be transported from one site to another, so the kidney is in better condition when it's transplanted.

- Living donation helps people waiting for kidneys from deceased donors by lowering the number of people on the waiting list.

Minority Donation

Diseases of the kidney are found more frequently in racial and ethnic minority populations in the United States than in the general population. African Americans, Asian Americans, Hispanic Americans, and Pacific Islander Americans are three times more likely to suffer from kidney failure than Americans of European descent. Successful transplantation is often enhanced if organs are matched between members of the same ethnic and racial group. A shortage of organs donated by minorities can contribute to longer waiting periods for transplants for minorities.

The National Minority Organ/Tissue Transplant Education Program (MOTTEP), with the support of the National Institutes of Health's (NIH's) Office of Research on Minority Health and NIDDK, is the first national program to empower minority communities to promote minority donation and transplantation, as well as good health habits. In turn, this effort should improve the chances for a well-matched organ among all those waiting for a transplant. [For information on MOTTEP and other issues related to organ and tissue donation, see http://www.healthgap.omhrc.gov/otdonation.htm.]

Resources

Government Agencies

A number of federal agencies are involved in various aspects of transplantation, including financing, procurement regulation and oversight, allocation policy development, donation promotion, and biomedical research.

The Centers for Medicare and Medicaid Services runs the Medicare and Medicaid programs. You can apply for Medicare through your local Social Security office. The national phone number for the Social Security Administration is 800-772-1213, and you can get additional information about Medicare health plans by calling 800-633-4227 (800-MEDICARE). The official U.S. government website for Medicare information can be found at http://www.medicare.gov on the internet.

The U.S. Department of Health and Human Services coordinates organ procurement and allocation activities through its Health Resources and Services Administration (HRSA).

Health Resources and Services Administration
Division of Transplantation
Room 16C-17, Parklawn Building
5600 Fishers Lane
Rockville, MD 20857
Phone: 301-443-7577
Website: http://www.hrsa.gov
E-mail: comments@hrsa.gov

HRSA also maintains a website devoted to organ donation at http://www.organdonor.gov on the internet.

HRSA's Division of Transplantation administers the OPTN through a contract with UNOS, whose website can be found at http://www.transplantliving.org on the internet. You can request a packet of information about kidney transplantation by calling UNOS at 888-894-6361 (888-TX-INFO-1).

Non-Government Organizations

Many national organizations—including government agencies, private foundations, and commercial industries—have joined the Coalition on Donation to promote organ and tissue donation through educational programs and campaigns conducted nationally and at the local level.

Coalition on Donation
700 North 4th Street
Richmond, VA 23219
Phone: 804-782-4920
Fax: 804-782-4643
Website: http://www.shareyourlife.org
E-mail: coalition@donatelife.net

TransWeb: All About Transplantation and Donation is a non-profit educational website (http://www.transweb.org) featuring answers to frequently asked questions, donor memorials, patient experiences, and a reference section.

Chapter 50

Financial Information for Dialysis and Transplant Patients

Chapter Contents

Section 50.1

Medicare Coverage of Kidney Dialysis and Kidney Transplant Services

Excerpted from "Medicare Coverage of Kidney Dialysis and Kidney Transplant Services," the U.S. Department of Health and Human Services, Centers for Medicare and Medicaid Services, Baltimore, MD. Pub. No. CMS-10128. Revised November 2004.

Introduction

This text explains how Medicare helps pay for kidney dialysis and kidney transplant services in the Original Medicare Plan, also known as "fee-for-service." [For more details on Medicare coverage please refer to the Centers for Medicare and Medicaid Services Publication No. CMS-10128 available for download online at http://www.medicare .gov/publications/pubs/pdf/10128.pdf or by calling 800-MEDICARE (800-633-4227). TTY users should call 877-486-2048.]

Medicare for People with Kidney Failure

Who Is Eligible?

You can get Medicare Part A no matter how old you are if your kidneys no longer work and you need regular dialysis or have had a kidney transplant, and:

- You have worked the required amount of time under Social Security, the Railroad Retirement Board, or as a government employee; or

- You are getting or are eligible for Social Security, Office of Personnel Management, or Railroad Retirement benefits; or

- You are the spouse or dependent child of a person who has worked the required amount of time under Social Security, the Railroad Retirement Board, or as a government employee or who is getting Social Security, Office of Personnel Management, or Railroad Retirement benefits.

550

If you get Medicare Part A you can also get Medicare Part B. Enrolling in Part B is your choice. You will need both Part A and Part B in order for Medicare to cover certain dialysis and kidney transplant services.

How to Sign Up for Medicare

If you need Medicare because of ESRD (permanent kidney failure), you can enroll in Medicare Part A and Part B based on ESRD at your local Social Security office. Call or visit your local Social Security office or call Social Security at 800-772-1213 to make an appointment to enroll in Medicare based on ESRD.

When Medicare Coverage Begins

When you enroll in Medicare based on ESRD (permanent kidney failure) and you are on dialysis, your Medicare coverage usually starts the fourth month of dialysis treatments. For example, if you start getting your hemodialysis treatments in July, your Medicare coverage would start on October 1. If you are covered by an employer group health plan, your Medicare coverage will still start the fourth month of dialysis treatments. Your employer group health plan will pay first on your healthcare bills and Medicare will pay second for a 30-month coordination period.

Important: Medicare will not cover surgery or other services that are needed to prepare for dialysis (such as surgery for a blood access) if it is done before Medicare coverage begins.

When Medicare Coverage Ends

If you have Medicare only because of kidney failure, your Medicare coverage will end:

- 12 months after the month you stop dialysis treatments, or
- 36 months after the month you have a successful kidney transplant.

Your Medicare coverage will not end if:

- You have to start dialysis again or you get a kidney transplant within 12 months after the month you stopped getting dialysis, or
- You start dialysis or get another kidney transplant within 36 months after a transplant.

Important: Remember, in order for Medicare to pay for kidney dialysis and some transplant services, you need both Medicare Part A and Part B. If you don't pay your Medicare Part B premium or if you choose to cancel it, your Medicare Part B will end.

Kidney Dialysis Services

Where to Get Dialysis Treatments

Dialysis can be done at home or in a medical facility. In order for Medicare to pay for your treatments, the facility must be approved to provide dialysis (even if they already provide other Medicare-covered healthcare services).

At the dialysis facility, a nurse or a trained technician may give you the treatment. At home, you can treat yourself with the help of a family member or friend. If you decide to do home dialysis, you and your helper will get special training.

How to Find a Dialysis Facility

In most cases, the facility your kidney doctor works with is where you will get dialysis treatments. However, you have the right to choose to get your treatments from another facility at any time. Keep in mind, this could mean changing doctors. You can also call your local ESRD Network to find a facility that is close to you. [See "End-stage Renal Disease (ESRD) Networks" at the end of this section.]

What You Pay for Dialysis Services

Dialysis in a hospital: If you are admitted to a hospital and get dialysis, your treatments will be covered by Medicare Part A as part of the costs of your covered in-patient hospital stay.

Self-dialysis training: Self-dialysis training is covered by Medicare Part B on an outpatient basis. Self-dialysis training costs more than dialysis treatments. The costs may be different from one dialysis facility to another, depending on the type of facility and where it's located.

Home dialysis: You have two payment options for home dialysis.

- *Dealing with your dialysis facility (Method 1):* Under Method 1, you must get all services, equipment, and supplies needed for home dialysis from your dialysis facility.

- *Dealing directly with a supplier (Method 2):* Under Method 2, you must get your dialysis equipment and supplies from one supplier. Your supplier must accept assignment. This means that if you are in the Original Medicare Plan, your supplier agrees to accept Medicare's fee as full payment. Your supplier must also

Table 50.1. Method 1 and Method 2 Payment Chart for Home Dialysis Equipment, Supplies, and Support Services in the Original Medicare Plan

Home Dialysis Equipment

Dealing with your dialysis facility (Method 1)

Medicare pays 80% of the facility's composite rate. You pay the 20% coinsurance.

Dealing directly with a supplier (Method 2)

If you buy or rent home dialysis equipment, Medicare Part B will cover it. You must pay the $110 Part B yearly deductible (see note below). Medicare Part B usually makes monthly payments.

If you buy the equipment, Medicare will pay 80% of the monthly payment purchase price. You pay the 20% coinsurance. The monthly Part B payment includes any interest or carrying charges.

If you rent the equipment, Medicare Part B pays 80% of the approved monthly rental charge. You pay the 20% coinsurance.

Home Dialysis Supplies

Dealing with your dialysis facility (Method 1)

Medicare pays 80% of the facility's composite rate. You pay the 20% coinsurance.

Dealing directly with a supplier (Method 2)

After you pay the $110 Part B yearly deductible (see note below), Medicare Part B pays 80% of the approved charges for all covered supplies. You pay the 20% coinsurance.

Home Dialysis Support Services

Dealing with your dialysis facility (Method 1)

Medicare pays 80% of the facility's composite rate. You pay the 20% coinsurance.

Dealing directly with a supplier (Method 2)

After you pay the $110 Part B yearly deductible (see note below), Medicare Part B pays the facility 80% of the approved charges for all covered services. You pay 20% coinsurance.

*Each year, you pay a total of one $110 Part B deductible.

have a written agreement with a dialysis facility to make sure that you will get all necessary home dialysis support services.

Under both Method 1 and Method 2, you must get your support services from your dialysis facility in order for Medicare to pay. Medicare will pay the facility directly for these services.

Home Dialysis Drugs Covered by Medicare

The most common drugs that Medicare Part B covers for home dialysis are:

- heparin,
- the antidote for heparin when medically necessary,
- topical anesthetics, and
- Epogen or Epoetin alfa.

How Long Will Medicare Pay for Home Dialysis Equipment?

Medicare Part B will pay for home dialysis equipment as long as you need dialysis at home. If you no longer need home dialysis, Part B will stop paying. For example, if you had a kidney transplant and no longer need home dialysis, then Part B would stop paying for your equipment.

If you buy your dialysis equipment, Part B payments will stop once the Medicare-approved purchase price is reached. For example, if Medicare agrees to pay $200 for your dialysis equipment, Part B payments will stop once Medicare pays $200.

Kidney Transplant Services

Where to Get a Kidney Transplant

Your kidney transplant must be done in a hospital that is approved by Medicare to do kidney transplants. **Note:** Medicare doesn't pay for the actual kidneys for a transplant. Buying or selling human organs is against the law.

Transplant Drugs (Called Immunosuppressive Drugs)

Immunosuppressive drugs are transplant drugs used to reduce the risk of your body rejecting your new kidney after your transplant. You will need to take these drugs for the rest of your life.

What if I Stop Taking My Transplant Drugs?

If you stop taking them, your body may reject your new kidney and the kidney could stop working. If that happens, you may have to start dialysis again. Talk to your doctor before you stop taking your transplant drugs.

How Long Will Medicare Pay for Transplant Drugs?

If you have Medicare only because of kidney failure, your Medicare will end 36 months after the month of the transplant.

Medicare will not pay for any services, including immunosuppressive drugs, for patients who are not entitled to Medicare. If you already had Medicare because of age or disability before you got ESRD, or if you became eligible for Medicare because of age or disability after receiving a transplant that was paid for by Medicare, or paid for by private insurance that paid primary to your Medicare Part A coverage, in a Medicare-certified facility, Medicare will continue to pay for your immunosuppressive drugs with no time limit.

What If I Can't Pay for the Transplant Drug?

Transplant drugs can be very costly. If you have Medicare because of kidney failure, your immunosuppressive drugs are only covered for 36 months after the month of the transplant. If you are worried about paying for them, talk to your doctor, nurse, or social worker. There may be other ways to help you pay for these drugs.

Do I Have to Pay for My Kidney Donor?

No. Medicare will pay the full cost of care for your kidney donor. There is no deductible, coinsurance, or other costs that you have to pay for your donor's hospital stay.

Where to Get More Information

End-Stage Renal Disease (ESRD) Networks

You can call your local ESRD Network Organization to get information about:

- Dialysis or kidney transplants.
- How to get help from other kidney-related agencies.

- Problems with your facility that are not solved after talking to the staff at the facility.

- Location of dialysis facilities and transplant centers.

Your ESRD Network makes sure that you are getting the best possible care, and uses mailings to keep your facility aware of important issues about kidney dialysis and transplants. To get the most updated phone numbers, call 800-MEDICARE (800-633-4227). TTY users should call 877-486-2048. Or, look on the web at http://www.medicare.gov/Contacts/Home.asp.

State Health Insurance Assistance Program (SHIP)

Call your State Health Insurance Assistance Program if you have questions about:

- Medigap Policies.

- Medicare health plan choices.

- Help with filing an appeal.

- Other general health insurance questions.

For the most up-to-date contact information for your state, go to the "Helpful Contacts" section of the Medicare website at http://www.medicare.gov/Contacts/Home.asp.

Section 50.2

Medigap Policies for People under Age 65 with a Disability or End-Stage Renal Disease

"Medigap Policies for People under Age 65 with a Disability or End-Stage Renal Disease (ESRD)," Department of Health and Human Services, Centers for Medicare and Medicaid Services, Baltimore, MD. Updated December 9, 2004.

You may have Medicare before age 65 due to the following:

- A disability, or

- ESRD (permanent kidney failure requiring dialysis or a kidney transplant)

If you are under age 65 and disabled or have ESRD, you may not be able to buy the Medigap policy you want until you turn 65. Federal law doesn't require insurance companies to sell Medigap policies to people under age 65. However, some states require insurance companies to sell you a policy, at certain times, even if you are under age 65.

During the first six months after you turn age 65 and are enrolled in Medicare Part B, you will get a Medigap open enrollment period. It doesn't matter that you have had Medicare Part B before you turned age 65. During this time:

- You can buy any Medigap policy (including those policies that help pay the cost of prescription drugs), and

- Insurance companies cannot refuse to sell you a Medigap policy due to a disability or other health problem, or charge you a higher premium than they charge other people who are 65 years old.

When you buy a policy during your Medigap open enrollment period, the insurance company must shorten the waiting period for pre-existing conditions by the amount of creditable coverage you have. If you had Medicare for more than six months before you turned 65 years old, you won't have a pre-existing condition waiting period because Medicare counts as creditable coverage.

Several states require Medigap insurance companies to offer a limited Medigap open enrollment period for people with Medicare Part B who are under age 65. The following states require insurance companies to offer at least one kind of Medigap policy during a special open enrollment period to people with Medicare under age 65:

- California
- Connecticut
- Kansas
- Louisiana
- Maine
- Maryland
- Massachusetts
- Michigan
- Minnesota
- Missouri
- Mississippi

- New Hampshire
- New Jersey
- New York
- North Carolina
- Oklahoma
- Oregon
- Pennsylvania
- South Dakota
- Texas
- Washington
- Wisconsin

Also, some insurance companies will sell Medigap policies to people with Medicare under age 65. However, these policies may cost you more. Remember, if you live in a state that has a Medigap open enrollment period for people under age 65, you will still get another Medigap open enrollment period when you turn age 65.

If you join a Medicare Advantage Plan (formerly Medicare + Choice) and your coverage ends, you may have the right to buy a Medigap policy. If you have questions, you should call your State Health Insurance Assistance Program.

Right to Suspend a Medigap Policy for Disabled People with Medicare

If you are under 65, have Medicare, and have a Medigap policy, you have a right to suspend your Medigap policy. You can suspend your Medigap policy benefits and premiums, without penalty, while you are enrolled in your or your spouse's employer group health plan.

If, for any reason, you lose your employer group health plan coverage, you can get your Medigap policy back. You must notify your

Medigap insurance company that you want your Medigap policy back within 90 days of losing your employer group health plan coverage.

Your Medigap benefits and premiums will start again on the day your employer group health plan coverage stops. The Medigap policy must have the same benefits and premiums it would have had if you had never suspended your coverage. Your Medigap insurance company can't refuse to cover care for any pre-existing conditions you have. So, if you are disabled and working, you can enjoy the benefits of your employer's insurance without giving up your Medigap policy.

Section 50.3

Financial Help for Treatment of Kidney Failure

National Kidney and Urologic Diseases Information Clearinghouse (NKUDIC), a service of the National Institute of Diabetes an Digestive and Kidney Diseases (NIDDK), National Institutes of Health (NIH), Pub. No. 05-4765, February 2005.

If you have permanent kidney failure, you may be worried about paying for the expensive treatments you need.

In 1972, Congress passed legislation making people of any age with permanent kidney failure eligible for Medicare, a program that helps people over 65 and people with disabilities pay for medical care, usually up to 80 percent. Other public and private resources can help with the remaining 20 percent. Your dialysis or transplant center has a social worker who can help you locate and apply for financial assistance.

Medicare

Medicare is a federally administered health insurance program for people 65 and older and people of any age with permanent kidney failure. To qualify for Medicare on the basis of kidney failure, you must need regular dialysis or have had a kidney transplant; and you must have worked under Social Security, the Railroad Retirement Board, or as a government employee (or be the child or spouse of someone who has), or you must already be receiving Social Security or Railroad Retirement benefits. You can enroll for Medicare at your local Social Security office (check the blue pages in your phone directory to locate the office). [For more information on Medicare's coverage for kidney dialysis and transplant services, see section 50.1.]

Contact your local Social Security office or call the nationwide toll-free number at 800-772-1213 if you want to apply for Medicare. Often, the social worker at your hospital or dialysis center will help you apply.

Private Insurance

Private insurance frequently pays for the entire cost of treatment. Or it may pay for the 20 percent that Medicare doesn't cover. Private insurance may also pay for your prescription drugs. Read your private health insurance policy carefully to make sure it covers kidney failure. Talk with your insurance agent or company benefits counselor if you have any questions about your benefits.

Medicaid

Medicaid is a state program. Your income must be below a certain level to receive Medicaid funds. If you aren't eligible for Medicare, Medicaid may pay for your treatments. In some states, it pays the 20 percent that Medicare doesn't cover. It may also pay for some of your medicines. To apply for Medicaid, talk with your social worker or contact your local department of human services or social services.

State Children's Health Insurance Program

The U.S. Department of Health and Human Services has established the State Children's Health Insurance Program (SCHIP) to help children without health insurance. SCHIP provides health coverage for children whose families earn too much to qualify for Medicaid but too little to afford private health insurance. Consumers can obtain information about the program by calling toll-free 877-KIDS-NOW (543-7669), or by checking http://www.insurekidsnow.gov.

Department of Veterans Affairs (VA) Benefits

If you're a veteran, the VA can help pay for treatment or provide other benefits. Contact your local VA office for more information, or call 800-827-1000 to reach the national office. If you're retired from the military, you may also call the Department of Defense at 800-538-9552.

Social Security Disability Income (SSDI) and Supplemental Security Income (SSI)

These benefits from the Social Security Administration help you with the costs of daily living. To receive Social Security Disability Income (SSDI), you must be unable to work and have earned the required number of work credits.

You can receive Supplemental Security Income (SSI) if you don't own much and have a low income. People who get SSI usually get food stamps and Medicaid, too. To find out if you qualify for SSDI and SSI, talk to your social worker or call your local Social Security office or the nationwide number, 800-772-1213.

Patient Assistance Programs from Prescription Drug Companies

Medicare pays for erythropoietin to treat anemia in kidney failure and for immunosuppressants to prevent rejection of a transplanted kidney. But other self-administered drugs that you need may not be covered by Medicare. If you have trouble paying for all the medications your doctor prescribes, you may qualify for assistance from private programs. Most drug manufacturers have patient assistance programs giving discounts to patients who can show that they can't afford the cost of their prescribed medications.

The Partnership for Prescription Assistance provides a website that directs patients, caregivers, and doctors to more than 275 public and private patient assistance programs, including more than 150 programs offered by pharmaceutical companies. The website features an application wizard that helps determine which programs might be available to you. The web address is https://www.pparx.org/Intro.php.

Additional Patient Assistance Programs

The United Network for Organ Sharing (UNOS) offers a website called Transplant Living, which includes a section on financing a transplant. The web address is http://www.transplantliving.org/before thetransplant/finance/finance.aspx. [For more information about UNOS, see Chapter 49, "Facts about Kidney Transplants," which is a reprint of the National Institute of Diabetes and Digestive and Kidney Diseases (NIDDK) booklet "Treatment Methods for Kidney Failure: Kidney Transplantation" or go to the UNOS listing in Chapter 53, "Directory of Urinary and Kidney Disorders Organizations."]

Part Eight

Additional Help and Information

Chapter 51

Glossary of Terms Related to the Urinary Tract and Kidney Disease

acute renal failure (ARF): Sudden and temporary loss of kidney function.[2]

albuminuria: Presence of protein in urine.[1]

amyloidosis: A condition in which a protein-like material builds up in one or more organs. This material cannot be broken down and interferes with the normal function of that organ. People who have been on dialysis for several years often develop amyloidosis because the artificial membranes used in dialysis fail to filter the protein-like material out of the blood.[2]

anemia: The condition of having too few red blood cells. Healthy red blood cells carry oxygen throughout the body. If the blood is low on red blood cells, the body does not get enough oxygen. People with anemia may be tired and pale and may feel their heartbeat change. Anemia is common in people with chronic kidney disease or those on dialysis.[2]

angiotensin-converting enzyme inhibitors (ACEI): A class of drugs used in the treatment of hypertension and congestive heart

---

The terms in this glossary marked "1" were excerpted from *Stedman's Electronic Medical Dictionary* v. 5.0, Copyright © 2000 Lippincott Williams and Wilkins. All rights reserved. Terms marked "2" are from documents produced by the National Kidney and Urologic Diseases Information Clearinghouse (NKUDIC), a service of the National Institute of Diabetes and Digestive and Kidney Diseases (NIDDK), and the National Cancer Institute (NCI), a part of the U.S. National Institutes of Health.

failure; they produce a reduction of peripheral arterial resistance, although the exact mechanism of action has not been fully determined; they block the conversion of angiotensin I to angiotensin II, a powerful vasoconstrictor.[1]

angiotensin receptor blockers (ARB): Agents, such as losartan, that bind with angiotensin receptors, thus preventing access of angiotensin II to the receptor and consequently reducing the vasoconstriction produced by this agonist; used in the treatment of hypertension.[1]

arteriovenous fistula: Surgical connection of an artery directly to a vein, usually in the forearm, created in patients who will need hemodialysis. The arteriovenous fistula causes the vein to grow thicker, allowing the repeated needle insertions required for hemodialysis.[2]

benign prostatic hyperplasia (BPH): Progressive enlargement of the prostate due to hyperplasia of both glandular and stromal components, typically beginning in the fifth decade and sometimes causing obstructive or irritative symptoms, or both; does not evolve into cancer.[1]

biopsy: The removal of cells or tissues for examination by a pathologist. The pathologist may study the tissue under a microscope or perform other tests on the cells or tissue. When only a sample of tissue is removed, the procedure is called an incisional biopsy. When an entire lump or suspicious area is removed, the procedure is called an excisional biopsy. When a sample of tissue or fluid is removed with a needle, the procedure is called a needle biopsy, core biopsy, or fine-needle aspiration.[2]

bladder: The balloon-shaped organ inside the pelvis that holds urine.[2]

bladder stone: Urinary tract calculi in the bladder. Throughout most of the history of humans, this was the predominant form of urinary tract stone disease, mentioned in the Hippocratic oath, and giving rise to the common ancient surgical procedure, lithotomy. In much of the world, bladder stone disease has become uncommon and renal and ureteral stones (which are usually of different origins) have become more common. Bladder stones are now typically seen in patients with neurogenic bladders, urinary tract reconstruction, or intravesical obstruction. Syn: bladder calculus.[1]

Bright disease: Nonsuppurative [not forming pus] nephritis with albuminuria and edema, associated in fatal cases with large white kidneys; or with hematuria and red kidneys; or with contracted granular kidneys, corresponding to the stages of glomerulonephritis now termed subacute or membranous, acute, and chronic, respectively.[1]

calculus (stone): A concretion formed in any part of the body, most commonly in the passages of the biliary and urinary tracts; usually composed of salts of inorganic or organic acids, or of other material such as cholesterol. Pl.: calculi.[1]

carcinoma in situ: Cancer that involves only cells in the tissue in which it began and that has not spread to nearby tissues.[2]

catheter: A tubular instrument to allow passage of fluid from or into a body cavity or blood vessel. Especially a catheter designed to be passed through the urethra into the bladder to drain it of retained urine.[1]

chronic kidney disease: Slow and progressive loss of kidney function over several years, resulting in permanent kidney failure. People with permanent kidney failure need dialysis or transplantation to replace the work of the kidneys.[2]

clinical trial: A type of research study that uses volunteers to test new methods of screening, prevention, diagnosis, or treatment of a disease. Also called a clinical study.[2]

congenital: Existing at birth, referring to certain mental or physical traits, anomalies, malformations, diseases, etc. which may be either hereditary or due to an influence occurring during gestation up to the moment of birth.[1]

continence: The ability to retain urine until a proper time for its discharge.[1]

creatinine: A waste product in the blood that results from the normal breakdown of muscle. Healthy kidneys filter creatinine from the blood.[2]

cystectomy: Surgery to remove all or part of the bladder.[2]

cystitis: Inflammation of the urinary bladder.[1]

diabetes: Either diabetes insipidus or diabetes mellitus, diseases having in common the symptom polyuria; when used without qualification, refers to diabetes mellitus.[1]

dialysate: That part of a mixture that passes through a dialyzing membrane; the material that does not pass through is referred to as the retentate.[1]

dialysis: The process of cleaning wastes from the blood artificially. This job is normally done by the kidneys. If the kidneys fail, the blood must be cleaned artificially with special equipment. The two major forms of dialysis are hemodialysis and peritoneal dialysis.[2]

dialyzer: The apparatus for performing dialysis; a membrane used in dialysis.[1]

dysuria: Difficulty or pain in urination.[1]

edema: Swelling caused by the accumulation of fluid in cells and tissues. In kidney failure, fluid may collect in the feet, hands, abdomen, or face.[2]

end-stage renal disease (ESRD): Total and permanent kidney failure. When the kidneys fail, the body retains fluid and harmful wastes build up. A person with ESRD needs treatment to replace the work of the failed kidneys.[2]

enuresis: Involuntary discharge or leakage of urine.[1]

erythropoietin: A hormone made by the kidneys to help form red blood cells. Lack of this hormone may lead to anemia.[2]

Escherichia coli (E. coli): A species that occurs normally in the intestines of humans and other vertebrates, is widely distributed in nature, and is a frequent cause of infections of the urogenital tract and of neonatal meningitis and diarrhea in infants.[1]

focal glomerulonephritis: Glomerulonephritis affecting a small proportion of renal glomeruli which commonly presents with hematuria and may be associated with acute upper respiratory infection in young males, not usually due to streptococci; associated with IgA deposits in the glomerular mesangium and may also be associated with systemic disease, as in Henoch-Schönlein purpura. Syn: Berger disease, Berger focal glomerulonephritis, focal nephritis, IgA nephropathy.[1]

fulguration: Destruction of tissue by means of a high-frequency electric current.[1]

genitourinary: Relating to the organs of reproduction and urination. Syn: urinogenital, urinosexual, urogenital.[1]

glomerulonephritis: Renal disease characterized by diffuse inflammatory changes in glomeruli that are not the acute response to infection of the kidneys.[1]

glomerulosclerosis: Hyaline deposits or scarring within the renal glomeruli, a degenerative process occurring in association with renal arteriosclerosis or diabetes.[1]

glomerulus: The tiny cluster of looping blood vessels in the nephron, where wastes are filtered from the blood.[2]

grade: The grade of a tumor depends on how abnormal the cancer cells look under a microscope and how quickly the tumor is likely to grow and spread. Grading systems are different fro each type of cancer.[2]

hematuria: Presence of blood or red blood cells in the urine.[1]

hemodialyzer: A machine for hemodialysis in acute or chronic renal failure; toxic substances in the blood are removed by exposure to dialyzing fluid across a semipermeable membrane.[1]

Hunner ulcer: a focal and often multiple lesion involving all layers of the bladder wall in chronic interstitial cystitis; the surface epithelium is destroyed by inflammation and the initially pale lesion cracks and bleeds with distention of the bladder.[1]

hypertension: High blood pressure, a condition that can cause kidney damage or be caused by kidney disease.[2]

idiopathic: A disease that occurs without a known cause.[2]

incontinence of urine: The involuntary voiding of urine.[1]

intravenous (I.V.): Into a vein.[2]

intravesical: Within the bladder.[2]

Kegel exercises: Alternate contraction and relaxation of perineal muscles for treatment of urinary stress incontinence.[1]

kidneys: A pair of organs in the abdomen that remove waste from the blood (as urine), produce erythropoietin (a substance that stimulates red blood cell production), and play a role in blood pressure regulation.[2]

minimally invasive surgery: Operative procedure performed in a manner derived to result in the smallest possible incision or no incision at all; includes laparoscopic, laparoscopically assisted, thoracoscopic, and endoscopic surgical procedures.[1]

nasogastric tube: A flexible tube passed through the nose and into the gastric pouch to decompress the stomach.[1]

naturopathy: A system of therapeutics in which neither surgical nor medicinal agents are used, dependence being placed only on natural (nonmedicinal) forces.[1]

nephrectomy: Surgical removal of the kidney.[2]

nephric: Relating to the kidney. Syn: renal.[1]

nephritis: Inflammation of the kidneys.[1]

nephron: One of a million tiny filtering units in each kidney. Each nephron is made up of both a glomerulus and a fluid-collecting tubule that processes extra water and wastes.[2]

nephropathy: Any disease of the kidney.[1]

nephrotoxic: Damaging to the kidneys.[2]

neuropathic bladder: Any defective functioning of bladder due to impaired innervation, e.g., cord bladder, neuropathic bladder. Syn: neurogenic bladder.[1]

oxalate calculus: A hard urinary calculus of calcium oxalate; some are covered with minute sharp spines that can abrade [scrape away] the renal pelvic epithelium, whereas others are smooth.[1]

percutaneous: Denoting the passage of substances through unbroken skin; also passage through the skin by needle puncture.[1]

pessary: An appliance of varied form, introduced into the vagina to support the uterus or to correct any displacement.[1]

polycystic kidney: A progressive disease characterized by formation of multiple cysts of varying size scattered diffusely throughout both kidneys, resulting in compression and destruction of renal parenchyma, usually with hypertension, gross hematuria, and uremia leading to progressive renal failure. There are two major types. Syn: polycystic disease of kidneys.[1]

polyuria: Excessive excretion of urine resulting in profuse and frequent micturition [urination].[1]

prostate: A gland in the male reproductive system just below the bladder. It surrounds part of the urethra, the canal that empties the bladder, and produces a fluid that forms part of semen.[2]

prostatitis: Inflammation of the prostate. The National Institutes of Health (NIH) consensus designates 4 categories of prostatitis: I, acute bacterial prostatitis; II, chronic bacterial prostatitis; III, chronic prostatitis/chronic pelvic pain syndrome: A, inflammatory and B, noninflammatory; and IV, asymptomatic inflammatory prostatitis.[1]

proteinuria: Large amounts of protein in the urine.[2]

renal: Of the kidneys. A renal disease is a disease of the kidneys. Renal failure means the kidneys have stopped working properly.[2]

renal agenesis: Absence of one or both kidneys.[1]

renal pelvis: The area at the center of the kidney. Urine collects here and is funneled into the ureter, the tube that connects the kidney to the bladder.[2]

renin: A hormone made by the kidneys that helps regulate the volume of fluid in the body and blood pressure.[2]

sclerotic: A disease in which tissues become hardened or scarred.[2]

stage: The extent of a cancer within the body. If the cancer has spread, the stage describes how far it has spread from the original site to other parts of the body.[2]

staging: Performing exams and tests to learn the extent of the cancer within the body, especially whether the disease has spread from the original site to other parts of the body. It is important to know the stage of the disease in order to plan the best treatment.[2]

stoma: An artificial opening between two cavities or canals, or between such and the surface of the body.[1]

struvite calculus: A calculus in which the crystalloid component consists of magnesium ammonium phosphate; usually associated with urinary tract infection caused by urease-producing bacteria.[1]

systemic: A disease that affects multiple parts of the body, often as a result of substances circulating in the blood.[2]

transitional cell: Any cell thought to represent a phase of development from one form to another.[1]

urea: A waste produce found in the blood and caused by the normal breakdown of protein in the liver. Urea is normally removed from the blood by the kidneys and then excreted in the urine. Urea accumulates in the body of people with renal failure.[2]

urease: An enzyme that catalyzes the hydrolysis of urea to carbon dioxide and ammonia; used as an antitumor enzyme; it is present in intestinal bacteria and accounts for most of the ammonia generated from urea in mammals.[1]

uremia: The illness associated with the buildup of urea in the blood because the kidneys are not working effectively. Symptoms include nausea, vomiting, loss of appetite, weakness, and mental confusion.[2]

ureter: The tube that conducts the urine from the renal pelvis to the bladder; it consists of an abdominal part and a pelvic part. [1]

urethra: The canal leading from the bladder, discharging the urine externally.[1]

urgency: A strong desire to void.[1]

urinary tract: The path that urine takes as it leaves the body. It includes the kidneys, ureters, bladder, and urethra.[2]

urinary tract infection (UTI): Microbial infection, usually bacterial, of any part of the urinary tract; can involve the parenchyma of the kidney, the renal pelvis, the ureter, the bladder, the urethra or combinations of these organs; often the entire urinary tract is affected; the most common organism causing such infection is *Escherichia coli*.[1]

urinate (void): To release urine from the bladder to the outside.[2]

urolithiasis: Presence of calculi in the urinary system.[1]

vascular: A general term to describe the area on the body where blood is drawn for circulation through a hemodialysis circuit. A vascular access may be an arteriovenous fistula, a graft, or a catheter.[2]

Chapter 52

Further Reading about Urinary and Kidney Diseases and Disorders

In this chapter, names of organizations are provided with information and a listing of the publications they offer. For contact information, see Chapter 53, "Directory of Kidney and Urologic Disorders Organizations."

American Association of Kidney Patients

AAKP Patient Plan, a series of booklets and newsletters that cover the different phases of learning about kidney failure, choosing a treatment, and adjusting to changes

Renalife (quarterly magazine)

Understanding Your Hemodialysis Access Options (booklet)

American Kidney Fund

Diet Guide for the CAPD Patient

"The Kid," a booklet written for children with kidney disease

Kidney Disease: A Guide for Patients and Their Families

Kidney Disease in Children; Kidneys for Kids

Resources listed in this chapter were compiled from several sources. Inclusion does not constitute endorsement. This list is not considered complete; it is merely intended to serve as a starting point for readers interested in pursuing additional information. Websites were all verified and accessed in May 2005.

American Prostate Society

Medication Versus Surgery (brochure)

What You Don't Know about Your Prostate Can Kill You

American Society of Transplantation

ASTP Newsletter (member newsletter)

ASTP Primer on Transplantation

Getting a New Kidney: Facts about Kidney Transplantation

Institute for Healthcare Improvement

The Fistula First Change Package: The Centers for Medicare and Medicaid Services (CMS), the End-Stage Renal Disease (ESRD) Networks, and the Institute for Healthcare Improvement (IHI) launched the National Vascular Access Improvement Initiative in 2003. Materials from the Fistula First Change Package are available through the IHI website, or by contacting the Institute for Healthcare Improvement.

Interstitial Cystitis Association of America, Inc. (ICA)

ICA (brochure)

ICA Update (quarterly newsletter)

Kidney Cancer Association

Kidney Cancer News (quarterly newsletter)

We Have Kidney Cancer (56-page booklet for patients)

National Association for Continence (NAFC)

Assorted educational leaflets on topics related to incontinence

Quality Care (quarterly newsletter)

The Resource Guide (annual directory of products and services for incontinence)

National Kidney Foundation, Inc. (NKF)

Patient education brochures include information on diet, work, and exercise. Booklets, newsletters, and journals also include the following topics:

Advances in Renal Replacement Therapy

American Journal of Kidney Diseases

Children with Chronic Kidney Disease: Tips for Parents

CRN News and Briefs (newsletter)

Family Focus (newsletter)

For Those Who Give and Grieve (newsletter)

Getting the Most from Your Treatment series: A series of brochures based on the National Kidney Foundation's Dialysis Outcomes Quality Initiatives (NKF-DOQI)

How to Increase Calories in Your Renal Diet (brochure)

Journal of Nephrology Social Work

Journal of Renal Nutrition

Nutrition and Hemodialysis (brochure)

Transplant Chronicles (newsletter)

National Kidney Foundation of Indiana, Inc.

Adventure at Riverside Park: A Story about Pediatric Dialysis: This story describes a young girl's experiences and emotions as a peritoneal dialysis patient. The book introduces the members of the health-care team and explains the role each plays in dialysis treatment.

North American Transplant Coordinators Organization

In Touch newsletter

Progress in Transplantation journal

Polycystic Kidney Disease Foundation

Autosomal Recessive PKD, Questions and Answers

The Family and ADPKD

Health Tips for Living with PKD

Polycystic Kidney Disease (patient manual)

PKD Progress (quarterly newsletter)

Renal Physicians Association

Appropriate Patient Preparation for Renal Replacement Therapy

ESRD in the Age of Managed Care: A Primer on Capitation

Capitation Models for ESRD: Methodology and Results

RPA Newsletter (bimonthly)

The Renal Physicians Guide to Nephrology Practice

Shared Decision Making in the Appropriate Initiation of and Withdrawal from Dialysis

The Simon Foundation for Continence

Several videos, slide presentations, and other educational materials

The Informer (quarterly newsletter)

Managing Incontinence: A Guide to Living with the Loss of Bladder Control

United Network for Organ Sharing

Financing Transplantation: What Every Patient Needs to Know, 2nd edition, 1996

Cookbooks for Dialysis Patients

Living Well on Dialysis Cookbook, a patient education program of the National Kidney Foundation, Inc. Developed by the Council on Renal Nutrition. Supported by an educational grant from Amgen Inc. http://www.epogen.com/patient/pdf/dialysis_cookbook.pdf.

The Cleveland Clinic Foundation Renal Diet Cookbooks: *Creative Cooking for Renal Diets*, ISBN 0-941511-00-6, and *Creative Cooking for Renal Diabetic Diets,* ISBN: 0-941511-01-4. Senay Publishing, Inc. For ordering information: 440-256-4435 or http://patientsupport.net/renal-diet-cookbooks.htm.

The Renal Gourmet: What to Eat When Your Kidneys Quit by Mardy Peters. ISBN: 0-9641730-0-X. For ordering information: 800-445-5653 or http://kidney-cookbook.com.

Southwest Cookbook for People on Dialysis, a project of the El Paso Chapter Council on Renal Nutrition and the National Kidney Foundation of Texas, Inc. Funded by an educational grant from Amgen Inc. http://www.epogen.com/patient/pdf/southwest_cookbook.pdf.

Websites

Several agencies and organizations maintain informative websites for people with urinary tract and kidney problems. The following resources are arranged by organization name or topic.

American Board of Medical Specialties® (ABMS)
http://www.abms.org

The American Board of Medical Specialties (ABMS), a not-for-profit organization comprising 24 medical specialty boards, is the pre-eminent entity overseeing physician certification in the United States. Their website contains a directory of board certified medical specialists.

Bladder Control for Women Campaign
http://www.kidney.niddk.nih.gov/kudiseases/pubs/bladdercontrol/index.htm

Let's Talk About Bladder Control for Women is a public health awareness campaign conducted by the National Kidney and Urologic Diseases Information Clearinghouse (NKUDIC), an information dissemination service of the National Institute of Diabetes and Digestive and Kidney Diseases (NIDDK), National Institutes of Health.

Cancer Incidence and Survival
http://seer.cancer.gov

The Surveillance, Epidemiology, and End Results (SEER) Program of the National Cancer Institute is an authoritative source of information on cancer incidence and survival in the United States.

Daily Bladder Diary
http://kidney.niddk.nih.gov/kudiseases/pubs/diary/index.htm

Contains links to pages that you can print out on your printer so that you have copies of a bladder diary.

Glomerular Filtration Rate Calculators
http://www.nkdep.nih.gov/healthprofessionals/tools/index.htm

The National Kidney Disease Education Program (NKDEP) "Information for Health Professionals" page links to calculators to estimate kidney function for adults and children.

Health Resources and Services Administration (HRSA)
http://www.hrsa.gov

The U.S. Department of Health and Human Services coordinates organ procurement and allocation activities through its Health Resources and Services Administration (HRSA). HRSA also maintains a website devoted to organ donation at http://www.organdonor.gov on the internet.

HRSA's Division of Transplantation administers the Organ Procurement and Transplantation Network (OPTN) through a contract with UNOS, whose website can be found at http://www.transplantliving.org on the internet. You can request a packet of information about kidney transplantation by calling UNOS at 888-894-6361 (888-TX-INFO-1).

The Kidney Failure Series
http://www.kidney.niddk.nih.gov/kudiseases/pubs/kidneyfailure/index.htm

The NIDDK Kidney Failure Series includes six booklets and seven fact sheets that can help you learn more about treatment methods for kidney failure, complications of dialysis, financial help for the treatment of kidney failure, and eating right on hemodialysis. For free single printed copies of this series, please contact the National Kidney and Urologic Diseases Information Clearinghouse.

Life Options Rehabilitation Resource Center
http://www.kidneyschool.org

The Life Options Rehabilitation Program has developed an interactive patient education website called Kidney School. Module 8 of this program deals with vascular access for hemodialysis. To view this module, log in to http://www.kidneyschool.org.

MEDLINEplus: Kidney Diseases (General)
http://www.nlm.nih.gov/medlineplus/kidneydiseasesgeneral.html

The National Library of Medicine maintains MEDLINEplus, a resource providing health information for consumers. The page on kidney diseases contains links to news articles and fact sheets about kidney diseases under many headings, including "Children."

The Nemours Foundation's KidsHealth.org
http://kidshealth.org/parent/medical/kidney/chronic_kidney_disease.html
http://kidshealth.org/kid/feel_better/things/dialysis.html

The Nemours Foundation supports children's hospitals in Delaware and Florida. The KidsHealth website includes articles on many health topics written for parents, teenagers, and young children. The pages listed above contain *When Your Child Has a Chronic Kidney Disease* and *What's the Deal with Dialysis?*—an article written for children. You can click on "Related Articles" and find several more KidsHealth pages devoted to kidney diseases and their treatments.

Nephkids Cyber-Support Group for Parents of Children with Kidney Disease
http://cnserver0.nkf.med.ualberta.ca/nephkids

Nephkids is a listserv, an interactive e-mail group for parents of children with various chronic kidney diseases.

National Cancer Institute Publications Locator
https://cissecure.nci.nih.gov/ncipubs

Use this site to view a list of, search for, or order National Cancer Institute publications.

National Cancer Institute (NCI) Cancer Information Database—Physician Data Query (PDQ®)
http://cancer.gov

PDQ is the National Cancer Institute's (NCI's) comprehensive cancer information database. Most of the information contained in PDQ is available online at NCI's website [click on PDQ® under "Cancer Topics"]. PDQ is provided as a service of the NCI. The NCI is part of the National Institutes of Health, the federal government's focal point for biomedical research.

The PDQ database contains summaries of the latest published information on cancer prevention, detection, genetics, treatment, supportive care, and complementary and alternative medicine. Most summaries are available in two versions. The health professional versions provide detailed information written in technical language. The patient versions are written in easy-to-understand, non-technical language. Both versions provide current and accurate cancer information.

The PDQ cancer information summaries are developed by cancer experts and reviewed regularly. Editorial Boards made up of experts in oncology and related specialties are responsible for writing and maintaining the cancer information summaries. The summaries are reviewed regularly and changes are made as new information becomes available. The date on each summary ("Date Last Modified") indicates the time of the most recent change.

PDQ also contains information on clinical trials. Before starting treatment, patients may want to think about taking part in a clinical trial. A clinical trial is a study to answer a scientific question, such as whether one treatment is better than another. Trials are based on past studies and what has been learned in the laboratory. Each trial answers certain scientific questions in order to find new and better ways to help cancer patients. During treatment clinical trials, information is collected about new treatments, the risks involved, and how well they do or do not work. If a clinical trial shows that a new treatment is better than one currently being used, the new treatment may become "standard."

Listings of clinical trials are included in PDQ and are available online at NCI's website. Descriptions of the trials are available in health professional and patient versions. Many cancer doctors who take part in clinical trials are also listed in PDQ. For more information, call the Cancer Information Service 800-4-CANCER (800-422-6237); TTY at 800-332-8615.

Organ Donation and Transplantation
http://www.shareyourlife.org

The Coalition on Donation, which is made up of many national organizations—including government agencies, private foundations, and commercial industries—promotes organ and tissue donation through educational programs and campaigns conducted nationally and at the local level.

Partnership for Prescription Assistance Program Overview
http://www.pparx.org

The Partnership for Prescription Assistance brings together America's pharmaceutical companies, doctors, other healthcare providers, patient advocacy organizations, and community groups to help qualifying patients who lack prescription coverage get the medicines they need through the public or private program that's right for them. Many will get them free or nearly free. Among the organizations collaborating on this program are the American Academy of Family Physicians, the American Autoimmune Related Diseases Association, the Lupus Foundation of America, the National Association for the Advancement of Colored People (NAACP), the National Alliance for Hispanic Health, and the National Medical Association. To access the Partnership for Prescription Assistance by phone, you can call toll-free, 888-4PPA-NOW (888-477-2669).

Prostate-Specific Antigen (PSA) Testing
http://cis.nci.nih.gov/fact/5_29.htm

National Cancer Institute (NCI) Fact Sheet, "The Prostate-Specific Antigen (PSA) Test: Questions and Answers" provides extensive information on PSA tests.

RenalInfo: Support and Resources for People with Kidney Disease
http://www.renalinfo.com/us

RenalInfo offers information about kidney disease—causes, symptoms, tests, and ideas to help maintain health and a comprehensive presentation of treatment choices.

Transplant Living
http://www.transplantliving.org

The Transplant Living site contains information for patients on organ donations and transplantation.

Transplantation and Donation
http://www.transweb.org

TransWeb: All about Transplantation and Donation is a non-profit educational website featuring answers to frequently asked questions, donor memorials, patient experiences, and a reference section.

Urologic Diseases in America: Interim Compendium (KU-188)
http://catalog.niddk.nih.gov/detail.cfm?ID=313&CH=NKUDIC

A report on the prevalence, incidence, treatment, and economic impact of urologic diseases in the United States by the National Institute of Diabetes and Digestive and Kidney Diseases (NIDDK). Single copies free.

United States Renal Data System (USRDS)
http://www.usrds.org/atlas.htm

Five central goals define the mission of the USRDS: to characterize the ESRD population; to describe the prevalence and incidence of ESRD along with trends in mortality and disease rates; to investigate relationships among patient demographics, treatment modalities, and morbidity; to identify new areas for special renal studies and support investigator-initiated research; and to provide data sets and samples of national data to support research by the Special Studies Centers.

What You Need to Know about Cancer Index
http://www.cancer.gov/cancerinfo/wyntk

The National Cancer Institute's What You Need To Know about™ Cancer publication series provides information on many types of cancer.

Chapter 53

Directory of Urinary and Kidney Disorders Organizations

Directory of Kidney and Urologic Diseases Organizations

This directory lists voluntary, governmental, and private organizations. Some of the organizations offer educational materials and other services to patients and the public; others primarily serve healthcare professionals.

Alport Syndrome Study
410 Chipeta Way
Room 155
University of Utah
Research Park
Salt Lake City, UT 84108-1297
Phone: 801-581-5479
Fax: 801-585-3233
Website: http://alport.cjb.net

American Association of Clinical Urologists
1111 North Plaza Drive
Suite 550
Schaumburg, IL 60173
Phone: 847-517-1050
Fax: 847-517-7229
Website: http://www.aacuweb.org
E-mail: info@aacuweb.org

Resources in this chapter were compiled from a variety of sources including, "Directory of Kidney and Urologic Diseases Organizations," April 2004, and "Other Sources for Statistics," undated, from the National Kidney and Urologic Diseases Information Clearinghouse (NKUDIC), a service of the National Institute of Diabetes and Digestive and Kidney Diseases (NIDDK), National Institutes of Health (NIH). All contact information was verified in May 2005. Inclusion does not constitute endorsement.

American Association of Genitourinary Surgeons
41 Mall Road
Burlington, MA 01805
Phone: 781-744-5796
Fax: 781-744-5767
Website: http://aagus.org

American Association of Kidney Patients
3505 East Frontage Road
Suite 315
Tampa, FL 33607
Toll-Free: 800-749-2257
Phone: 813-636-8100
Fax: 813-636-8122
Website: http://www.aakp.org
E-mail: info@aakp.org

American Board of Urology
2216 Ivy Road
Suite 210
Charlottesville, VA 22903
Phone: 434-979-0059
Fax: 434-979-0266
Website: http://www.abu.org

American Foundation for Urologic Disease
1000 Corporate Boulevard
Suite 410
Linthicum, MD 21090
Toll-Free: 800-828-7866
Phone: 410-689-3990
Fax: 410-689-3998
Website: http://www.afud.org
E-mail: admin@afud.org

American Kidney Fund
6110 Executive Boulevard
Suite 1010
Rockville, MD 20852
Toll-Free: 800-638-8299
Phone: 301-881-3052
Fax: 301-881-0898
Website: http://www.kidneyfund.org
E-mail: helpline@akfinc.org

American Lithotripsy Society
305 Second Avenue
Suite 200
Waltham, MA 02451
Phone: 781-895-9098
Fax: 781-895-9088
Website: http://www.lithotripsy.org
E-mail: als@lithotripsy.org

American Nephrology Nurses' Association
East Holly Avenue, Box 56
Pitman, NJ 08071-0056
Toll-Free: 888-600-2662
Phone: 856-256-2320
Fax: 856-589-7463
Website: http://www.annanurse.org
E-mail: anna@ajj.com

American Prostate Society
1327 Ashton Road
Hanover, MD 21076
Toll-Free: 800-308-1106 (Information Line)
Phone: 410-859-3735
Fax: 410-850-0818
Website: http://www.ameripros.org
E-mail: ameripros@mindspring.com

American Society for Artificial Internal Organs Inc.
National Office
P.O. Box C
Boca Raton, FL 33429-0468
Phone: 561-391-8589
Fax: 561-368-9153
Website: http://www.asaio.com
E-mail: info@asaio.com

American Society for Histocompatibility and Immunogenetics
15000 Commerce Parkway
Suite C
Mt. Laurel, NJ 08054
Phone: 856-638-0428
Fax: 856-439-0525
Website: http://www.ashi-hla.org
E-mail: info@ashi-hla.org

American Society of Nephrology
1725 I Street NW, Suite 510
Washington, DC 20006-2403
Phone: 202-659-0599
Fax: 202-659-0709
Website: http://www.asn-online.org
E-mail: email@asn-online.org

American Society of Pediatric Nephrology
Northwestern University
Feinberg School of Medicine
Pediatrics W140
303 East Chicago Avenue
Chicago, IL 60611-3008
Phone: 312-503-4000
Fax: 312-503-1181
Website: http://www.aspneph.com
E-mail: aspn@northwestern.edu

American Society of Transplant Surgeons
1020 North Fairfax Street
Suite 200
Alexandria, VA 22314
Toll-Free: 888-990-2787
Fax: 703-684-6303
Website: http://www.asts.org
E-mail: asts@asts.org

American Society of Transplantation
15000 Commerce Parkway
Suite C
Mt. Laurel, NJ 08054
Phone: 856-439-9986
Fax: 856-439-9982
Website: http://www.a-s-t.org
E-mail: ast@ahint.com

American Urogynecologic Society
2025 M Street NW
Suite 800
Washington, DC 20036
Phone: 202-367-1167
Fax: 202-367-2167
Website: http://www.augs.org
E-mail: info@augs.org

American Urological Association Inc.
1000 Corporate Boulevard
Linthicum, MD 21090
Toll-Free: 866-RING-AUA (746-4282)
Phone: 410-689-3700
Fax: 410-689-3800
Website: http://www.auanet.org
E-mail: aua@auanet.org

Cystinuria Support Network
21001 NE 36th Street
Sammamish, WA 98074
Phone: 425-868-2996
Fax: 425-897-8675
Website: http://
www.cystinuria.com
E-mail: Cystinuria@aol.com

The Diabetes Insipidus Foundation, Inc.
5203 New Prospect Drive
Ellicott City, MD 21043
Phone: 410-247-3953
Fax: 410-247-5584
Website: http://
www.diabetesinsipidus.org
E-mail:
info@diabetesinsipidus.org

Endourological Society
c/o Department of Urology
Long Island Jewish Medical
Center
270-05 76th Avenue
New Hyde Park, NY 11042
Phone: 718-470-3900
Fax: 718-343-6254

Hereditary Nephritis Foundation
1390 West 6690 South
#202H
Murray, UT 84123
Phone: 801-262-5901
Fax: 801-262-5901
Website: http://www.cc.utah.edu/
~cla6202/HNF.htm

IgA Nephropathy Support Network
9 G Street, Apt. B
Turner Falls, MA 01376
Phone: 413-863-8663
Website: http://www.igan.ca
E-mail: info@igan.ca

International Pediatric Nephrology Association
Children's Hospital and Medical
Center
4800 Sand Point Way NE
Seattle, WA 98105-0371
Phone: 206-987-4572
Fax: 206-527-3836
Website: http://www.ipna-
online.org

International Society of Nephrology
Washington University School of
Medicine
Barnes-Jewish Hospital
216 South Kingshighway Blvd.
Suite 4300
St. Louis, MO 63110
Phone: 314-454-7107
Fax: 314-454-5110
Website: http://www.isn-online.org

International Transplant Nurses Society
1739 E Carson Street
Box 351
Pittsburgh, PA 15203-1700
Phone: 412-343-ITNS (4867)
Fax: 412-343-3959
Website: http://www.itns.org
E-mail: itns@msn.com

Interstitial Cystitis Association of America, Inc. (ICA)
110 North Washington Street
Suite 340
Rockville, MD 20850
Toll-Free: 800-HELP-ICA (435-7422)
Phone: 301-610-5300
Fax: 301-610-5308
Website: http://www.ichelp.org
E-mail: icamail@ichelp.org

Kidney Cancer Association
1234 Sherman Avenue, Suite 203
Evanston, IL 60202-1378
Toll-Free: 800-850-9132
Phone: 847-332-1051
Fax: 847-332-2978
Website: http://www.curekidneycancer.org
E-mail: office@curekidneycancer.org

Lupus Foundation of America, Inc.
2000 L Street NW, Suite 710
Washington, DC 20036
Toll-Free: 800-558-0121
Phone: 202-349-1155
Fax: 202-349-1156
Website: http://www.lupus.org
E-mail: lupusinfo@lupus.org

Medical Education Institute, Inc.
414 D'Onofrio Drive, Suite 200
Madison, WI 53719
Phone: 608-833-8033
Fax: 608-833-8366
Website: http://www.meiresearch.org
E-mail: schatell@meiresearch.org

National Association for Continence (NAFC)
P.O. Box 1019
Charleston, SC 29402-1019
Toll-Free: 800-BLADDER (252-3337)
Phone: 843-377-0900
Fax: 843-377-0905
Website: http://www.nafc.org
E-mail: memberservices@nafc.org

National Association of Nephrology Technicians/ Technologists
11 West Monument Avenue, Suite 510
P.O. Box 2307
Dayton, OH 45401-2307
Toll-Free: 877-607-NANT (6268)
Phone: 937-586-3705
Fax: 937-586-3699
Website: http://www.dialysistech.org and http://www.nant.biz
E-mail: nant@nant.meinet.com

National Bladder Foundation
P.O. Box 1095
Ridgefield, CT 06877
Toll-Free: 877-BLADDER (252-3337)
Fax: 203-431-0008

National Foundation for Transplants
(formerly the Organ Transplant Fund)
1102 Brookfield Road
Suite 200
Memphis, TN 38119
Toll-Free: 800-489-3863
Phone: 901-684-1697
Fax: 901-684-1128
Website: http://
www.transplants.org
E-mail: info@transplants.org

National Kidney Foundation (NKF)
30 East 33rd Street
New York, NY 10016
Toll-Free: 800-622-9010
Phone: 212-889-2210
Fax: 212-689-9261
Website: http://www.kidney.org
E-mail: info@kidney.org

National Organization for Rare Disorders Inc. (NORD)
55 Kenosia Avenue
P.O. Box 1968
Danbury, CT 06813-1968
Toll-Free: 800-999-6673
Phone: 203-744-0100
Fax: 203-798-2291
TDD: 203-797-9590
Website: http://
www.rarediseases.org
E-mail:
orphan@rarediseases.org

The NephCure Foundation
15 Waterloo Avenue
Suite 200
Berwyn, PA 19312
Toll-Free: 866-637-4287
Phone: 610-540-0186
Fax: 610-540-0190
Website: http://
www.nephcure.org
E-mail: info@nephcure.org

Nephrogenic Diabetes Insipidus Foundation
Main Street
P.O. Box 1390
Eastsound, WA 98245
Toll-Free: 888-376-6343
Fax: 888-376-6356
Website: http://www.ndif.org
E-mail: info@ndif.org

North American Society for Dialysis and Transplantation
4010 Bentley Drive
Pearland, TX 77584
Phone: 281-997-1944
Fax: 281-997-0733
Website: http://www.nasdat.org

North American Transplant Coordinators Organization
P.O. Box 15384
Lenexa, KS 66285-5384
Phone: 913-492-3600
Fax: 913-599-5340
Website: http://www.natco1.org
E-mail: natco-info@goAMP.com

Oxalosis and Hyperoxaluria Foundation (OHF)

201 East 19th Street
Suite 12E
New York, NY 10003
Toll-Free: 800-643-8699
Phone: 212-777-0470
Fax: 212-777-0471
Website: http://www.ohf.org
E-mail: execdirector@ohf.org

Polycystic Kidney Disease Foundation

9221 Ward Parkway
Suite 400
Kansas City, MO 64114-3367
Toll-Free: 800-PKD-CURE (753-2873)
Phone: 816-931-2600
Fax: 816-931-8655
Website: http://www.pkdcure.org
E-mail: pkdcure@pkdcure.org

The Prostatitis Foundation

1063 30th Street, Box 8
Smithshire, IL 61478
Toll-Free: 888-891-4200
Fax: 309-325-7184
Website: http://www.prostatitis.org
E-mail: mcapstone@aol.com

Renal Physicians Association

1700 Rockville Pike
Suite 220
Rockville, MD 20852
Phone: 301-468-3515
Fax: 301-468-3511
Website: http://www.renalmd.org
E-mail: rpa@renalmd.org

The Simon Foundation for Continence

P.O. Box 835
Wilmette, IL 60091
Toll-Free: 800-23-SIMON
Phone: 847-864-3913
Fax: 847-864-9758
Website: http://www.simonfoundation.org
E-mail: simoninfo@simonfoundation.org

The Society for Urodynamics and Female Urology

1111 North Plaza Drive, Suite 550
Shaumberg, IL 60173-4950
Phone: 847-517-7225
Fax: 847-517-7229
Website: http://www.sufuorg.com
E-mail: sufu@wjweiser.com

Society of Government Service Urologists

P.O. Box 681965
San Antonio, TX 78268-7202
Phone: 210-681-5800
Fax: 210-680-7725
Website: http://home.satx.rr.com/sgsu
E-mail: sgsu@txdirect.net

Society of University Urologists

Ohio State University Medical Center
Division of Urology
4980 University Hospitals Clinic
456 West 10th Avenue
Columbus, OH 43210-1228
Phone: 614-293-3648
Fax: 614-293-3565

Society of Urologic Nurses and Associates
East Holly Avenue, Box 56
Pitman, NJ 08071-0056
Toll-Free: 888-TAP-SUNA (827-7862)
Phone: 856-256-2335
Fax: 856-589-7463
Website: http://www.suna.org
E-mail: suna@ajj.com

Transplant Recipients International Organization (TRIO)
2100 M Street NW, #170-353
Washington, DC 20037-1233
Toll-Free: 800-TRIO-386
Phone: 202-293-0980
Website: http://www.trioweb.org
E-mail: info@trioweb.org

The Transplantation Society
Central Business Office
Edifice Place du Quartier
1111 St. Urbain Street, Suite 108
Montreal, QC, Canada H2Z 1Y6
Phone: 514-874-1717
Fax: 514-874-1716
Website: http://www.transplantation-soc.org
E-mail: info@transplantation-soc.org

United Network for Organ Sharing (UNOS)
P.O. Box 2484
Richmond, VA 23218
Toll-Free: 888-894-6361 (Patient Hotline)
Phone: 804-782-4800
Fax: 804-782-4817
Website: http://www.unos.org

United Ostomy Association Inc. (UOA)
19772 MacArthur Boulevard, Suite 200
Irvine, CA 92612
Toll-Free: 800-826-0826
Phone: 949-660-8624
Fax: 949-660-9262
Website: http://www.uoa.org
E-mail: info@uoa.org

Other Sources for Statistics

For additional statistical information on kidney diseases, please contact the following organizations:

American Foundation for Urologic Disease, Inc.
1000 Corporate Boulevard
Suite 410
Linthicum, MD 21090
Toll-Free: 800-828-7866
Phone: 410-689-3990
Website: http://www.afud.org

American Society of Nephrology (ASN)
2025 M Street NW
Suite 800
Washington, DC 20036
Phone: 202-659-0599
Fax: 202-367-2190
Website: http://www.asn-online.org
E-mail: email@asn-online.org

American Urological Association (AUA)

1000 Corporate Boulevard
Linthicum, MD 21090
Toll-Free: 866-RING-AUA
Phone: 410-689-3700
Fax: 410-689-3800
Website: http://www.auanet.org
E-mail: aua@auanet.org

Center for Medicare and Medicaid Services

7500 Security Boulevard
Baltimore, MD 21244
Toll-Free: 877-267-2323
Phone: 410-786-3000
TTY Toll-Free: 866-226-1819
TTY: 410-786-0727
Website: http://www.cms.hhs.gov

Centers for Disease Control and Prevention (CDC)

1600 Clifton Road NE, Mail Stop G37
Atlanta, GA 30333
Toll-Free: 800-311-3435
Phone: 404-639-3311 (Public Inquiries)
Website: http://www.cdc.gov

Interstitial Cystitis Association (ICA)

110 N Washington Street
Suite 340
Rockville, MD 20850
Toll-Free: 800-HELP-ICA (435-7422)
Phone: 301-610-5300
Fax: 301-610-5308
Website: http://www.ichelp.org
E-mail: icamail@ichelp.org

National Association for Continence (NAFC)

P.O. Box 1019
Spartanburg, SC 29402-1019
Toll-Free: 800-BLADDER (252-3337)
Phone: 864-579-7900 (Business Office)
Fax: 864-579-7902
Website: http://www.nafc.org

National Center for Health Statistics

Hyattsville, MD 20782-2003
Phone: 301-458-4000
Website: http://www.cdc.gov/nchs

National Kidney Foundation (NKF)

30 East 33rd Street
New York, NY 10016
Toll-Free: 800-622-9010
Phone: 212-889-2210
Fax: 212-689-9261
Website: http://www.kidney.org
E-mail: info@kidney.org

Polycystic Kidney Disease Foundation

9221 Ward Parkway
Suite 400
Kansas City, MO 64114-3367
Toll-Free: 800-PKD-CURE (753-2873)
Phone: 816-931-2600
Fax: 816-931-8655
Website: http://www.pkdcure.org
E-mail: pkdcure@pkdcure.org

The Simon Foundation for Continence

P.O. Box 815
Wilmette, IL 60091
Toll-Free: 800-23-SIMON (237-4666)
Phone: 847-864-3913
Fax: 847-864-9758
Website: http://www.simonfoundation.org
E-mail: simoninfo@simonfoundation.org

Transplant Recipient International Organization (TRIO)

2100 M Street NW, #170-353
Washington, DC 20037-1233
Toll-Free: 800-TRIO-386 (874-6386)
Phone: 202-293-0980
Fax: 202-296-0973
Website: http://www.trioweb.org
E-mail: info@trioweb.org

United Network for Organ Sharing (UNOS)

P.O. Box 2484
Richmond, VA 23218
Phone: 804-782-4800
Fax: 804-782-4817
Website: http://www.unos.org

United States Renal Data System (USRDS) Coordinating Center

914 South 8th Street, Suite D206
Minneapolis, MN 55404
Toll-Free: 888-99-USRDS (998-7737)
Phone: 612-347-7776
Fax: 612-347-5878
Website: http://www.usrds.org

Additional Resources

American College of Obstetricians and Gynecologists (ACOG) Resource Center

409 12th Street, SW
P.O. Box 96920
Washington, DC 20090-6920
Phone: 202-638-5577
Website: http://www.acog.org

Amyloidosis Network International, Inc.

7118 Cole Creek Drive
Houston, TX 77092-1421
Toll-Free: 888-AMYLOID

The Cleveland Clinic Foundation

9500 Euclid Avenue
Cleveland, OH 44195
Phone: 216-444-5000

Coalition on Donation

700 North 4th Street
Richmond, VA 23219
Phone: 804-782-4920
Fax: 804-782-4643
Website: http://www.shareyourlife.org
E-mail: coalition@donatelife.net

The Diabetes Insipidus and Related Disorders Network

535 Echo Court
Saline, MI 48176-1270
Phone: 734-944-0078
Fax: 734-944-0078

Lois Joy Galler Foundation for Hemolytic-Uremic Syndrome
734 Walt Whitman Road
Suite 300
Melville, NY 11747
Phone: 516-673-3017

Health Resources and Services Administration
Division of Transplantation
Parklawn Building
Room 16C-17
5600 Fishers Lane
Rockville, MD 20857
Phone: 301-443-7577
Website: http://www.hrsa.gov
E-mail: comments@hrsa.gov

Institute for Healthcare Improvement (IHI)
20 University Road, 7th Floor
Cambridge, MA 02138
Toll-Free: 866-787-0831
Phone: 617-301-4800
Fax: 617-301-4848
Website: http://www.ihi.org
E-mail: info@ihi.org

The Medicine Program
P.O. Box 1089
Poplar Bluff, MO 63901-1089
Toll-Free: 866-694-3893
Website: http://
www.themedicineprogram.com

National Cancer Institute (NCI)
Cancer Information Service
6116 Executive Boulevard
MSC 8322
Suite 3036A
Bethesda, MD 20892-8322
Toll-Free: 800-4-CANCER (800-422-6237)
TTY: 800-332-8615
Website: http://www.nci.nih.gov
E-mail:
cancermail@icicc.nci.nih.gov

National Heart, Lung, and Blood Institute Health Information Center (NHLBI)
P.O. Box 30105
Bethesda, MD 20824-0105
Phone: 301-592-8573
TTY: 240-629-3255
Fax: 240-629-3246
Website: http://
www.nhlbi.nih.gov
E-mail: nhlbiinfo@nhlbi.nih.gov

National Institute of Arthritis and Musculoskeletal and Skin Diseases (NIAMS) Information Clearinghouse
National Institutes of Health
1 AMS Circle
Bethesda, MD 20892-3675
Toll-Free: 877-22-NIAMS
Phone: 301-495-4484
TTY: 301-565-2966
Website: http://
www.niams.nih.gov

National Kidney Foundation of Indiana, Inc.

911 East 86th Street
Suite 100
Indianapolis, IN 46240-1840
Toll-Free: 800-382-9971
Phone: 317-722-5640
Fax: 317-722-5650
Website: http://
www.kidneyindiana.org
E-mail: nkfi@myvine.com

National Kidney and Urologic Diseases Information Clearinghouse (NKUDIC)

3 Information Way
Bethesda, MD 20892-3580
Toll-Free: 800-891-5390
Phone: 301-654-4415
Fax: 301-907-8906
Website: http://
kidney.niddk.nih.gov
E-mail:
nkudic@info.niddk.nih.gov

National Kidney Disease Education Program (NKDEP)

3 Kidney Information Way
Bethesda, MD 20892
Toll-Free 866-4-KIDNEY (866-454-3639)
Fax: 301-897-9587
Website: http://
www.nkdep.nih.gov
E-mail:
nkdep@info.niddk.nih.gov

National Women's Health Information Center (NWHIC)

8550 Arlington Boulevard
Suite 300
Fairfax, VA 22031
Toll-Free: 800-994-WOMAN
(800-994-9626)
TDD: 888-220-5446
Website: http://
www.4woman.gov

Partnership for Caring: America's Voices for the Dying

1620 Eye Street NW
Suite 202
Washington, DC 20006
Toll-Free: 800-989-9455
Phone: 202-296-8071
Website: http://
www.partnershipforcaring.org
E-mail:
pfc@partnershipforcaring.org

Pharmaceutical Research and Manufacturers of America

1100 Fifteenth Street NW
Washington, DC 20005
Phone: 202-835-3400
Fax: 202-835-3414
Website: http://www.phrma.org

Prostate Cancer Research Institute (PCRI)
5777 W Century Boulevard, Suite 800
Los Angeles, CA 90045
Toll-Free: 800-641-7274 (Helpline)
Phone: 310-743-2116
Fax: 310-743-2113
Website: http://www.pcri.org
E-mail: info@pcri.org

Us Too International, Inc. (Prostate Cancer Survivors)
5003 Fairview Avenue
Downers Grove, IL 60515
Toll-Free: 800-808-7866
Phone: 630-795-1002
Fax: 630-795-1602
Website: http://www.ustoo.org
E-mail: ustoo@ustoo.org

Index

Index

S

Health Reference Series
COMPLETE CATALOG
List price $87 per volume. **School and library price $78 per volume.**

Adolescent Health Sourcebook

Basic Consumer Health Information about Common Medical, Mental, and Emotional Concerns in Adolescents, Including Facts about Acne, Body Piercing, Mononucleosis, Nutrition, Eating Disorders, Stress, Depression, Behavior Problems, Peer Pressure, Violence, Gangs, Drug Use, Puberty, Sexuality, Pregnancy, Learning Disabilities, and More

Along with a Glossary of Terms and Other Resources for Further Help and Information

Edited by Chad T. Kimball. 658 pages. 2002. 0-7808-0248-9.

"It is written in clear, nontechnical language aimed at general readers. . . . Recommended for public libraries, community colleges, and other agencies serving health care consumers."
— *American Reference Books Annual, 2003*

"Recommended for school and public libraries. Parents and professionals dealing with teens will appreciate the easy-to-follow format and the clearly written text. This could become a 'must have' for every high school teacher." — *E-Streams, Jan '03*

"A good starting point for information related to common medical, mental, and emotional concerns of adolescents." — *School Library Journal, Nov '02*

"This book provides accurate information in an easy to access format. It addresses topics that parents and caregivers might not be aware of and provides practical, useable information." — *Doody's Health Sciences Book Review Journal, Sep-Oct '02*

"Recommended reference source."
— *Booklist, American Library Association, Sep '02*

AIDS Sourcebook, 3rd Edition

Basic Consumer Health Information about Acquired Immune Deficiency Syndrome (AIDS) and Human Immunodeficiency Virus (HIV) Infection, Including Facts about Transmission, Prevention, Diagnosis, Treatment, Opportunistic Infections, and Other Complications, with a Section for Women and Children, Including Details about Associated Gynecological Concerns, Pregnancy, and Pediatric Care

Along with Updated Statistical Information, Reports on Current Research Initiatives, a Glossary, and Directories of Internet, Hotline, and Other Resources

Edited by Dawn D. Matthews. 664 pages. 2003. 0-7808-0631-X.

ALSO AVAILABLE: AIDS Sourcebook, 1st Edition. Edited by Karen Bellenir and Peter D. Dresser. 831 pages. 1995. 0-7808-0031-1.

AIDS Sourcebook, 2nd Edition. Edited by Karen Bellenir. 751 pages. 1999. 0-7808-0225-X.

"The 3rd edition of the *AIDS Sourcebook*, part of Omnigraphics' *Health Reference Series*, is a welcome update. . . . This resource is highly recommended for academic and public libraries."
— *American Reference Books Annual, 2004*

"Excellent sourcebook. This continues to be a highly recommended book. There is no other book that provides as much information as this book provides."
— *AIDS Book Review Journal, Dec-Jan 2000*

"Recommended reference source."
— *Booklist, American Library Association, Dec '99*

"A solid text for college-level health libraries."
— *The Bookwatch, Aug '99*

Cited in *Reference Sources for Small and Medium-Sized Libraries, American Library Association, 1999*

Alcoholism Sourcebook

Basic Consumer Health Information about the Physical and Mental Consequences of Alcohol Abuse, Including Liver Disease, Pancreatitis, Wernicke-Korsakoff Syndrome (Alcoholic Dementia), Fetal Alcohol Syndrome, Heart Disease, Kidney Disorders, Gastrointestinal Problems, and Immune System Compromise and Featuring Facts about Addiction, Detoxification, Alcohol Withdrawal, Recovery, and the Maintenance of Sobriety

Along with a Glossary and Directories of Resources for Further Help and Information

Edited by Karen Bellenir. 613 pages. 2000. 0-7808-0325-6.

"This title is one of the few reference works on alcoholism for general readers. For some readers this will be a welcome complement to the many self-help books on the market. Recommended for collections serving general readers and consumer health collections."
— *E-Streams, Mar '01*

"This book is an excellent choice for public and academic libraries."
— *American Reference Books Annual, 2001*

"Recommended reference source."
— *Booklist, American Library Association, Dec '00*

"Presents a wealth of information on alcohol use and abuse and its effects on the body and mind, treatment, and prevention." — *SciTech Book News, Dec '00*

"Important new health guide which packs in the latest consumer information about the problems of alcoholism." — *Reviewer's Bookwatch, Nov '00*

SEE ALSO Drug Abuse Sourcebook, Substance Abuse Sourcebook

623

Allergies Sourcebook, 2nd Edition

Basic Consumer Health Information about Allergic Disorders, Triggers, Reactions, and Related Symptoms, Including Anaphylaxis, Rhinitis, Sinusitis, Asthma, Dermatitis, Conjunctivitis, and Multiple Chemical Sensitivity

Along with Tips on Diagnosis, Prevention, and Treatment, Statistical Data, a Glossary, and a Directory of Sources for Further Help and Information

Edited by Annemarie S. Muth. 598 pages. 2002. 0-7808-0376-0.

ALSO AVAILABLE: *Allergies Sourcebook, 1st Edition.* Edited by Allan R. Cook. 611 pages. 1997. 0-7808-0036-2.

"This book brings a great deal of useful material together.... This is an excellent addition to public and consumer health library collections."
— *American Reference Books Annual, 2003*

"This second edition would be useful to laypersons with little or advanced knowledge of the subject matter. This book would also serve as a resource for nursing and other health care professions students. It would be useful in public, academic, and hospital libraries with consumer health collections." — *E-Streams, Jul '02*

▪

Alternative Medicine Sourcebook, 2nd Edition

Basic Consumer Health Information about Alternative and Complementary Medical Practices, Including Acupuncture, Chiropractic, Herbal Medicine, Homeopathy, Naturopathic Medicine, Mind-Body Interventions, Ayurveda, and Other Non-Western Medical Traditions

Along with Facts about such Specific Therapies as Massage Therapy, Aromatherapy, Qigong, Hypnosis, Prayer, Dance, and Art Therapies, a Glossary, and Resources for Further Information

Edited by Dawn D. Matthews. 618 pages. 2002. 0-7808-0605-0.

ALSO AVAILABLE: *Alternative Medicine Sourcebook, 1st Edition.* Edited by Allan R. Cook. 737 pages. 1999. 0-7808-0200-4.

"Recommended for public, high school, and academic libraries that have consumer health collections. Hospital libraries that also serve the public will find this to be a useful resource." — *E-Streams, Feb '03*

"Recommended reference source."
— *Booklist, American Library Association, Jan '03*

"An important alternate health reference."
— *MBR Bookwatch, Oct '02*

"A great addition to the reference collection of every type of library." — *American Reference Books Annual, 2000*

Alzheimer's Disease Sourcebook, 3rd Edition

Basic Consumer Health Information about Alzheimer's Disease, Other Dementias, and Related Disorders, Including Multi-Infarct Dementia, AIDS Dementia Complex, Dementia with Lewy Bodies, Huntington's Disease, Wernicke-Korsakoff Syndrome (Alcohol-Reated Dementia), Delirium, and Confusional States

Along with Information for People Newly Diagnosed with Alzheimer's Disease and Caregivers, Reports Detailing Current Research Efforts in Prevention, Diagnosis, and Treatment, Facts about Long-Term Care Issues, and Listings of Sources for Additional Information

Edited by Karen Bellenir. 645 pages. 2003. 0-7808-0666-2.

ALSO AVAILABLE: *Alzheimer's, Stroke & 29 Other Neurological Disorders Sourcebook, 1st Edition.* Edited by Frank E. Bair. 579 pages. 1993. 1-55888-748-2.

ALSO AVAILABLE: *Alzheimer's Disease Sourcebook, 2nd Edition.* Edited by Karen Bellenir. 524 pages. 1999. 0-7808-0223-3.

"This very informative and valuable tool will be a great addition to any library serving consumers, students and health care workers."
— *American Reference Books Annual, 2004*

"This is a valuable resource for people affected by dementias such as Alzheimer's. It is easy to navigate and includes important information and resources."
— *Doody's Review Service, Feb. 2004*

"Recommended reference source."
— *Booklist, American Library Association, Oct '99*

SEE ALSO *Brain Disorders Sourcebook*

▪

Arthritis Sourcebook, 2nd Edition

Basic Consumer Health Information about Osteoarthritis, Rheumatoid Arthritis, Other Rheumatic Disorders, Infectious Forms of Arthritis, and Diseases with Symptoms Linked to Arthritis, Featuring Facts about Diagnosis, Pain Management, and Surgical Therapies

Along with Coping Strategies, Research Updates, a Glossary, and Resources for Additional Help and Information

Edited by Amy L. Sutton. 593 pages. 2004. 0-7808-0667-0.

ALSO AVAILABLE: *Arthritis Sourcebook, 1st Edition.* Edited by Allan R. Cook. 550 pages. 1998. 0-7808-0201-2.

"... accessible to the layperson."
— *Reference and Research Book News, Feb '99*

▪

Asthma Sourcebook

Basic Consumer Health Information about Asthma, Including Symptoms, Traditional and Nontraditional Remedies, Treatment Advances, Quality-of-Life Aids,

Medical Research Updates, and the Role of Allergies, Exercise, Age, the Environment, and Genetics in the Development of Asthma

Along with Statistical Data, a Glossary, and Directories of Support Groups, and Other Resources for Further Information

Edited by Annemarie S. Muth. 628 pages. 2000. 0-7808-0381-7.

"A worthwhile reference acquisition for public libraries and academic medical libraries whose readers desire a quick introduction to the wide range of asthma information." *— Choice, Association of College & Research Libraries, Jun '01*

"Recommended reference source." *—Booklist, American Library Association, Feb '01*

"Highly recommended." *— The Bookwatch, Jan '01*

"There is much good information for patients and their families who deal with asthma daily." *— American Medical Writers Association Journal, Winter '01*

"This informative text is recommended for consumer health collections in public, secondary school, and community college libraries and the libraries of universities with a large undergraduate population." *— American Reference Books Annual, 2001*

Attention Deficit Disorder Sourcebook

Basic Consumer Health Information about Attention Deficit/Hyperactivity Disorder in Children and Adults, Including Facts about Causes, Symptoms, Diagnostic Criteria, and Treatment Options Such as Medications, Behavior Therapy, Coaching, and Homeopathy

Along with Reports on Current Research Initiatives, Legal Issues, and Government Regulations, and Featuring a Glossary of Related Terms, Internet Resources, and a List of Additional Reading Material

Edited by Dawn D. Matthews. 470 pages. 2002. 0-7808-0624-7.

"Recommended reference source." *—Booklist, American Library Association, Jan '03*

"This book is recommended for all school libraries and the reference or consumer health sections of public libraries." *— American Reference Books Annual, 2003*

Back & Neck Sourcebook, 2nd Edition

Basic Consumer Health Information about Spinal Pain, Spinal Cord Injuries, and Related Disorders, Such as Degenerative Disk Disease, Osteoarthritis, Scoliosis, Sciatica, Spina Bifida, and Spinal Stenosis, and Featuring Facts about Maintaining Spinal Health, Self-Care, Pain Management, Rehabilitative Care, Chiropractic Care, Spinal Surgeries, and Complementary Therapies

Along with Suggestions for Preventing Back and Neck Pain, a Glossary of Related Terms, and a Directory of Resources

Edited by Amy L. Sutton. 633 pages. 2004. 0-7808-0738-3

ALSO AVAILABLE: *Back & Neck Disorders Sourcebook, 1st Edition.* Edited by Karen Bellenir. 548 pages. 1997. 0-7808-0202-0.

"The strength of this work is its basic, easy-to-read format. Recommended." *— Reference and User Services Quarterly, American Library Association, Winter '97*

Blood & Circulatory Disorders Sourcebook, 2nd Edition

Basic Consumer Health Information about the Blood and Circulatory System and Related Disorders, Such as Anemia and Other Hemoglobin Diseases, Cancer of the Blood and Associated Bone Marrow Disorders, Clotting and Bleeding Problems, and Conditions That Affect the Veins, Blood Vessels, and Arteries, Including Facts about the Donation and Transplantation of Bone Marrow, Stem Cells, and Blood and Tips for Keeping the Blood and Circulatory System Healthy

Along with a Glossary of Related Terms and Resources for Additional Help and Information

Edited by Amy L. Sutton. 659 pages. 2005. 0-7808-0746-4.

ALSO AVAILABLE: *Blood and Circulatory Disorders Sourcebook, 1st Edition.* Edited by Karen Bellenir and Linda M. Shin. 554 pages. 1998. 0-7808-0203-9.

"Recommended reference source." *—Booklist, American Library Association, Feb '99*

"An important reference sourcebook written in simple language for everyday, non-technical users. " *— Reviewer's Bookwatch, Jan '99*

Brain Disorders Sourcebook, 2nd Edition

Basic Consumer Health Information about Acquired and Traumatic Brain Injuries, Infections of the Brain, Epilepsy and Seizure Disorders, Cerebral Palsy, and Degenerative Neurological Disorders, Including Amyotrophic Lateral Sclerosis (ALS), Dementias, Multiple Sclerosis, and More

Along with Information on the Brain's Structure and Function, Treatment and Rehabilitation Options, Reports on Current Research Initiatives, a Glossary of Terms Related to Brain Disorders and Injuries, and a Directory of Sources for Further Help and Information

Edited by Sandra J. Judd. 625 pages. 2005. 0-7808-0744-8.

ALSO AVAILABLE: *Brain Disorders Sourcebook, 1st Edition.* Edited by Karen Bellenir. 481 pages. 1999. 0-7808-0229-2.

"Belongs on the shelves of any library with a consumer health collection." *— E-Streams, Mar '00*

Breast Cancer Sourcebook, 2nd Edition

Basic Consumer Health Information about Breast Cancer, Including Facts about Risk Factors, Prevention, Screening and Diagnostic Methods, Treatment Options, Complementary and Alternative Therapies, Post-Treatment Concerns, Clinical Trials, Special Risk Populations, and New Developments in Breast Cancer Research

Along with Breast Cancer Statistics, a Glossary of Related Terms, and a Directory of Resources for Additional Help and Information

Edited by Sandra J. Judd. 595 pages. 2004. 0-7808-0668-9.

ALSO AVAILABLE: Breast Cancer Sourcebook, 1st Edition. Edited by Edward J. Prucha and Karen Bellenir. 580 pages. 2001. 0-7808-0244-6.

SEE ALSO Cancer Sourcebook for Women, Women's Health Concerns Sourcebook

Breastfeeding Sourcebook

Basic Consumer Health Information about the Benefits of Breastmilk, Preparing to Breastfeed, Breastfeeding as a Baby Grows, Nutrition, and More, Including Information on Special Situations and Concerns Such as Mastitis, Illness, Medications, Allergies, Multiple Births, Prematurity, Special Needs, and Adoption

Along with a Glossary and Resources for Additional Help and Information

Edited by Jenni Lynn Colson. 388 pages. 2002. 0-7808-0332-9.

SEE ALSO Pregnancy & Birth Sourcebook

Burns Sourcebook

Basic Consumer Health Information about Various Types of Burns and Scalds, Including Flame, Heat, Cold, Electrical, Chemical, and Sun Burns

Along with Information on Short-Term and Long-Term Treatments, Tissue Reconstruction, Plastic Surgery, Prevention Suggestions, and First Aid

Edited by Allan R. Cook. 604 pages. 1999. 0-7808-0204-7.

SEE ALSO Skin Disorders Sourcebook

Cancer Sourcebook, 4th Edition

Basic Consumer Health Information about Major Forms and Stages of Cancer, Featuring Facts about Head and Neck Cancers, Lung Cancers, Gastrointestinal Cancers, Genitourinary Cancers, Lymphomas, Blood Cell Cancers, Endocrine Cancers, Skin Cancers, Bone Cancers, Sarcomas, and Others, and Including Information about Cancer Treatments and Therapies, Identifying and Reducing Cancer Risks, and Strategies for Coping with Cancer and the Side Effects of Treatment

Along with a Cancer Glossary, Statistical and Demographic Data, and a Directory of Sources for Additional Help and Information

Edited by Karen Bellenir. 1,119 pages. 2003. 0-7808-0633-6.

ALSO AVAILABLE: Cancer Sourcebook, 1st Edition. Edited by Frank E. Bair. 932 pages. 1990. 1-55888-888-8.

New Cancer Sourcebook, 2nd Edition. Edited by Allan R. Cook. 1,313 pages. 1996. 0-7808-0041-9.

Cancer Sourcebook, 3rd Edition. Edited by Edward J. Prucha. 1,069 pages. 2000. 0-7808-0227-6.

"With cancer being the second leading cause of death for Americans, a prodigious work such as this one, which locates centrally so much cancer-related information, is clearly an asset to this nation's citizens and others."
—*Journal of the National Medical Association, 2004*

"This title is recommended for health sciences and public libraries with consumer health collections."
—*E-Streams, Feb '01*

"... can be effectively used by cancer patients and their families who are looking for answers in a language they can understand. Public and hospital libraries should have it on their shelves."
—*American Reference Books Annual, 2001*

"Recommended reference source."
—*Booklist, American Library Association, Dec '00*

Cited in *Reference Sources for Small and Medium-Sized Libraries*, American Library Association, 1999

"The amount of factual and useful information is extensive. The writing is very clear, geared to general readers. Recommended for all levels."
—*Choice, Association of College & Research Libraries, Jan '97*

SEE ALSO *Breast Cancer Sourcebook, Cancer Sourcebook for Women, Pediatric Cancer Sourcebook, Prostate Cancer Sourcebook*

Cancer Sourcebook for Women, 2nd Edition

Basic Consumer Health Information about Gynecologic Cancers and Related Concerns, Including Cervical Cancer, Endometrial Cancer, Gestational Trophoblastic Tumor, Ovarian Cancer, Uterine Cancer, Vaginal Cancer, Vulvar Cancer, Breast Cancer, and Common Non-Cancerous Uterine Conditions, with Facts about Cancer Risk Factors, Screening and Prevention, Treatment Options, and Reports on Current Research Initiatives

Along with a Glossary of Cancer Terms and a Directory of Resources for Additional Help and Information

Edited by Karen Bellenir. 604 pages. 2002. 0-7808-0226-8.

ALSO AVAILABLE: *Cancer Sourcebook for Women, 1st Edition.* Edited by Allan R. Cook and Peter D. Dresser. 524 pages. 1996. 0-7808-0076-1.

"An excellent addition to collections in public, consumer health, and women's health libraries."
—*American Reference Books Annual, 2003*

"Overall, the information is excellent, and complex topics are clearly explained. As a reference book for the consumer it is a valuable resource to assist them to make informed decisions about cancer and its treatments."
—*Cancer Forum, Nov '02*

"Highly recommended for academic and medical reference collections."
—*Library Bookwatch, Sep '02*

"This is a highly recommended book for any public or consumer library, being reader friendly and containing accurate and helpful information."
—*E-Streams, Aug '02*

"Recommended reference source."
—*Booklist, American Library Association, Jul '02*

SEE ALSO *Breast Cancer Sourcebook, Women's Health Concerns Sourcebook*

Cardiovascular Diseases & Disorders Sourcebook, 3rd Edition

Basic Consumer Health Information about Heart and Vascular Diseases and Disorders, Such as Angina, Heart Attacks, Arrhythmias, Cardiomyopathy, Valve Disease, Atherosclerosis, and Aneurysms, with Information about Managing Cardiovascular Risk Factors and Maintaining Heart Health, Medications and Procedures Used to Treat Cardiovascular Disorders, and Concerns of Special Significance to Women

long with Reports on Current Research Initiatives, a Glossary of Related Medical Terms, and a Directory of Sources for Further Help and Information

Edited by Sandra J. Judd. 713 pages. 2005. 0-7808-0739-1.

ALSO AVAILABLE: *Heart Diseases & Disorders Sourcebook, 2nd Edition.* Edited by Karen Bellenir. 612 pages. 2000. 0-7808-0238-1.

Cardiovascular Diseases & Disorders Sourcebook, 1st Edition. Edited by Karen Bellenir and Peter D. Dresser. 683 pages. 1995. 0-7808-0032-X.

"This work stands out as an imminently accessible resource for the general public. It is recommended for the reference and circulating shelves of school, public, and academic libraries."
—*American Reference Books Annual, 2001*

"Recommended reference source."
—*Booklist, American Library Association, Dec '00*

"Provides comprehensive coverage of matters related to the heart. This title is recommended for health sciences and public libraries with consumer health collections."
—*E-Streams, Oct '00*

SEE ALSO *Healthy Heart Sourcebook for Women*

Caregiving Sourcebook

Basic Consumer Health Information for Caregivers, Including a Profile of Caregivers, Caregiving Responsibilities and Concerns, Tips for Specific Conditions, Care Environments, and the Effects of Caregiving

Along with Facts about Legal Issues, Financial Information, and Future Planning, a Glossary, and a Listing of Additional Resources

Edited by Joyce Brennfleck Shannon. 600 pages. 2001. 0-7808-0331-0.

"Essential for most collections."
—*Library Journal, Apr 1, 2002*

"An ideal addition to the reference collection of any public library. Health sciences information professionals may also want to acquire the *Caregiving Source-*

book for their hospital or academic library for use as a ready reference tool by health care workers interested in aging and caregiving." —*E-Streams, Jan '02*

"Recommended reference source."
—*Booklist, American Library Association, Oct '01*

Child Abuse Sourcebook

Basic Consumer Health Information about the Physical, Sexual, and Emotional Abuse of Children, with Additional Facts about Neglect, Munchausen Syndrome by Proxy (MSBP), Shaken Baby Syndrome, and Controversial Issues Related to Child Abuse, Such as Withholding Medical Care, Corporal Punishment, and Child Maltreatment in Youth Sports, and Featuring Facts about Child Protective Services, Foster Care, Adoption, Parenting Challenges, and Other Abuse Prevention Efforts

Along with a Glossary of Related Terms and Resources for Additional Help and Information

Edited by Dawn D. Matthews. 620 pages. 2004. 0-7808-0705-7.

Childhood Diseases & Disorders Sourcebook

Basic Consumer Health Information about Medical Problems Often Encountered in Pre-Adolescent Children, Including Respiratory Tract Ailments, Ear Infections, Sore Throats, Disorders of the Skin and Scalp, Digestive and Genitourinary Diseases, Infectious Diseases, Inflammatory Disorders, Chronic Physical and Developmental Disorders, Allergies, and More

Along with Information about Diagnostic Tests, Common Childhood Surgeries, and Frequently Used Medications, with a Glossary of Important Terms and Resource Directory

Edited by Chad T. Kimball. 662 pages. 2003. 0-7808-0458-9.

"This is an excellent book for new parents and should be included in all health care and public libraries."
—*American Reference Books Annual, 2004*

Colds, Flu & Other Common Ailments Sourcebook

Basic Consumer Health Information about Common Ailments and Injuries, Including Colds, Coughs, the Flu, Sinus Problems, Headaches, Fever, Nausea and Vomiting, Menstrual Cramps, Diarrhea, Constipation, Hemorrhoids, Back Pain, Dandruff, Dry and Itchy Skin, Cuts, Scrapes, Sprains, Bruises, and More

Along with Information about Prevention, Self-Care, Choosing a Doctor, Over-the-Counter Medications, Folk Remedies, and Alternative Therapies, and Including a Glossary of Important Terms and a Directory of Resources for Further Help and Information

Edited by Chad T. Kimball. 638 pages. 2001. 0-7808-0435-X.

"A good starting point for research on common illnesses. It will be a useful addition to public and consumer health library collections."
— *American Reference Books Annual 2002*

"Will prove valuable to any library seeking to maintain a current, comprehensive reference collection of health resources. . . . Excellent reference."
— *The Bookwatch, Aug '01*

"Recommended reference source."
— *Booklist, American Library Association, July '01*

Communication Disorders Sourcebook

Basic Information about Deafness and Hearing Loss, Speech and Language Disorders, Voice Disorders, Balance and Vestibular Disorders, and Disorders of Smell, Taste, and Touch

Edited by Linda M. Ross. 533 pages. 1996. 0-7808-0077-X.

"This is skillfully edited and is a welcome resource for the layperson. It should be found in every public and medical library." — *Booklist Health Sciences Supplement, American Library Association, Oct '97*

Congenital Disorders Sourcebook

Basic Information about Disorders Acquired during Gestation, Including Spina Bifida, Hydrocephalus, Cerebral Palsy, Heart Defects, Craniofacial Abnormalities, Fetal Alcohol Syndrome, and More

Along with Current Treatment Options and Statistical Data

Edited by Karen Bellenir. 607 pages. 1997. 0-7808-0205-5.

"Recommended reference source."
— *Booklist, American Library Association, Oct '97*

SEE ALSO Pregnancy & Birth Sourcebook

Consumer Issues in Health Care Sourcebook

Basic Information about Health Care Fundamentals and Related Consumer Issues, Including Exams and Screening Tests, Physician Specialties, Choosing a Doctor, Using Prescription and Over-the-Counter Medications Safely, Avoiding Health Scams, Managing Common Health Risks in the Home, Care Options for Chronically or Terminally Ill Patients, and a List of Resources for Obtaining Help and Further Information

Edited by Karen Bellenir. 618 pages. 1998. 0-7808-0221-7.

"Both public and academic libraries will want to have a copy in their collection for readers who are interested in self-education on health issues."
—*American Reference Books Annual, 2000*

Contagious Diseases Sourcebook

Basic Consumer Health Information about Infectious Diseases Spread by Person-to-Person Contact through Direct Touch, Airborne Transmission, Sexual Contact, or Contact with Blood or Other Body Fluids, Including Hepatitis, Herpes, Influenza, Lice, Measles, Mumps, Pinworm, Ringworm, Severe Acute Respiratory Syndrome (SARS), Streptococcal Infections, Tuberculosis, and Others

Along with Facts about Disease Transmission, Antimicrobial Resistance, and Vaccines, with a Glossary and Directories of Resources for More Information

Edited by Karen Bellenir. 643 pages. 2004. 0-7808-0736-7.

Contagious & Non-Contagious Infectious Diseases Sourcebook

Basic Information about Contagious Diseases like Measles, Polio, Hepatitis B, and Infectious Mononucleosis, and Non-Contagious Infectious Diseases like Tetanus and Toxic Shock Syndrome, and Diseases Occurring as Secondary Infections Such as Shingles and Reye Syndrome

Along with Vaccination, Prevention, and Treatment Information, and a Section Describing Emerging Infectious Disease Threats

Edited by Karen Bellenir and Peter D. Dresser. 566 pages. 1996. 0-7808-0075-3.

Death & Dying Sourcebook

Basic Consumer Health Information for the Layperson about End-of-Life Care and Related Ethical and Legal Issues, Including Chief Causes of Death, Autopsies, Pain Management for the Terminally Ill, Life Support Systems, Insurance, Euthanasia, Assisted Suicide, Hospice Programs, Living Wills, Funeral Planning, Counseling, Mourning, Organ Donation, and Physician Training

Along with Statistical Data, a Glossary, and Listings of Sources for Further Help and Information

Edited by Annemarie S. Muth. 641 pages. 1999. 0-7808-0230-6.

Dental Care & Oral Health Sourcebook, 2nd Edition

Basic Consumer Health Information about Dental Care, Including Oral Hygiene, Dental Visits, Pain Management, Cavities, Crowns, Bridges, Dental Implants, and Fillings, and Other Oral Health Concerns, Such as Gum Disease, Bad Breath, Dry Mouth, Genetic and Developmental Abnormalities, Oral Cancers, Orthodontics, and Temporomandibular Disorders

Along with Updates on Current Research in Oral Health, a Glossary, a Directory of Dental and Oral Health Organizations, and Resources for People with Dental and Oral Health Disorders

Edited by Amy L. Sutton. 609 pages. 2003. 0-7808-0634-4.

ALSO AVAILABLE: *Oral Health Sourcebook, 1st Edition.* Edited by Allan R. Cook. 558 pages. 1997. 0-7808-0082-6.

Depression Sourcebook

Basic Consumer Health Information about Unipolar Depression, Bipolar Disorder, Postpartum Depression, Seasonal Affective Disorder, and Other Types of Depression in Children, Adolescents, Women, Men, the Elderly, and Other Selected Populations

Along with Facts about Causes, Risk Factors, Diagnostic Criteria, Treatment Options, Coping Strategies, Suicide Prevention, a Glossary, and a Directory of Sources for Additional Help and Information

Edited by Karen Belleni. 602 pages. 2002. 0-7808-0611-5.

Dermatological Disorders Sourcebook, 2nd Edition

Basic Consumer Health Information about Conditions and Disorders Affecting the Skin, Hair, and Nails, Such as Acne, Rosacea, Rashes, Dermatitis, Pigmentation Disorders, Birthmarks, Skin Cancer, Skin Injuries, Psoriasis, Scleroderma, and Hair Loss, Including Facts about Medications and Treatments for Dermatological Disorders and Tips for Maintaining Healthy Skin, Hair, and Nails

Along with Information about How Aging Affects the Skin, a Glossary of Related Terms, and a Directory of Resources for Additional Help and Information

Edited by Amy L. Sutton. 600 pages. 2005. 0-7808-0795-2.

ALSO AVAILABLE: *Skin Disorders Sourcebook, 1st Edition.* Edited by Allan R. Cook. 647 pages. 1997. 0-7808-0080-X.

". . . comprehensive, easily read reference book."
—*Doody's Health Sciences Book Reviews, Oct '97*

■

Diabetes Sourcebook, 3rd Edition

Basic Consumer Health Information about Type 1 Diabetes (Insulin-Dependent or Juvenile-Onset Diabetes), Type 2 Diabetes (Noninsulin-Dependent or Adult-Onset Diabetes), Gestational Diabetes, Impaired Glucose Tolerance (IGT), and Related Complications, Such as Amputation, Eye Disease, Gum Disease, Nerve Damage, and End-Stage Renal Disease, Including Facts about Insulin, Oral Diabetes Medications, Blood Sugar Testing, and the Role of Exercise and Nutrition in the Control of Diabetes

Along with a Glossary and Resources for Further Help and Information

Edited by Dawn D. Matthews. 622 pages. 2003. 0-7808-0629-8.

ALSO AVAILABLE: *Diabetes Sourcebook, 1st Edition.* Edited by Karen Bellenir and Peter D. Dresser. 827 pages. 1994. 1-55888-751-2.

Diabetes Sourcebook, 2nd Edition. Edited by Karen Bellenir. 688 pages. 1998. 0-7808-0224-1.

"This edition is even more helpful than earlier versions. . . . It is a truly valuable tool for anyone seeking readable and authoritative information on diabetes."
—*American Reference Books Annual, 2004*

"An invaluable reference." —*Library Journal, May '00*

Selected as one of the 250 "Best Health Sciences Books of 1999." —*Doody's Rating Service, Mar-Apr 2000*

"Provides useful information for the general public."
—*Healthlines, University of Michigan Health Management Research Center, Sep/Oct '99*

". . . provides reliable mainstream medical information . . . belongs on the shelves of any library with a consumer health collection." —*E-Streams, Sep '99*

"Recommended reference source."
—*Booklist, American Library Association, Feb '99*

Diet & Nutrition Sourcebook, 2nd Edition

Basic Consumer Health Information about Dietary Guidelines, Recommended Daily Intake Values, Vitamins, Minerals, Fiber, Fat, Weight Control, Dietary Supplements, and Food Additives

Along with Special Sections on Nutrition Needs throughout Life and Nutrition for People with Such Specific Medical Concerns as Allergies, High Blood Cholesterol, Hypertension, Diabetes, Celiac Disease, Seizure Disorders, Phenylketonuria (PKU), Cancer, and Eating Disorders, and Including Reports on Current Nutrition Research and Source Listings for Additional Help and Information

Edited by Karen Bellenir. 650 pages. 1999. 0-7808-0228-4.

ALSO AVAILABLE: *Diet & Nutrition Sourcebook, 1st Edition.* Edited by Dan R. Harris. 662 pages. 1996. 0-7808-0084-2.

"This book is an excellent source of basic diet and nutrition information." —*Booklist Health Sciences Supplement, American Library Association, Dec '00*

"This reference document should be in any public library, but it would be a very good guide for beginning students in the health sciences. If the other books in this publisher's series are as good as this, they should all be in the health sciences collections."
—*American Reference Books Annual, 2000*

"This book is an excellent general nutrition reference for consumers who desire to take an active role in their health care for prevention. Consumers of all ages who select this book can feel confident they are receiving current and accurate information." —*Journal of Nutrition for the Elderly, Vol. 19, No. 4, '00*

"Recommended reference source."
—*Booklist, American Library Association, Dec '99*

SEE ALSO *Digestive Diseases & Disorders Sourcebook, Eating Disorders Sourcebook, Gastrointestinal Diseases & Disorders Sourcebook, Vegetarian Sourcebook*

■

Digestive Diseases & Disorders Sourcebook

Basic Consumer Health Information about Diseases and Disorders that Impact the Upper and Lower Digestive System, Including Celiac Disease, Constipation, Crohn's Disease, Cyclic Vomiting Syndrome, Diarrhea, Diverticulosis and Diverticulitis, Gallstones, Heartburn, Hemorrhoids, Hernias, Indigestion (Dyspepsia), Irritable Bowel Syndrome, Lactose Intolerance, Ulcers, and More

Along with Information about Medications and Other Treatments, Tips for Maintaining a Healthy Digestive Tract, a Glossary, and Directory of Digestive Diseases Organizations

Edited by Karen Bellenir. 335 pages. 2000. 0-7808-0327-2.

"This title would be an excellent addition to all public or patient-research libraries."
—*American Reference Books Annual, 2001*

"This title is recommended for public, hospital, and health sciences libraries with consumer health collections." —E-Streams, Jul-Aug '00

"Recommended reference source."
—Booklist, American Library Association, May '00

SEE ALSO Diet & Nutrition Sourcebook, Eating Disorders Sourcebook, Gastrointestinal Diseases & Disorders Sourcebook

■

Disabilities Sourcebook

Basic Consumer Health Information about Physical and Psychiatric Disabilities, Including Descriptions of Major Causes of Disability, Assistive and Adaptive Aids, Workplace Issues, and Accessibility Concerns

Along with Information about the Americans with Disabilities Act, a Glossary, and Resources for Additional Help and Information

Edited by Dawn D. Matthews. 616 pages. 2000. 0-7808-0389-2.

"It is a must for libraries with a consumer health section." —American Reference Books Annual 2002

"A much needed addition to the Omnigraphics *Health Reference Series*. A current reference work to provide people with disabilities, their families, caregivers or those who work with them, a broad range of information in one volume, has not been available until now. . . . It is recommended for all public and academic library reference collections." —E-Streams, May '01

"An excellent source book in easy-to-read format covering many current topics; highly recommended for all libraries." —Choice, Association of College and Research Libraries, Jan '01

"Recommended reference source."
—Booklist, American Library Association, Jul '00

■

Domestic Violence Sourcebook, 2nd Edition

Basic Consumer Health Information about the Causes and Consequences of Abusive Relationships, Including Physical Violence, Sexual Assault, Battery, Stalking, and Emotional Abuse, and Facts about the Effects of Violence on Women, Men, Young Adults, and the Elderly, with Reports about Domestic Violence in Selected Populations, and Featuring Facts about Medical Care, Victim Assistance and Protection, Prevention Strategies, Mental Health Services, and Legal Issues

Along with a Glossary of Related Terms and Resources for Additional Help and Information

Edited by Dawn D. Matthews. 628 pages. 2004. 0-7808-0669-7.

ALSO AVAILABLE: Domestic Violence & Child Abuse Sourcebook, 1st Edition. Edited by Helene Henderson. 1,064 pages. 2001. 0-7808-0235-7.

"Interested lay persons should find the book extremely beneficial. . . . A copy of Domestic Violence and Child

Abuse Sourcebook should be in every public library in the United States." —Social Science & Medicine, No. 56, 2003

"This is important information. The Web has many resources but this sourcebook fills an important societal need. I am not aware of any other resources of this type." —Doody's Review Service, Sep '01

"Recommended for all libraries, scholars, and practitioners." —Choice, Association of College & Research Libraries, Jul '01

"Recommended reference source."
—Booklist, American Library Association, Apr '01

"Important pick for college-level health reference libraries." —The Bookwatch, Mar '01

"Because this problem is so widespread and because this book includes a lot of issues within one volume, this work is recommended for all public libraries." —American Reference Books Annual, 2001

■

Drug Abuse Sourcebook, 2nd Edition

Basic Consumer Health Information about Illicit Substances of Abuse and the Misuse of Prescription and Over-the-Counter Medications, Including Depressants, Hallucinogens, Inhalants, Marijuana, Stimulants, and Anabolic Steroids

Along with Facts about Related Health Risks, Treatment Programs, Prevention Programs, a Glossary of Abuse and Addiction Terms, a Glossary of Drug-Related Street Terms, and a Directory of Resources for More Information

Edited by Catherine Ginther. 607 pages. 2004. 0-7808-0740-5.

ALSO AVAILABLE: Drug Abuse Sourcebook, 1st Edition. Edited by Karen Bellenir. 629 pages. 2000. 0-7808-0242-X.

"Containing a wealth of information . . . . This resource belongs in libraries that serve a lower-division undergraduate or community college clientele as well as the general public." —Choice, Association of College and Research Libraries, Jun '01

"Recommended reference source."
—Booklist, American Library Association, Feb '01

"Highly recommended." —The Bookwatch, Jan '01

"Even though there is a plethora of books on drug abuse, this volume is recommended for school, public, and college libraries." —American Reference Books Annual, 2001

SEE ALSO Alcoholism Sourcebook, Substance Abuse Sourcebook

Ear, Nose & Throat Disorders Sourcebook

Basic Information about Disorders of the Ears, Nose, Sinus Cavities, Pharynx, and Larynx, Including Ear Infections, Tinnitus, Vestibular Disorders, Allergic and Non-Allergic Rhinitis, Sore Throats, Tonsillitis, and Cancers That Affect the Ears, Nose, Sinuses, and Throat

Along with Reports on Current Research Initiatives, a Glossary of Related Medical Terms, and a Directory of Sources for Further Help and Information

Edited by Karen Bellenir and Linda M. Shin. 576 pages. 1998. 0-7808-0206-3.

"Overall, this sourcebook is helpful for the consumer seeking information on ENT issues. It is recommended for public libraries."
— *American Reference Books Annual, 1999*

"Recommended reference source."
— *Booklist, American Library Association, Dec '98*

■

Eating Disorders Sourcebook

Basic Consumer Health Information about Eating Disorders, Including Information about Anorexia Nervosa, Bulimia Nervosa, Binge Eating, Body Dysmorphic Disorder, Pica, Laxative Abuse, and Night Eating Syndrome

Along with Information about Causes, Adverse Effects, and Treatment and Prevention Issues, and Featuring a Section on Concerns Specific to Children and Adolescents, a Glossary, and Resources for Further Help and Information

Edited by Dawn D. Matthews. 322 pages. 2001. 0-7808-0335-3.

"Recommended for health science libraries that are open to the public, as well as hospital libraries. This book is a good resource for the consumer who is concerned about eating disorders." — *E-Streams, Mar '02*

"This volume is another convenient collection of excerpted articles. Recommended for school and public library patrons; lower-division undergraduates; and two-year technical program students." — *Choice, Association of College & Research Libraries, Jan '02*

"Recommended reference source." — *Booklist, American Library Association, Oct '01*

SEE ALSO *Diet & Nutrition Sourcebook, Digestive Diseases & Disorders Sourcebook, Gastrointestinal Diseases & Disorders Sourcebook*

■

Emergency Medical Services Sourcebook

Basic Consumer Health Information about Preventing, Preparing for, and Managing Emergency Situations, When and Who to Call for Help, What to Expect in the Emergency Room, the Emergency Medical Team, Patient Issues, and Current Topics in Emergency Medicine

Along with Statistical Data, a Glossary, and Sources of Additional Help and Information

Edited by Jenni Lynn Colson. 494 pages. 2002. 0-7808-0420-1.

"Handy and convenient for home, public, school, and college libraries. Recommended."
— *Choice, Association of College and Research Libraries, Apr '03*

"This reference can provide the consumer with answers to most questions about emergency care in the United States, or it will direct them to a resource where the answer can be found."
— *American Reference Books Annual, 2003*

"Recommended reference source."
— *Booklist, American Library Association, Feb '03*

■

Endocrine & Metabolic Disorders Sourcebook

Basic Information for the Layperson about Pancreatic and Insulin-Related Disorders Such as Pancreatitis, Diabetes, and Hypoglycemia; Adrenal Gland Disorders Such as Cushing's Syndrome, Addison's Disease, and Congenital Adrenal Hyperplasia; Pituitary Gland Disorders Such as Growth Hormone Deficiency, Acromegaly, and Pituitary Tumors; Thyroid Disorders Such as Hypothyroidism, Graves' Disease, Hashimoto's Disease, and Goiter; Hyperparathyroidism; and Other Diseases and Syndromes of Hormone Imbalance or Metabolic Dysfunction

Along with Reports on Current Research Initiatives

Edited by Linda M. Shin. 574 pages. 1998. 0-7808-0207-1.

"Omnigraphics has produced another needed resource for health information consumers."
— *American Reference Books Annual, 2000*

"Recommended reference source."
— *Booklist, American Library Association, Dec '98*

■

Environmental Health Sourcebook, 2nd Edition

Basic Consumer Health Information about the Environment and Its Effect on Human Health, Including the Effects of Air Pollution, Water Pollution, Hazardous Chemicals, Food Hazards, Radiation Hazards, Biological Agents, Household Hazards, Such as Radon, Asbestos, Carbon Monoxide, and Mold, and Information about Associated Diseases and Disorders, Including Cancer, Allergies, Respiratory Problems, and Skin Disorders

Along with Information about Environmental Concerns for Specific Populations, a Glossary of Related Terms, and Resources for Further Help and Information

Edited by Dawn D. Matthews. 673 pages. 2003. 0-7808-0632-8.

ALSO AVAILABLE: *Environmentally Induced Disorders Sourcebook, 1st Edition.* Edited by Allan R. Cook. 620 pages. 1997. 0-7808-0083-4.

"This recently updated edition continues the level of quality and the reputation of the numerous other volumes in Omnigraphics' *Health Reference Series*."
— *American Reference Books Annual, 2004*

"Recommended reference source."
— *Booklist, American Library Association, Sep '98*

"This book will be a useful addition to anyone's library." — *Choice Health Sciences Supplement, Association of College and Research Libraries, May '98*

". . . a good survey of numerous environmentally induced physical disorders . . . a useful addition to anyone's library."
— *Doody's Health Sciences Book Reviews, Jan '98*

". . . provide[s] introductory information from the best authorities around. Since this volume covers topics that potentially affect everyone, it will surely be one of the most frequently consulted volumes in the *Health Reference Series*." — *Rettig on Reference, Nov '97*

Environmentally Induced Disorders Sourcebook, 1st Edition

SEE *Environmental Health Sourcebook, 2nd Edition*

Ethnic Diseases Sourcebook

Basic Consumer Health Information for Ethnic and Racial Minority Groups in the United States, Including General Health Indicators and Behaviors, Ethnic Diseases, Genetic Testing, the Impact of Chronic Diseases, Women's Health, Mental Health Issues, and Preventive Health Care Services

Along with a Glossary and a Listing of Additional Resources

Edited by Joyce Brennfleck Shannon. 664 pages. 2001. 0-7808-0336-1.

"Recommended for health sciences libraries where public health programs are a priority."
— *E-Streams, Jan '02*

"Not many books have been written on this topic to date, and the *Ethnic Diseases Sourcebook* is a strong addition to the list. It will be an important introductory resource for health consumers, students, health care personnel, and social scientists. It is recommended for public, academic, and large hospital libraries."
— *American Reference Books Annual 2002*

"Recommended reference source."
— *Booklist, American Library Association, Oct '01*

"Will prove valuable to any library seeking to maintain a current, comprehensive reference collection of health resources. . . . An excellent source of health information about genetic disorders which affect particular ethnic and racial minorities in the U.S."
— *The Bookwatch, Aug '01*

Eye Care Sourcebook, 2nd Edition

Basic Consumer Health Information about Eye Care and Eye Disorders, Including Facts about the Diagnosis, Prevention, and Treatment of Common Refractive Problems Such as Myopia, Hyperopia, Astigmatism, and Presbyopia, and Eye Diseases, Including Glaucoma, Cataract, Age-Related Macular Degeneration, and Diabetic Retinopathy

Along with a Section on Vision Correction and Refractive Surgeries, Including LASIK and LASEK, a Glossary, and Directories of Resources for Additional Help and Information

Edited by Amy L. Sutton. 543 pages. 2003. 0-7808-0635-2.

ALSO AVAILABLE: *Ophthalmic Disorders Sourcebook, 1st Edition.* Edited by Linda M. Ross. 631 pages. 1996. 0-7808-0081-8.

". . . a solid reference tool for eye care and a valuable addition to a collection."
— *American Reference Books Annual, 2004*

Family Planning Sourcebook

Basic Consumer Health Information about Planning for Pregnancy and Contraception, Including Traditional Methods, Barrier Methods, Hormonal Methods, Permanent Methods, Future Methods, Emergency Contraception, and Birth Control Choices for Women at Each Stage of Life

Along with Statistics, a Glossary, and Sources of Additional Information

Edited by Amy Marcaccio Keyzer. 520 pages. 2001. 0-7808-0379-5.

"Recommended for public, health, and undergraduate libraries as part of the circulating collection."
— *E-Streams, Mar '02*

"Information is presented in an unbiased, readable manner, and the sourcebook will certainly be a necessary addition to those public and high school libraries where Internet access is restricted or otherwise problematic." — *American Reference Books Annual 2002*

"Recommended reference source."
— *Booklist, American Library Association, Oct '01*

"Will prove valuable to any library seeking to maintain a current, comprehensive reference collection of health resources. . . . Excellent reference."
— *The Bookwatch, Aug '01*

SEE ALSO *Pregnancy & Birth Sourcebook*

Fitness & Exercise Sourcebook, 2nd Edition

Basic Consumer Health Information about the Fundamentals of Fitness and Exercise, Including How to Begin and Maintain a Fitness Program, Fitness as a Lifestyle, the Link between Fitness and Diet, Advice for Specific Groups of People, Exercise as It Relates to Specific Medical Conditions, and Recent Research in Fitness and Exercise

Along with a Glossary of Important Terms and Resources for Additional Help and Information

Edited by Kristen M. Gledhill. 646 pages. 2001. 0-7808-0334-5.

ALSO AVAILABLE: Fitness & Exercise Sourcebook, 1st Edition. Edited by Dan R. Harris. 663 pages. 1996. 0-7808-0186-5.

"This work is recommended for all general reference collections."
— *American Reference Books Annual 2002*

"Highly recommended for public, consumer, and school grades fourth through college."
—*E-Streams, Nov '01*

"Recommended reference source." — *Booklist, American Library Association, Oct '01*

"The information appears quite comprehensive and is considered reliable. . . . This second edition is a welcomed addition to the series."
—*Doody's Review Service, Sep '01*

"This reference is a valuable choice for those who desire a broad source of information on exercise, fitness, and chronic-disease prevention through a healthy lifestyle." —*American Medical Writers Association Journal, Fall '01*

"Will prove valuable to any library seeking to maintain a current, comprehensive reference collection of health resources. . . . Excellent reference."
— *The Bookwatch, Aug '01*

Food & Animal Borne Diseases Sourcebook

Basic Information about Diseases That Can Be Spread to Humans through the Ingestion of Contaminated Food or Water or by Contact with Infected Animals and Insects, Such as Botulism, E. Coli, Hepatitis A, Trichinosis, Lyme Disease, and Rabies

Along with Information Regarding Prevention and Treatment Methods, and Including a Special Section for International Travelers Describing Diseases Such as Cholera, Malaria, Travelers' Diarrhea, and Yellow Fever, and Offering Recommendations for Avoiding Illness

Edited by Karen Bellenir and Peter D. Dresser. 535 pages. 1995. 0-7808-0033-8.

"Targeting general readers and providing them with a single, comprehensive source of information on selected topics, this book continues, with the excellent caliber of its predecessors, to catalog topical information on health matters of general interest. Readable and thorough, this valuable resource is highly recommended for all libraries."
— *Academic Library Book Review, Summer '96*

"A comprehensive collection of authoritative information." — *Emergency Medical Services, Oct '95*

Food Safety Sourcebook

Basic Consumer Health Information about the Safe Handling of Meat, Poultry, Seafood, Eggs, Fruit Juices, and Other Food Items, and Facts about Pesticides, Drinking Water, Food Safety Overseas, and the Onset, Duration, and Symptoms of Foodborne Illnesses, Including Types of Pathogenic Bacteria, Parasitic Protozoa, Worms, Viruses, and Natural Toxins

Along with the Role of the Consumer, the Food Handler, and the Government in Food Safety; a Glossary, and Resources for Additional Help and Information

Edited by Dawn D. Matthews. 339 pages. 1999. 0-7808-0326-4.

"This book is recommended for public libraries and universities with home economic and food science programs." — *E-Streams, Nov '00*

"Recommended reference source."
—*Booklist, American Library Association, May '00*

"This book takes the complex issues of food safety and foodborne pathogens and presents them in an easily understood manner. [It does] an excellent job of covering a large and often confusing topic."
—*American Reference Books Annual, 2000*

Forensic Medicine Sourcebook

Basic Consumer Information for the Layperson about Forensic Medicine, Including Crime Scene Investigation, Evidence Collection and Analysis, Expert Testimony, Computer-Aided Criminal Identification, Digital Imaging in the Courtroom, DNA Profiling, Accident Reconstruction, Autopsies, Ballistics, Drugs and Explosives Detection, Latent Fingerprints, Product Tampering, and Questioned Document Examination

Along with Statistical Data, a Glossary of Forensics Terminology, and Listings of Sources for Further Help and Information

Edited by Annemarie S. Muth. 574 pages. 1999. 0-7808-0232-2.

"Given the expected widespread interest in its content and its easy to read style, this book is recommended for most public and all college and university libraries." — *E-Streams, Feb '01*

"Recommended for public libraries."
—*Reference & User Services Quarterly, American Library Association, Spring 2000*

"Recommended reference source."
—*Booklist, American Library Association, Feb '00*

"A wealth of information, useful statistics, references are up-to-date and extremely complete. This wonderful collection of data will help students who are interested in a career in any type of forensic field. It is a great resource for attorneys who need information about types of expert witnesses needed in a particular case. It also offers useful information for fiction and nonfiction writers whose work involves a crime. A fascinating compilation. All levels." — *Choice, Association of College and Research Libraries, Jan 2000*

"There are several items that make this book attractive to consumers who are seeking certain forensic data.... This is a useful current source for those seeking general forensic medical answers."
—American Reference Books Annual, 2000

Gastrointestinal Diseases & Disorders Sourcebook

Basic Information about Gastroesophageal Reflux Disease (Heartburn), Ulcers, Diverticulosis, Irritable Bowel Syndrome, Crohn's Disease, Ulcerative Colitis, Diarrhea, Constipation, Lactose Intolerance, Hemorrhoids, Hepatitis, Cirrhosis, and Other Digestive Problems, Featuring Statistics, Descriptions of Symptoms, and Current Treatment Methods of Interest for Persons Living with Upper and Lower Gastrointestinal Maladies

Edited by Linda M. Ross. 413 pages. 1996. 0-7808-0078-8.

". . . very readable form. The successful editorial work that brought this material together into a useful and understandable reference makes accessible to all readers information that can help them more effectively understand and obtain help for digestive tract problems."
— Choice, Association of College & Research Libraries, Feb '97

SEE ALSO *Diet & Nutrition Sourcebook, Digestive Diseases & Disorders, Eating Disorders Sourcebook*

Genetic Disorders Sourcebook, 3rd Edition

Basic Consumer Health Information about Hereditary Diseases and Disorders, Including Facts about the Human Genome, Genetic Inheritance Patterns, Disorders Associated with Specific Genes, Such as Sickle Cell Disease, Hemophilia, and Cystic Fibrosis, Chromosome Disorders, Such as Down Syndrome, Fragile X Syndrome, and Turner Syndrome, and Complex Diseases and Disorders Resulting from the Interaction of Environmental and Genetic Factors, Such as Allergies, Cancer, and Obesity

Along with Facts about Genetic Testing, Suggestions for Parents of Children with Special Needs, Reports on Current Research Initiatives, a Glossary of Genetic Terminology, and Resources for Additional Help and Information

Edited by Karen Bellenir. 777 pages. 2004. 0-7808-0742-1.

ALSO AVAILABLE: *Genetic Disorders Sourcebook, 1st Edition.* Edited by Karen Bellenir. 642 pages. 1996. 0-7808-0034-6.

Genetic Disorders Sourcebook, 2nd Edition. Edited by Kathy Massimini. 768 pages. 2001. 0-7808-0241-1.

"Recommended for public libraries and medical and hospital libraries with consumer health collections."
— E-Streams, May '01

"Recommended reference source."
— Booklist, American Library Association, Apr '01

"Important pick for college-level health reference libraries."
— The Bookwatch, Mar '01

"Provides essential medical information to both the general public and those diagnosed with a serious or fatal genetic disease or disorder."
—Choice, Association of College and Research Libraries, Jan '97

Head Trauma Sourcebook

Basic Information for the Layperson about Open-Head and Closed-Head Injuries, Treatment Advances, Recovery, and Rehabilitation

Along with Reports on Current Research Initiatives

Edited by Karen Bellenir. 414 pages. 1997. 0-7808-0208-X.

Headache Sourcebook

Basic Consumer Health Information about Migraine, Tension, Cluster, Rebound and Other Types of Headaches, with Facts about the Cause and Prevention of Headaches, the Effects of Stress and the Environment, Headaches during Pregnancy and Menopause, and Childhood Headaches

Along with a Glossary and Other Resources for Additional Help and Information

Edited by Dawn D. Matthews. 362 pages. 2002. 0-7808-0337-X.

"Highly recommended for academic and medical reference collections." — Library Bookwatch, Sep '02

Health Insurance Sourcebook

Basic Information about Managed Care Organizations, Traditional Fee-for-Service Insurance, Insurance Portability and Pre-Existing Conditions Clauses, Medicare, Medicaid, Social Security, and Military Health Care

Along with Information about Insurance Fraud

Edited by Wendy Wilcox. 530 pages. 1997. 0-7808-0222-5.

"Particularly useful because it brings much of this information together in one volume. This book will be a handy reference source in the health sciences library, hospital library, college and university library, and medium to large public library."
— Medical Reference Services Quarterly, Fall '98

Awarded "Books of the Year Award"
— American Journal of Nursing, 1997

"The layout of the book is particularly helpful as it provides easy access to reference material. A most useful addition to the vast amount of information about health insurance. The use of data from U.S. government agencies is most commendable. Useful in a library or learning center for healthcare professional students."
— Doody's Health Sciences Book Reviews, Nov '97

Health Reference Series Cumulative Index 1999

A Comprehensive Index to the Individual Volumes of the Health Reference Series, Including a Subject Index, Name Index, Organization Index, and Publication Index

Along with a Master List of Acronyms and Abbreviations

Edited by Edward J. Prucha, Anne Holmes, and Robert Rudnick. 990 pages. 2000. 0-7808-0382-5.

"This volume will be most helpful in libraries that have a relatively complete collection of the Health Reference Series." —*American Reference Books Annual, 2001*

"Essential for collections that hold any of the numerous *Health Reference Series* titles."
— *Choice, Association of College and Research Libraries, Nov '00*

■

Healthy Aging Sourcebook

Basic Consumer Health Information about Maintaining Health through the Aging Process, Including Advice on Nutrition, Exercise, and Sleep, Help in Making Decisions about Midlife Issues and Retirement, and Guidance Concerning Practical and Informed Choices in Health Consumerism

Along with Data Concerning the Theories of Aging, Different Experiences in Aging by Minority Groups, and Facts about Aging Now and Aging in the Future; and Featuring a Glossary, a Guide to Consumer Help, Additional Suggested Reading, and Practical Resource Directory

Edited by Jenifer Swanson. 536 pages. 1999. 0-7808-0390-6.

"Recommended reference source."
—*Booklist, American Library Association, Feb '00*

SEE ALSO Physical & Mental Issues in Aging Sourcebook

■

Healthy Children Sourcebook

Basic Consumer Health Information about the Physical and Mental Development of Children between the Ages of 3 and 12, Including Routine Health Care, Preventative Health Services, Safety and First Aid, Healthy Sleep, Dental Care, Nutrition, and Fitness, and Featuring Parenting Tips on Such Topics as Bedwetting, Choosing Day Care, Monitoring TV and Other Media, and Establishing a Foundation for Substance Abuse Prevention

Along with a Glossary of Commonly Used Pediatric Terms and Resources for Additional Help and Information.

Edited by Chad T. Kimball. 647 pages. 2003. 0-7808-0247-0.

"It is hard to imagine that any other single resource exists that would provide such a comprehensive guide of timely information on health promotion and disease prevention for children aged 3 to 12."

—American Reference Books Annual, 2004

"The strengths of this book are many. It is clearly written, presented and structured."
—*Journal of the National Medical Association, 2004*

■

Healthy Heart Sourcebook for Women

Basic Consumer Health Information about Cardiac Issues Specific to Women, Including Facts about Major Risk Factors and Prevention, Treatment and Control Strategies, and Important Dietary Issues

Along with a Special Section Regarding the Pros and Cons of Hormone Replacement Therapy and Its Impact on Heart Health, and Additional Help, Including Recipes, a Glossary, and a Directory of Resources

Edited by Dawn D. Matthews. 336 pages. 2000. 0-7808-0329-9.

"A good reference source and recommended for all public, academic, medical, and hospital libraries."
— *Medical Reference Services Quarterly, Summer '01*

"Because of the lack of information specific to women on this topic, this book is recommended for public libraries and consumer libraries."
—*American Reference Books Annual, 2001*

"Contains very important information about coronary artery disease that all women should know. The information is current and presented in an easy-to-read format. The book will make a good addition to any library." — *American Medical Writers Association Journal, Summer '00*

"Important, basic reference."
— *Reviewer's Bookwatch, Jul '00*

SEE ALSO Heart Diseases & Disorders Sourcebook, Women's Health Concerns Sourcebook

■

Heart Diseases & Disorders Sourcebook, 2nd Edition

SEE Cardiovascular Diseases & Disorders Sourcebook, 3rd Edition

■

Hepatitis Sourcebook

Basic Consumer Health Information about Hepatitis A, Hepatitis B, Hepatitis C, and Other Forms of Hepatitis, Including Autoimmune Hepatitis, Alcoholic Hepatitis, Nonalcoholic Steatohepatitis, and Toxic Hepatitis, with Facts about Risk Factors, Screening Methods, Diagnostic Tests, and Treatment Options

Along with Information on Liver Health, Tips for People Living with Chronic Hepatitis, Reports on Current Research Initiatives, a Glossary of Terms Related to Hepatitis, and a Directory of Sources for Further Help and Information

Edited by Sandra J. Judd. 597 pages. 2005. 0-7808-0749-9.

Household Safety Sourcebook

Basic Consumer Health Information about Household Safety, Including Information about Poisons, Chemicals, Fire, and Water Hazards in the Home

Along with Advice about the Safe Use of Home Maintenance Equipment, Choosing Toys and Nursery Furniture, Holiday and Recreation Safety, a Glossary, and Resources for Further Help and Information

Edited by Dawn D. Matthews. 606 pages. 2002. 0-7808-0338-8.

"This work will be useful in public libraries with large consumer health and wellness departments."
— *American Reference Books Annual, 2003*

"As a sourcebook on household safety this book meets its mark. It is encyclopedic in scope and covers a wide range of safety issues that are commonly seen in the home." — *E-Streams, Jul '02*

Hypertension Sourcebook

Basic Consumer Health Information about the Causes, Diagnosis, and Treatment of High Blood Pressure, with Facts about Consequences, Complications, and Co-Occurring Disorders, Such as Coronary Heart Disease, Diabetes, Stroke, Kidney Disease, and Hypertensive Retinopathy, and Issues in Blood Pressure Control, Including Dietary Choices, Stress Management, and Medications

Along with Reports on Current Research Initiatives and Clinical Trials, a Glossary, and Resources for Additional Help and Information

Edited by Dawn D. Matthews and Karen Bellenir. 613 pages. 2004. 0-7808-0674-3.

Immune System Disorders Sourcebook, 2nd Edition

Basic Consumer Health Information about Disorders of the Immune System, Including Immune System Function and Response, Diagnosis of Immune Disorders, Information about Inherited Immune Disease, Acquired Immune Disease, and Autoimmune Diseases, Including Primary Immune Deficiency, Acquired Immunodeficiency Syndrome (AIDS), Lupus, Multiple Sclerosis, Type 1 Diabetes, Rheumatoid Arthritis, and Graves Disease

Along with Treatments, Tips for Coping with Immune Disorders, a Glossary, and a Directory of Additional Resources

Edited by Joyce Brennfleck Shannon. 671 pages. 2005. 0-7808-0748-0.

ALSO AVAILABLE: *Immune System Disorders Sourcebook.* Edited by Allan R. Cook. 608 pages. 1997. 0-7808-0209-8.

Infant & Toddler Health Sourcebook

Basic Consumer Health Information about the Physical and Mental Development of Newborns, Infants, and Toddlers, Including Neonatal Concerns, Nutrition Recommendations, Immunization Schedules, Common Pediatric Disorders, Assessments and Milestones, Safety Tips, and Advice for Parents and Other Caregivers

Along with a Glossary of Terms and Resource Listings for Additional Help

Edited by Jenifer Swanson. 585 pages. 2000. 0-7808-0246-2.

"As a reference for the general public, this would be useful in any library." — *E-Streams, May '01*

"Recommended reference source." — *Booklist, American Library Association, Feb '01*

"This is a good source for general use." — *American Reference Books Annual, 2001*

Infectious Diseases Sourcebook

Basic Consumer Health Information about Non-Contagious Bacterial, Viral, Prion, Fungal, and Parasitic Diseases Spread by Food and Water, Insects and Animals, or Environmental Contact, Including Botulism, E. Coli, Encephalitis, Legionnaires' Disease, Lyme Disease, Malaria, Plague, Rabies, Salmonella, Tetanus, and Others, and Facts about Newly Emerging Diseases, Such as Hantavirus, Mad Cow Disease, Monkeypox, and West Nile Virus

Along with Information about Preventing Disease Transmission, the Threat of Bioterrorism, and Current Research Initiatives, with a Glossary and Directory of Resources for More Information

Edited by Karen Bellenir. 634 pages. 2004. 0-7808-0675-1.

Injury & Trauma Sourcebook

Basic Consumer Health Information about the Impact of Injury, the Diagnosis and Treatment of Common and Traumatic Injuries, Emergency Care, and Specific Injuries Related to Home, Community, Workplace, Transportation, and Recreation

Along with Guidelines for Injury Prevention, a Glossary, and a Directory of Additional Resources

Edited by Joyce Brennfleck Shannon. 696 pages. 2002. 0-7808-0421-X.

"This publication is the most comprehensive work of its kind about injury and trauma." — *American Reference Books Annual, 2003*

"This sourcebook provides concise, easily readable, basic health information about injuries. . . . This book is well organized and an easy to use reference resource suitable for hospital, health sciences and public libraries with consumer health collections." — *E-Streams, Nov '02*

"Practitioners should be aware of guides such as this in order to facilitate their use by patients and their families." —*Doody's Health Sciences Book Review Journal, Sep-Oct '02*

"Recommended reference source." —*Booklist, American Library Association, Sep '02*

"Highly recommended for academic and medical reference collections." —*Library Bookwatch, Sep '02*

◼

Kidney & Urinary Tract Diseases & Disorders Sourcebook, 1st Edition

SEE *Urinary Tract & Kidney Diseases & Disorders Sourcebook, 2nd Edition*

◼

Learning Disabilities Sourcebook, 2nd Edition

Basic Consumer Health Information about Learning Disabilities, Including Dyslexia, Developmental Speech and Language Disabilities, Non-Verbal Learning Disorders, Developmental Arithmetic Disorder, Developmental Writing Disorder, and Other Conditions That Impede Learning Such as Attention Deficit/ Hyperactivity Disorder, Brain Injury, Hearing Impairment, Klinefelter Syndrome, Dyspraxia, and Tourette Syndrome

Along with Facts about Educational Issues and Assistive Technology, Coping Strategies, a Glossary of Related Terms, and Resources for Further Help and Information

Edited by Dawn D. Matthews. 621 pages. 2003. 0-7808-0626-3.

ALSO AVAILABLE: *Learning Disabilities Sourcebook, 1st Edition.* Edited by Linda M. Shin. 579 pages. 1998. 0-7808-0210-1.

"The second edition of *Learning Disabilities Sourcebook* far surpasses the earlier edition in that it is more focused on information that will be useful as a consumer health resource." —*American Reference Books Annual, 2004*

"Teachers as well as consumers will find this an essential guide to understanding various syndromes and their latest treatments. [An] invaluable reference for public and school library collections alike." —*Library Bookwatch, Apr '03*

Named "Outstanding Reference Book of 1999." —*New York Public Library, Feb 2000*

"An excellent candidate for inclusion in a public library reference section. It's a great source of information. Teachers will also find the book useful. Definitely worth reading." —*Journal of Adolescent & Adult Literacy, Feb 2000*

"Readable . . . provides a solid base of information regarding successful techniques used with individuals who have learning disabilities, as well as practical suggestions for educators and family members. Clear lan-

guage, concise descriptions, and pertinent information for contacting multiple resources add to the strength of this book as a useful tool." —*Choice, Association of College and Research Libraries, Feb '99*

"Recommended reference source." —*Booklist, American Library Association, Sep '98*

"A useful resource for libraries and for those who don't have the time to identify and locate the individual publications." —*Disability Resources Monthly, Sep '98*

◼

Leukemia Sourcebook

Basic Consumer Health Information about Adult and Childhood Leukemias, Including Acute Lymphocytic Leukemia (ALL), Chronic Lymphocytic Leukemia (CLL), Acute Myelogenous Leukemia (AML), Chronic Myelogenous Leukemia (CML), and Hairy Cell Leukemia, and Treatments Such as Chemotherapy, Radiation Therapy, Peripheral Blood Stem Cell and Marrow Transplantation, and Immunotherapy

Along with Tips for Life During and After Treatment, a Glossary, and Directories of Additional Resources

Edited by Joyce Brennfleck Shannon. 587 pages. 2003. 0-7808-0627-1.

"Unlike other medical books for the layperson, . . . the language does not talk down to the reader. . . . This volume is highly recommended for all libraries." —*American Reference Books Annual, 2004*

◼

Liver Disorders Sourcebook

Basic Consumer Health Information about the Liver and How It Works; Liver Diseases, Including Cancer, Cirrhosis, Hepatitis, and Toxic and Drug Related Diseases; Tips for Maintaining a Healthy Liver; Laboratory Tests, Radiology Tests, and Facts about Liver Transplantation

Along with a Section on Support Groups, a Glossary, and Resource Listings

Edited by Joyce Brennfleck Shannon. 591 pages. 2000. 0-7808-0383-3.

"A valuable resource." —*American Reference Books Annual, 2001*

"This title is recommended for health sciences and public libraries with consumer health collections." —*E-Streams, Oct '00*

"Recommended reference source." —*Booklist, American Library Association, Jun '00*

◼

Lung Disorders Sourcebook

Basic Consumer Health Information about Emphysema, Pneumonia, Tuberculosis, Asthma, Cystic Fibrosis, and Other Lung Disorders, Including Facts about Diagnostic Procedures, Treatment Strategies, Disease Prevention Efforts, and Such Risk Factors as Smoking, Air Pollution, and Exposure to Asbestos, Radon, and Other Agents

Along with a Glossary and Resources for Additional Help and Information

Edited by Dawn D. Matthews. 678 pages. 2002. 0-7808-0339-6.

"This title is a great addition for public and school libraries because it provides concise health information on the lungs."
— American Reference Books Annual, 2003

"Highly recommended for academic and medical reference collections." — Library Bookwatch, Sep '02

Medical Tests Sourcebook, 2nd Edition

Basic Consumer Health Information about Medical Tests, Including Age-Specific Health Tests, Important Health Screenings and Exams, Home-Use Tests, Blood and Specimen Tests, Electrical Tests, Scope Tests, Genetic Testing, and Imaging Tests, Such as X-Rays, Ultrasound, Computed Tomography, Magnetic Resonance Imaging, Angiography, and Nuclear Medicine

Along with a Glossary and Directory of Additional Resources

Edited by Joyce Brennfleck Shannon. 654 pages. 2004. 0-7808-0670-0.

ALSO AVAILABLE: Medical Tests, 1st Edition. Edited by Joyce Brennfleck Shannon. 691 pages. 1999. 0-7808-0243-8.

"Recommended for hospital and health sciences libraries with consumer health collections."
— E-Streams, Mar '00

"This is an overall excellent reference with a wealth of general knowledge that may aid those who are reluctant to get vital tests performed."
— Today's Librarian, Jan 2000

"A valuable reference guide."
—American Reference Books Annual, 2000

Men's Health Concerns Sourcebook, 2nd Edition

Basic Consumer Health Information about the Medical and Mental Concerns of Men, Including Theories about the Shorter Male Lifespan, the Leading Causes of Death and Disability, Physical Concerns of Special Significance to Men, Reproductive and Sexual Concerns, Sexually Transmitted Diseases, Men's Mental and Emotional Health, and Lifestyle Choices That Affect Wellness, Such as Nutrition, Fitness, and Substance Use

Along with a Glossary of Related Terms and a Directory of Organizational Resources in Men's Health

Edited by Robert Aquinas McNally. 644 pages. 2004. 0-7808-0671-9.

ALSO AVAILABLE: Men's Health Concerns Sourcebook, 1st Edition. Edited by Allan R. Cook. 738 pages. 1998. 0-7808-0212-8.

"This comprehensive resource and the series are highly recommended."
—American Reference Books Annual, 2000

"Recommended reference source."
— Booklist, American Library Association, Dec '98

Mental Health Disorders Sourcebook, 3rd Edition

Basic Consumer Health Information about Mental and Emotional Health and Mental Illness, Including Facts about Depression, Bipolar Disorder, and Other Mood Disorders, Phobias, Post-Traumatic Stress Disorder (PTSD), Obsessive-Compulsive Disorder, and Other Anxiety Disorders, Impulse Control Disorders, Eating Disorders, Personality Disorders, and Psychotic Disorders, Including Schizophrenia and Dissociative Disorders

Along with Statistical Information, a Special Section Concerning Mental Health Issues in Children and Adolescents, a Glossary, and Directories of Resources for Additional Help and Information

Edited by Karen Bellenir. 661 pages. 2005. 0-7808-0747-2.

ALSO AVAILABLE: Mental Health Disorders Sourcebook, 1st Edition. Edited by Karen Bellenir. 548 pages. 1995. 0-7808-0040-0.

ALSO AVAILABLE: Mental Health Disorders Sourcebook, 2nd Edition. Edited by Karen Bellenir. 605 pages. 2000. 0-7808-0240-3.

"Well organized and well written."
—American Reference Books Annual, 2001

"Recommended reference source."
—Booklist, American Library Association, Jun '00

Mental Retardation Sourcebook

Basic Consumer Health Information about Mental Retardation and Its Causes, Including Down Syndrome, Fetal Alcohol Syndrome, Fragile X Syndrome, Genetic Conditions, Injury, and Environmental Sources

Along with Preventive Strategies, Parenting Issues, Educational Implications, Health Care Needs, Employment and Economic Matters, Legal Issues, a Glossary, and a Resource Listing for Additional Help and Information

Edited by Joyce Brennfleck Shannon. 642 pages. 2000. 0-7808-0377-9.

"Public libraries will find the book useful for reference and as a beginning research point for students, parents, and caregivers."
—American Reference Books Annual, 2001

"The strength of this work is that it compiles many basic fact sheets and addresses for further information in one volume. It is intended and suitable for the general public. This sourcebook is relevant to any collection providing health information to the general public."
—E-Streams, Nov '00

"From preventing retardation to parenting and family challenges, this covers health, social and legal issues and will prove an invaluable overview."
—Reviewer's Bookwatch, Jul '00

Movement Disorders Sourcebook

Basic Consumer Health Information about Neurological Movement Disorders, Including Essential Tremor, Parkinson's Disease, Dystonia, Cerebral Palsy, Huntington's Disease, Myasthenia Gravis, Multiple Sclerosis, and Other Early-Onset and Adult-Onset Movement Disorders, Their Symptoms and Causes, Diagnostic Tests, and Treatments

Along with Mobility and Assistive Technology Information, a Glossary, and a Directory of Additional Resources

Edited by Joyce Brennfleck Shannon. 655 pages. 2003. 0-7808-0628-X.

". . . a good resource for consumers and recommended for public, community college and undergraduate libraries."
— *American Reference Books Annual, 2004*

■

Muscular Dystrophy Sourcebook

Basic Consumer Health Information about Congenital, Childhood-Onset, and Adult-Onset Forms of Muscular Dystrophy, Such as Duchenne, Becker, Emery-Dreifuss, Distal, Limb-Girdle, Facioscapulohumeral (FSHD), Myotonic, and Ophthalmoplegic Muscular Dystrophies, Including Facts about Diagnostic Tests, Medical and Physical Therapies, Management of Co-Occurring Conditions, and Parenting Guidelines

Along with Practical Tips for Home Care, a Glossary, and Directories of Additional Resources

Edited by Joyce Brennfleck Shannon. 577 pages. 2004. 0-7808-0676-X.

■

Obesity Sourcebook

Basic Consumer Health Information about Diseases and Other Problems Associated with Obesity, and Including Facts about Risk Factors, Prevention Issues, and Management Approaches

Along with Statistical and Demographic Data, Information about Special Populations, Research Updates, a Glossary, and Source Listings for Further Help and Information

Edited by Wilma Caldwell and Chad T. Kimball. 376 pages. 2001. 0-7808-0333-7.

"The book synthesizes the reliable medical literature on obesity into one easy-to-read and useful resource for the general public."
— *American Reference Books Annual 2002*

"This is a very useful resource book for the lay public."
—*Doody's Review Service, Nov '01*

"Well suited for the health reference collection of a public library or an academic health science library that serves the general population." —*E-Streams, Sep '01*

"Recommended reference source."
—*Booklist, American Library Association, Apr '01*

" Recommended pick both for specialty health library collections and any general consumer health reference collection." — *The Bookwatch, Apr '01*

Ophthalmic Disorders Sourcebook, 1st Edition

SEE Eye Care Sourcebook, 2nd Edition

■

Oral Health Sourcebook

SEE Dental Care & Oral Health Sourcebook, 2nd Ed.

■

Osteoporosis Sourcebook

Basic Consumer Health Information about Primary and Secondary Osteoporosis and Juvenile Osteoporosis and Related Conditions, Including Fibrous Dysplasia, Gaucher Disease, Hyperthyroidism, Hypophosphatasia, Myeloma, Osteopetrosis, Osteogenesis Imperfecta, and Paget's Disease

Along with Information about Risk Factors, Treatments, Traditional and Non-Traditional Pain Management, a Glossary of Related Terms, and a Directory of Resources

Edited by Allan R. Cook. 584 pages. 2001. 0-7808-0239-X.

"This would be a book to be kept in a staff or patient library. The targeted audience is the layperson, but the therapist who needs a quick bit of information on a particular topic will also find the book useful."
— *Physical Therapy, Jan '02*

"This resource is recommended as a great reference source for public, health, and academic libraries, and is another triumph for the editors of Omnigraphics."
— *American Reference Books Annual 2002*

"Recommended for all public libraries and general health collections, especially those supporting patient education or consumer health programs."
— *E-Streams, Nov '01*

"Will prove valuable to any library seeking to maintain a current, comprehensive reference collection of health resources. . . . From prevention to treatment and associated conditions, this provides an excellent survey."
— *The Bookwatch, Aug '01*

"Recommended reference source."
— *Booklist, American Library Association, July '01*

SEE ALSO Women's Health Concerns Sourcebook

■

Pain Sourcebook, 2nd Edition

Basic Consumer Health Information about Specific Forms of Acute and Chronic Pain, Including Muscle and Skeletal Pain, Nerve Pain, Cancer Pain, and Disorders Characterized by Pain, Such as Fibromyalgia, Shingles, Angina, Arthritis, and Headaches

Along with Information about Pain Medications and Management Techniques, Complementary and Alternative Pain Relief Options, Tips for People Living with Chronic Pain, a Glossary, and a Directory of Sources for Further Information

Edited by Karen Bellenir. 670 pages. 2002. 0-7808-0612-3.

ALSO AVAILABLE: *Pain Sourcebook, 1st Edition.* Edited by Allan R. Cook. 667 pages. 1997. 0-7808-0213-6.

"A source of valuable information. . . . This book offers help to nonmedical people who need information about pain and pain management. It is also an excellent reference for those who participate in patient education."
— *Doody's Review Service, Sep '02*

"The text is readable, easily understood, and well indexed. This excellent volume belongs in all patient education libraries, consumer health sections of public libraries, and many personal collections."
— *American Reference Books Annual, 1999*

"A beneficial reference." — *Booklist Health Sciences Supplement, American Library Association, Oct '98*

"The information is basic in terms of scholarship and is appropriate for general readers. Written in journalistic style . . . intended for non-professionals. Quite thorough in its coverage of different pain conditions and summarizes the latest clinical information regarding pain treatment." — *Choice, Association of College and Research Libraries, Jun '98*

"Recommended reference source."
— *Booklist, American Library Association, Mar '98*

■

Pediatric Cancer Sourcebook

Basic Consumer Health Information about Leukemias, Brain Tumors, Sarcomas, Lymphomas, and Other Cancers in Infants, Children, and Adolescents, Including Descriptions of Cancers, Treatments, and Coping Strategies

Along with Suggestions for Parents, Caregivers, and Concerned Relatives, a Glossary of Cancer Terms, and Resource Listings

Edited by Edward J. Prucha. 587 pages. 1999. 0-7808-0245-4.

"An excellent source of information. Recommended for public, hospital, and health science libraries with consumer health collections." — *E-Streams, Jun '00*

"Recommended reference source."
— *Booklist, American Library Association, Feb '00*

"A valuable addition to all libraries specializing in health services and many public libraries."
— *American Reference Books Annual, 2000*

■

Physical & Mental Issues in Aging Sourcebook

Basic Consumer Health Information on Physical and Mental Disorders Associated with the Aging Process, Including Concerns about Cardiovascular Disease, Pulmonary Disease, Oral Health, Digestive Disorders, Musculoskeletal and Skin Disorders, Metabolic Changes, Sexual and Reproductive Issues, and Changes in Vision, Hearing, and Other Senses

Along with Data about Longevity and Causes of Death, Information on Acute and Chronic Pain, Descriptions of Mental Concerns, a Glossary of Terms, and Resource Listings for Additional Help

Edited by Jenifer Swanson. 660 pages. 1999. 0-7808-0233-0.

"This is a treasure of health information for the layperson." — *Choice Health Sciences Supplement, Association of College & Research Libraries, May 2000*

"Recommended for public libraries."
— *American Reference Books Annual, 2000*

"Recommended reference source."
— *Booklist, American Library Association, Oct '99*

SEE ALSO *Healthy Aging Sourcebook*

■

Podiatry Sourcebook

Basic Consumer Health Information about Foot Conditions, Diseases, and Injuries, Including Bunions, Corns, Calluses, Athlete's Foot, Plantar Warts, Hammertoes and Clawtoes, Clubfoot, Heel Pain, Gout, and More

Along with Facts about Foot Care, Disease Prevention, Foot Safety, Choosing a Foot Care Specialist, a Glossary of Terms, and Resource Listings for Additional Information

Edited by M. Lisa Weatherford. 380 pages. 2001. 0-7808-0215-2.

"Recommended reference source."
— *Booklist, American Library Association, Feb '02*

"There is a lot of information presented here on a topic that is usually only covered sparingly in most larger comprehensive medical encyclopedias."
— *American Reference Books Annual 2002*

■

Pregnancy & Birth Sourcebook, 2nd Edition

Basic Consumer Health Information about Conception and Pregnancy, Including Facts about Fertility, Infertility, Pregnancy Symptoms and Complications, Fetal Growth and Development, Labor, Delivery, and the Postpartum Period, as Well as Information about Maintaining Health and Wellness during Pregnancy and Caring for a Newborn

Along with Information about Public Health Assistance for Low-Income Pregnant Women, a Glossary, and Directories of Agencies and Organizations Providing Help and Support

Edited by Amy L. Sutton. 626 pages. 2004. 0-7808-0672-7.

ALSO AVAILABLE: *Pregnancy & Birth Sourcebook, 1st Edition.* Edited by Heather E. Aldred. 737 pages. 1997. 0-7808-0216-0.

"A well-organized handbook. Recommended."
— *Choice, Association of College and Research Libraries, Apr '98*

"Recommended reference source."
— *Booklist, American Library Association, Mar '98*

"Recommended for public libraries."
— *American Reference Books Annual, 1998*

SEE ALSO *Congenital Disorders Sourcebook, Family Planning Sourcebook*

Prostate Cancer Sourcebook

Basic Consumer Health Information about Prostate Cancer, Including Information about the Associated Risk Factors, Detection, Diagnosis, and Treatment of Prostate Cancer

Along with Information on Non-Malignant Prostate Conditions, and Featuring a Section Listing Support and Treatment Centers and a Glossary of Related Terms

Edited by Dawn D. Matthews. 358 pages. 2001. 0-7808-0324-8.

"Recommended reference source."
— Booklist, American Library Association, Jan '02

"A valuable resource for health care consumers seeking information on the subject. . . .All text is written in a clear, easy-to-understand language that avoids technical jargon. Any library that collects consumer health resources would strengthen their collection with the addition of the *Prostate Cancer Sourcebook.*"
— American Reference Books Annual 2002

Public Health Sourcebook

Basic Information about Government Health Agencies, Including National Health Statistics and Trends, Healthy People 2000 Program Goals and Objectives, the Centers for Disease Control and Prevention, the Food and Drug Administration, and the National Institutes of Health

Along with Full Contact Information for Each Agency

Edited by Wendy Wilcox. 698 pages. 1998. 0-7808-0220-9.

"Recommended reference source."
— Booklist, American Library Association, Sep '98

"This consumer guide provides welcome assistance in navigating the maze of federal health agencies and their data on public health concerns."
— SciTech Book News, Sep '98

Reconstructive & Cosmetic Surgery Sourcebook

Basic Consumer Health Information on Cosmetic and Reconstructive Plastic Surgery, Including Statistical Information about Different Surgical Procedures, Things to Consider Prior to Surgery, Plastic Surgery Techniques and Tools, Emotional and Psychological Considerations, and Procedure-Specific Information

Along with a Glossary of Terms and a Listing of Resources for Additional Help and Information

Edited by M. Lisa Weatherford. 374 pages. 2001. 0-7808-0214-4.

"An excellent reference that addresses cosmetic and medically necessary reconstructive surgeries. . . . The style of the prose is calm and reassuring, discussing the many positive outcomes now available due to advances in surgical techniques."
— American Reference Books Annual 2002

"Recommended for health science libraries that are open to the public, as well as hospital libraries that are open to the patients. This book is a good resource for the consumer interested in plastic surgery."
— E-Streams, Dec '01

"Recommended reference source."
— Booklist, American Library Association, July '01

Rehabilitation Sourcebook

Basic Consumer Health Information about Rehabilitation for People Recovering from Heart Surgery, Spinal Cord Injury, Stroke, Orthopedic Impairments, Amputation, Pulmonary Impairments, Traumatic Injury, and More, Including Physical Therapy, Occupational Therapy, Speech/ Language Therapy, Massage Therapy, Dance Therapy, Art Therapy, and Recreational Therapy

Along with Information on Assistive and Adaptive Devices, a Glossary, and Resources for Additional Help and Information

Edited by Dawn D. Matthews. 531 pages. 1999. 0-7808-0236-5.

"This is an excellent resource for public library reference and health collections."
— American Reference Books Annual, 2001

"Recommended reference source."
— Booklist, American Library Association, May '00

Respiratory Diseases & Disorders Sourcebook

Basic Information about Respiratory Diseases and Disorders, Including Asthma, Cystic Fibrosis, Pneumonia, the Common Cold, Influenza, and Others, Featuring Facts about the Respiratory System, Statistical and Demographic Data, Treatments, Self-Help Management Suggestions, and Current Research Initiatives

Edited by Allan R. Cook and Peter D. Dresser. 771 pages. 1995. 0-7808-0037-0.

"Designed for the layperson and for patients and their families coping with respiratory illness. . . . an extensive array of information on diagnosis, treatment, management, and prevention of respiratory illnesses for the general reader."
— Choice, Association of College and Research Libraries, Jun '96

"A highly recommended text for all collections. It is a comforting reminder of the power of knowledge that good books carry between their covers."
— Academic Library Book Review, Spring '96

"A comprehensive collection of authoritative information presented in a nontechnical, humanitarian style for patients, families, and caregivers."
— Association of Operating Room Nurses, Sep/Oct '95

SEE ALSO Lung Disorders Sourcebook

Sexually Transmitted Diseases Sourcebook, 2nd Edition

Basic Consumer Health Information about Sexually Transmitted Diseases, Including Information on the Diagnosis and Treatment of Chlamydia, Gonorrhea, Hepatitis, Herpes, HIV, Mononucleosis, Syphilis, and Others

Along with Information on Prevention, Such as Condom Use, Vaccines, and STD Education; And Featuring a Section on Issues Related to Youth and Adolescents, a Glossary, and Resources for Additional Help and Information

Edited by Dawn D. Matthews. 538 pages. 2001. 0-7808-0249-7.

ALSO AVAILABLE: *Sexually Transmitted Diseases Sourcebook, 1st Edition.* Edited by Linda M. Ross. 550 pages. 1997. 0-7808-0217-9.

"Recommended for consumer health collections in public libraries, and secondary school and community college libraries."
— *American Reference Books Annual 2002*

"Every school and public library should have a copy of this comprehensive and user-friendly reference book."
— *Choice, Association of College & Research Libraries, Sep '01*

"This is a highly recommended book. This is an especially important book for all school and public libraries." — *AIDS Book Review Journal, Jul-Aug '01*

"Recommended reference source."
— *Booklist, American Library Association, Apr '01*

"Recommended pick both for specialty health library collections and any general consumer health reference collection." — *The Bookwatch, Apr '01*

Skin Disorders Sourcebook, 1st Edition

SEE *Dermatological Disorders Sourcebook, 2nd Edition*

Sleep Disorders Sourcebook, 2nd Edition

Basic Consumer Health Information about Sleep and Sleep Disorders, Including Insomnia, Sleep Apnea, Restless Legs Syndrome, Narcolepsy, Parasomnias, and Other Health Problems That Affect Sleep, Plus Facts about Diagnostic Procedures, Treatment Strategies, Sleep Medications, and Tips for Improving Sleep Quality

Along with a Glossary of Related Terms and Resources for Additional Help and Information

Edited by Amy L. Sutton. 567 pages. 2005. 0-7808-0745-6.

ALSO AVAILABLE: *Sleep Disorders Sourcebook, 1st Edition.* Edited by Jenifer Swanson. 439 pages. 1998. 0-7808-0234-9.

"This text will complement any home or medical library. It is user-friendly and ideal for the adult reader."
— *American Reference Books Annual, 2000*

"A useful resource that provides accurate, relevant, and accessible information on sleep to the general public. Health care providers who deal with sleep disorders patients may also find it helpful in being prepared to answer some of the questions patients ask."
— *Respiratory Care, Jul '99*

"Recommended reference source."
— *Booklist, American Library Association, Feb '99*

Smoking Concerns Sourcebook

Basic Consumer Health Information about Nicotine Addiction and Smoking Cessation, Featuring Facts about the Health Effects of Tobacco Use, Including Lung and Other Cancers, Heart Disease, Stroke, and Respiratory Disorders, Such as Emphysema and Chronic Bronchitis

Along with Information about Smoking Prevention Programs, Suggestions for Achieving and Maintaining a Smoke-Free Lifestyle, Statistics about Tobacco Use, Reports on Current Research Initiatives, a Glossary of Related Terms, and Directories of Resources for Additional Help and Information

Edited by Karen Bellenir. 621 pages. 2004. 0-7808-0323-X.

Sports Injuries Sourcebook, 2nd Edition

Basic Consumer Health Information about the Diagnosis, Treatment, and Rehabilitation of Common Sports-Related Injuries in Children and Adults

Along with Suggestions for Conditioning and Training, Information and Prevention Tips for Injuries Frequently Associated with Specific Sports and Special Populations, a Glossary, and a Directory of Additional Resources

Edited by Joyce Brennfleck Shannon. 614 pages. 2002. 0-7808-0604-2.

ALSO AVAILABLE: *Sports Injuries Sourcebook, 1st Edition.* Edited by Heather E. Aldred. 624 pages. 1999. 0-7808-0218-7.

"This is an excellent reference for consumers and it is recommended for public, community college, and undergraduate libraries."
— *American Reference Books Annual, 2003*

"Recommended reference source."
— *Booklist, American Library Association, Feb '03*

Stress-Related Disorders Sourcebook

Basic Consumer Health Information about Stress and Stress-Related Disorders, Including Stress Origins and Signals, Environmental Stress at Work and Home, Mental and Emotional Stress Associated with Depression, Post-Traumatic Stress Disorder, Panic Disorder, Suicide, and the Physical Effects of Stress on the Cardiovascular, Immune, and Nervous Systems

Along with Stress Management Techniques, a Glossary, and a Listing of Additional Resources

Edited by Joyce Brennfleck Shannon. 610 pages. 2002. 0-7808-0560-7.

"Well written for a general readership, the *Stress-Related Disorders Sourcebook* is a useful addition to the health reference literature."
— *American Reference Books Annual, 2003*

"I am impressed by the amount of information. It offers a thorough overview of the causes and consequences of stress for the layperson. . . . A well-done and thorough reference guide for professionals and nonprofessionals alike." — *Doody's Review Service, Dec '02*

■

Stroke Sourcebook

Basic Consumer Health Information about Stroke, Including Ischemic, Hemorrhagic, Transient Ischemic Attack (TIA), and Pediatric Stroke, Stroke Triggers and Risks, Diagnostic Tests, Treatments, and Rehabilitation Information

Along with Stroke Prevention Guidelines, Legal and Financial Information, a Glossary, and a Directory of Additional Resources

Edited by Joyce Brennfleck Shannon. 606 pages. 2003. 0-7808-0630-1.

"This volume is highly recommended and should be in every medical, hospital, and public library."
— *American Reference Books Annual, 2004*

■

Substance Abuse Sourcebook

Basic Health-Related Information about the Abuse of Legal and Illegal Substances Such as Alcohol, Tobacco, Prescription Drugs, Marijuana, Cocaine, and Heroin; and Including Facts about Substance Abuse Prevention Strategies, Intervention Methods, Treatment and Recovery Programs, and a Section Addressing the Special Problems Related to Substance Abuse during Pregnancy

Edited by Karen Bellenir. 573 pages. 1996. 0-7808-0038-9.

"A valuable addition to any health reference section. Highly recommended."
— *The Book Report, Mar/Apr '97*

". . . a comprehensive collection of substance abuse information that's both highly readable and compact. Families and caregivers of substance abusers will find the information enlightening and helpful, while teachers, social workers and journalists should benefit from the concise format. Recommended."
— *Drug Abuse Update, Winter '96/'97*

SEE ALSO *Alcoholism Sourcebook, Drug Abuse Sourcebook*

Surgery Sourcebook

Basic Consumer Health Information about Inpatient and Outpatient Surgeries, Including Cardiac, Vascular, Orthopedic, Ocular, Reconstructive, Cosmetic, Gynecologic, and Ear, Nose, and Throat Procedures and More

Along with Information about Operating Room Policies and Instruments, Laser Surgery Techniques, Hospital Errors, Statistical Data, a Glossary, and Listings of Sources for Further Help and Information

Edited by Annemarie S. Muth and Karen Bellenir. 596 pages. 2002. 0-7808-0380-9.

"Large public libraries and medical libraries would benefit from this material in their reference collections."
— *American Reference Books Annual, 2004*

"Invaluable reference for public and school library collections alike." — *Library Bookwatch, Apr '03*

■

Thyroid Disorders Sourcebook

Basic Consumer Health Information about Disorders of the Thyroid and Parathyroid Glands, Including Hypothyroidism, Hyperthyroidism, Graves Disease, Hashimoto Thyroiditis, Thyroid Cancer, and Parathyroid Disorders, Featuring Facts about Symptoms, Risk Factors, Tests, and Treatments

Along with Information about the Effects of Thyroid Imbalance on Other Body Systems, Environmental Factors That Affect the Thyroid Gland, a Glossary, and a Directory of Additional Resources

Edited by Joyce Brennfleck Shannon. 599 pages. 2005. 0-7808-0745-6.

■

Transplantation Sourcebook

Basic Consumer Health Information about Organ and Tissue Transplantation, Including Physical and Financial Preparations, Procedures and Issues Relating to Specific Solid Organ and Tissue Transplants, Rehabilitation, Pediatric Transplant Information, the Future of Transplantation, and Organ and Tissue Donation

Along with a Glossary and Listings of Additional Resources

Edited by Joyce Brennfleck Shannon. 628 pages. 2002. 0-7808-0322-1.

"Along with these advances [in transplantation technology] have come a number of daunting questions for potential transplant patients, their families, and their health care providers. This reference text is the best single tool to address many of these questions. . . . It will be a much-needed addition to the reference collections in health care, academic, and large public libraries."
— *American Reference Books Annual, 2003*

"Recommended for libraries with an interest in offering consumer health information." — *E-Streams, Jul '02*

"This is a unique and valuable resource for patients facing transplantation and their families."
— *Doody's Review Service, Jun '02*

Traveler's Health Sourcebook

Basic Consumer Health Information for Travelers, Including Physical and Medical Preparations, Transportation Health and Safety, Essential Information about Food and Water, Sun Exposure, Insect and Snake Bites, Camping and Wilderness Medicine, and Travel with Physical or Medical Disabilities

Along with International Travel Tips, Vaccination Recommendations, Geographical Health Issues, Disease Risks, a Glossary, and a Listing of Additional Resources

Edited by Joyce Brennfleck Shannon. 613 pages. 2000. 0-7808-0384-1.

"Recommended reference source."
— Booklist, American Library Association, Feb '01

"This book is recommended for any public library, any travel collection, and especially any collection for the physically disabled."
—American Reference Books Annual, 2001

■

Urinary Tract & Kidney Diseases & Disorders Sourcebook, 2nd Edition

Basic Consumer Health Information about the Urinary System, Including the Bladder, Urethra, Ureters, and Kidneys, with Facts about Urinary Tract Infections, Incontinence, Congenital Disorders, Kidney Stones, Cancers of the Urinary Tract and Kidneys, Kidney Failure, Dialysis, and Kidney Transplantation

Along with Statistical and Demographic Information, Reports on Current Research in Kidney and Urologic Health, a Summary of Commonly Used Diagnostic Tests, a Glossary of Related Terms, and a Directory of Resources for Additional Help and Information

Edited by Ivy L. Alexander. 649 pages. 2005. 0-7808-0750-2.

ALSO AVAILABLE: Kidney & Urinary Tract Diseases & Disorders Sourcebook, 1st Ed. Edited by Linda M. Ross. 602 pages. 1997. 0-7808-0079-6.

■

Vegetarian Sourcebook

Basic Consumer Health Information about Vegetarian Diets, Lifestyle, and Philosophy, Including Definitions of Vegetarianism and Veganism, Tips about Adopting Vegetarianism, Creating a Vegetarian Pantry, and Meeting Nutritional Needs of Vegetarians, with Facts Regarding Vegetarianism's Effect on Pregnant and Lactating Women, Children, Athletes, and Senior Citizens

Along with a Glossary of Commonly Used Vegetarian Terms and Resources for Additional Help and Information

Edited by Chad T. Kimball. 360 pages. 2002. 0-7808-0439-2.

"Organizes into one concise volume the answers to the most common questions concerning vegetarian diets and lifestyles. This title is recommended for public and secondary school libraries." — E-Streams, Apr '03

"Invaluable reference for public and school library collections alike." — Library Bookwatch, Apr '03

"The articles in this volume are easy to read and come from authoritative sources. The book does not necessarily support the vegetarian diet but instead provides the pros and cons of this important decision. The *Vegetarian Sourcebook* is recommended for public libraries and consumer health libraries."
— American Reference Books Annual, 2003

■

Women's Health Concerns Sourcebook, 2nd Edition

Basic Consumer Health Information about the Medical and Mental Concerns of Women, Including Maintaining Health and Wellness, Gynecological Concerns, Breast Health, Sexuality and Reproductive Issues, Menopause, Cancer in Women, the Leading Causes of Death and Disability among Women, Physical Concerns of Special Significance to Women, and Women's Mental and Emotional Health

Along with a Glossary of Related Terms and Directories of Resources for Additional Help and Information

Edited by Amy L. Sutton. 748 pages. 2004. 0-7808-0673-5.

ALSO AVAILABLE: Women's Health Concerns Sourcebook, 1st Edition. Edited by Heather E. Aldred. 567 pages. 1997. 0-7808-0219-5.

"Handy compilation. There is an impressive range of diseases, devices, disorders, procedures, and other physical and emotional issues covered . . . well organized, illustrated, and indexed." — Choice, Association of College and Research Libraries, Jan '98

SEE ALSO Breast Cancer Sourcebook, Cancer Sourcebook for Women, Healthy Heart Sourcebook for Women, Osteoporosis Sourcebook

■

Workplace Health & Safety Sourcebook

Basic Consumer Health Information about Workplace Health and Safety, Including the Effect of Workplace Hazards on the Lungs, Skin, Heart, Ears, Eyes, Brain, Reproductive Organs, Musculoskeletal System, and Other Organs and Body Parts

Along with Information about Occupational Cancer, Personal Protective Equipment, Toxic and Hazardous Chemicals, Child Labor, Stress, and Workplace Violence

Edited by Chad T. Kimball. 626 pages. 2000. 0-7808-0231-4.

"As a reference for the general public, this would be useful in any library." —E-Streams, Jun '01

"Provides helpful information for primary care physicians and other caregivers interested in occupational medicine. . . . General readers; professionals."
— Choice, Association of College & Research Libraries, May '01

"Recommended reference source."
— Booklist, American Library Association, Feb '01

"Highly recommended." — The Bookwatch, Jan '01

Worldwide Health Sourcebook

Basic Information about Global Health Issues, Including Malnutrition, Reproductive Health, Disease Dispersion and Prevention, Emerging Diseases, Risky Health Behaviors, and the Leading Causes of Death

Along with Global Health Concerns for Children, Women, and the Elderly, Mental Health Issues, Research and Technology Advancements, and Economic, Environmental, and Political Health Implications, a Glossary, and a Resource Listing for Additional Help and Information

Edited by Joyce Brennfleck Shannon. 614 pages. 2001. 0-7808-0330-2.

"**Named an Outstanding Academic Title.**" —*Choice, Association of College & Research Libraries, Jan '02*

"**Yet another handy but also unique compilation in the extensive Health Reference Series, this is a useful work because many of the international publications reprinted or excerpted are not readily available. Highly recommended.**" —*Choice, Association of College & Research Libraries, Nov '01*

"**Recommended reference source.**" —*Booklist, American Library Association, Oct '01*

Teen Health Series

Helping Young Adults Understand, Manage, and Avoid Serious Illness

List price $65 per volume. **School and library price $58 per volume.**

Alcohol Information for Teens
Health Tips about Alcohol and Alcoholism

Including Facts about Underage Drinking, Preventing Teen Alcohol Use, Alcohol's Effects on the Brain and the Body, Alcohol Abuse Treatment, Help for Children of Alcoholics, and More

Edited by Joyce Brennfleck Shannon. 370 pages. 2005. 0-7808-0741-3.

Asthma Information for Teens
Health Tips about Managing Asthma and Related Concerns

Including Facts about Asthma Causes, Triggers, Symptoms, Diagnosis, and Treatment

Edited by Karen Bellenir. 386 pages. 2005. 0-7808-0770-7.

Cancer Information for Teens
Health Tips about Cancer Awareness, Prevention, Diagnosis, and Treatment

Including Facts about Frequently Occurring Cancers, Cancer Risk Factors, and Coping Strategies for Teens Fighting Cancer or Dealing with Cancer in Friends or Family Members

Edited by Wilma R. Caldwell. 428 pages. 2004. 0-7808-0678-6.

"Recommended for school libraries, or consumer libraries that see a lot of use by teens."
— E-Streams, May 2005

"A valuable educational tool."
— American Reference Books Annual, 2005

"Young adults and their parents alike will find this new addition to the *Teen Health Series* an important reference to cancer in teens."
— Children's Bookwatch, February 2005

Diet Information for Teens
Health Tips about Diet and Nutrition

Including Facts about Nutrients, Dietary Guidelines, Breakfasts, School Lunches, Snacks, Party Food, Weight Control, Eating Disorders, and More

Edited by Karen Bellenir. 399 pages. 2001. 0-7808-0441-4.

"Full of helpful insights and facts throughout the book. . . . An excellent resource to be placed in public libraries or even in personal collections."
— American Reference Books Annual 2002

"Recommended for middle and high school libraries and media centers as well as academic libraries that educate future teachers of teenagers. It is also a suitable addition to health science libraries that serve patrons who are interested in teen health promotion and education."
— E-Streams, Oct '01

"This comprehensive book would be beneficial to collections that need information about nutrition, dietary guidelines, meal planning, and weight control. . . . This reference is so easy to use that its purchase is recommended."
— The Book Report, Sep-Oct '01

"This book is written in an easy to understand format describing issues that many teens face every day, and then provides thoughtful explanations so that teens can make informed decisions. This is an interesting book that provides important facts and information for today's teens."
— Doody's Health Sciences Book Review Journal, Jul-Aug '01

"A comprehensive compendium of diet and nutrition. The information is presented in a straightforward, plain-spoken manner. This title will be useful to those working on reports on a variety of topics, as well as to general readers concerned about their dietary health."
— School Library Journal, Jun '01

Drug Information for Teens
Health Tips about the Physical and Mental Effects of Substance Abuse

Including Facts about Alcohol, Anabolic Steroids, Club Drugs, Cocaine, Depressants, Hallucinogens, Herbal Products, Inhalants, Marijuana, Narcotics, Stimulants, Tobacco, and More

Edited by Karen Bellenir. 452 pages. 2002. 0-7808-0444-9.

"A clearly written resource for general readers and researchers alike."
— School Library Journal

"The chapters are quick to make a connection to their teenage reading audience. The prose is straightforward and the book lends itself to spot reading. It should be useful both for practical information and for research, and it is suitable for public and school libraries."
— American Reference Books Annual, 2003

"Recommended reference source."
— Booklist, American Library Association, Feb '03

"This is an excellent resource for teens and their parents. Education about drugs and substances is key to discouraging teen drug abuse and this book provides this much needed information in a way that is interesting and factual." —*Doody's Review Service, Dec '02*

Eating Disorders Information for Teens

Health Tips about Anorexia, Bulimia, Binge Eating, and Other Eating Disorders

Including Information on the Causes, Prevention, and Treatment of Eating Disorders, and Such Other Issues as Maintaining Healthy Eating and Exercise Habits

Edited by Sandra Augustyn Lawton. 337 pages. 2005. 0-7808-0783-9.

Fitness Information for Teens

Health Tips about Exercise, Physical Well-Being, and Health Maintenance

Including Facts about Aerobic and Anaerobic Conditioning, Stretching, Body Shape and Body Image, Sports Training, Nutrition, and Activities for Non-Athletes

Edited by Karen Bellenir. 425 pages. 2004. 0-7808-0679-4.

"This book will be a great addition to any public, junior high, senior high, or secondary school library." —*American Reference Books Annual, 2005*

Learning Disabilities Information for Teens

Health Tips about Academic Skills Disorders and Other Disabilities That Affect Learning

Including Information about Common Signs of Learning Disabilities, School Issues, Learning to Live with a Learning Disability, and Other Related Issues

Edited by Sandra Augustyn Lawton. 337 pages. 2005. 0-7808-0796-0.

Mental Health Information for Teens

Health Tips about Mental Health and Mental Illness

Including Facts about Anxiety, Depression, Suicide, Eating Disorders, Obsessive-Compulsive Disorders, Panic Attacks, Phobias, Schizophrenia, and More

Edited by Karen Bellenir. 406 pages. 2001. 0-7808-0442-2.

"In both language and approach, this user-friendly entry in the *Teen Health Series* is on target for teens needing information on mental health concerns." —*Booklist, American Library Association, Jan '02*

"Readers will find the material accessible and informative, with the shaded notes, facts, and embedded glossary insets adding appropriately to the already interesting and succinct presentation."
—*School Library Journal, Jan '02*

"This title is highly recommended for any library that serves adolescents and parents/caregivers of adolescents." —*E-Streams, Jan '02*

"Recommended for high school libraries and young adult collections in public libraries. Both health professionals and teenagers will find this book useful." —*American Reference Books Annual 2002*

"This is a nice book written to enlighten the society, primarily teenagers, about common teen mental health issues. It is highly recommended to teachers and parents as well as adolescents." —*Doody's Review Service, Dec '01*

Sexual Health Information for Teens

Health Tips about Sexual Development, Human Reproduction, and Sexually Transmitted Diseases

Including Facts about Puberty, Reproductive Health, Chlamydia, Human Papillomavirus, Pelvic Inflammatory Disease, Herpes, AIDS, Contraception, Pregnancy, and More

Edited by Deborah A. Stanley. 391 pages. 2003. 0-7808-0445-7.

"This work should be included in all high school libraries and many larger public libraries. . . . highly recommended." —*American Reference Books Annual 2004*

"Sexual Health approaches its subject with appropriate seriousness and offers easily accessible advice and information." —*School Library Journal, Feb. 2004*

Skin Health Information for Teens

Health Tips about Dermatological Concerns and Skin Cancer Risks

Including Facts about Acne, Warts, Hives, and Other Conditions and Lifestyle Choices, Such as Tanning, Tattooing, and Piercing, That Affect the Skin, Nails, Scalp, and Hair

Edited by Robert Aquinas McNally. 429 pages. 2003. 0-7808-0446-5.

"This volume, as with others in the series, will be a useful addition to school and public library collections." —*American Reference Books Annual 2004*

"This volume serves as a one-stop source and should be a necessity for any health collection." —*Library Media Connection*

Sports Injuries Information for Teens

Health Tips about Sports Injuries and Injury Protection

Including Facts about Specific Injuries, Emergency Treatment, Rehabilitation, Sports Safety, Competition Stress, Fitness, Sports Nutrition, Steroid Risks, and More

Edited by Joyce Brennfleck Shannon. 405 pages. 2003. 0-7808-0447-3.

"This work will be useful in the young adult collections of public libraries as well as high school libraries."
— *American Reference Books Annual 2004*

Suicide Information for Teens

Health Tips about Suicide Causes and Prevention

Including Facts about Depression, Risk Factors, Getting Help, Survivor Support, and More

Edited by Joyce Brennfleck Shannon. 368 pages. 2005. 0-7808-0737-5.

Health Reference Series

Adolescent Health Sourcebook

AIDS Sourcebook, 3rd Edition

Alcoholism Sourcebook

Allergies Sourcebook, 2nd Edition

Alternative Medicine Sourcebook,
2nd Edition

Alzheimer's Disease Sourcebook,
3rd Edition

Arthritis Sourcebook, 2nd Edition

Asthma Sourcebook

Attention Deficit Disorder Sourcebook

Back & Neck Sourcebook, 2nd Edition

Blood & Circulatory Disorders
Sourcebook, 2nd Edition

Brain Disorders Sourcebook, 2nd Edition

Breast Cancer Sourcebook, 2nd Edition

Breastfeeding Sourcebook

Burns Sourcebook

Cancer Sourcebook, 4th Edition

Cancer Sourcebook for Women,
2nd Edition

Cardiovascular Diseases & Disorders
Sourcebook, 3rd Edition

Caregiving Sourcebook

Child Abuse Sourcebook

Childhood Diseases & Disorders
Sourcebook

Colds, Flu & Other Common Ailments
Sourcebook

Communication Disorders
Sourcebook

Congenital Disorders Sourcebook

Consumer Issues in Health Care
Sourcebook

Contagious & Non-Contagious
Infectious Diseases Sourcebook

Contagious Diseases Sourcebook

Death & Dying Sourcebook

Dental Care & Oral Health Sourcebook,
2nd Edition

Depression Sourcebook

Diabetes Sourcebook, 3rd Edition

Diet & Nutrition Sourcebook,
2nd Edition

Digestive Diseases & Disorder
Sourcebook

Disabilities Sourcebook

Domestic Violence Sourcebook,
2nd Edition

Drug Abuse Sourcebook, 2nd Edition

Ear, Nose & Throat Disorders
Sourcebook

Eating Disorders Sourcebook

Emergency Medical Services
Sourcebook

Endocrine & Metabolic Disorders
Sourcebook

Environmentally Health Sourcebook,
2nd Edition

Ethnic Diseases Sourcebook

Eye Care Sourcebook, 2nd Edition

Family Planning Sourcebook

Fitness & Exercise Sourcebook,
2nd Edition

Food & Animal Borne Diseases
Sourcebook

Food Safety Sourcebook

Forensic Medicine Sourcebook

Gastrointestinal Diseases & Disorders
Sourcebook

Genetic Disorders Sourcebook,
2nd Edition

Head Trauma Sourcebook

Headache Sourcebook

Health Insurance Sourcebook

Health Reference Series Cumulative
Index 1999

Healthy Aging Sourcebook

Healthy Children Sourcebook

Healthy Heart Sourcebook for Women